Division of Nuclear Medicine
The Johns Hopkins Medical Institutions
Baltimore, Maryland 21205

Practical Nuclear Medicine

MEDCOM MEDICAL UPDATE SERIES

Practical Nuclear Medicine

Editor

Fuad S. Ashkar, MD
Assistant Professor of Radiology and Medicine
University of Miami School of Medicine;
Director of Nuclear Metabolic Section
Division of Nuclear Medicine
Jackson Memorial Hospital, Miami, Florida and
Mount Sinai Hospital, Miami Beach, Florida

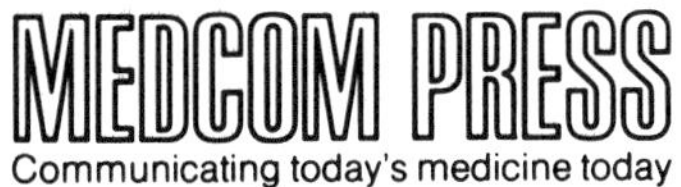

The science of medicine changes very quickly. And clinical research rapidly leads to expanded knowledge about drug therapy. Although the physicians who prepared this book and the MEDCOM staff have carefully given you accurate information on dosages, precautions and contraindications as of the time of publication, some dosages mentioned have been given in an investigational setting only; therefore, you are strongly urged to check the product information contained in the package of each drug prescribed. Only then can you be certain of obtaining the current official prescribing information for proper dosage recommendations, particularly for new or infrequently used drugs.

MEDCOM®

World leader in multimedia medical education programs
2 Hammarskjöld Plaza
New York, New York 10017 (212) 832-1400

Printed in the United States of America.

Library of Congress CIP Data

Ashkar, Fuad S
Practical nuclear medicine.

(Medcom medical update series)
1. Radiology, Medical. I. Title.
[DNLM: 1. Nuclear medicine. WN440 A825p 1973]
RM847.A8 616.07'57 73-13794

ISBN 0-8463-0126-1

First edition

Dedicated to Anda and all the young people—our hope for the future

Contents

About the Editor xi

Contributors xiii

Introduction xv
FUAD S. ASHKAR

Preface xvii
WILLIAM H. BEIERWALTES

1 **Instruments for Imaging Procedures** 1
PETER J. KENNY

The scintillation camera and the rectilinear scanner are the two imaging instruments used in nuclear medicine. Dr. Kenny discusses these systems in terms of the three major components common to each: the collimator, detector and associated electronics, and display.

2 **Radiopharmaceuticals for Clinical Use** 6
HOMER B. HUPF

Dr. Hupf describes the four classifications of radiopharmaceuticals—compounds, complexes, colloids, and generators—and explains preparation methods. He specifies clinical applications, including uptake mechanisms for the brain . . . thyroid . . . liver . . . lungs . . . and kidneys.

3 **Data and the Computer** 12
R. ROGER SANKEY

A small digital computer system, plus the hardware and software requirements for interfacing a computer to an Anger camera, are explained by Dr. Sankey. He discusses the most common imaging procedures.

4 **The Central Nervous System** 23
WILLIAM M. SMOAK III AND ALBERT J. GILSON

This survey emphasizes the spectrum of nervous system diseases detectable by both dynamic and static scintigraphy. Drs. Smoak and Gilson extensively discuss the normal and abnormal procedures and findings covering vascular traumatic . . . infectious . . . and neoplastic diseases.

5 **The Thyroid, Parathyroids and Adrenals** 38
FUAD S. ASHKAR

Dr. Ashkar explains all aspects of thyroid imaging and function tests—in vivo and in vitro techniques . . . the dynamic thyroid study . . . thyroid differential scanning methods . . . normal and pathological thyroid regulation . . . goiter evaluation . . . and the work-up of functioning and nonfunctioning nodules. Parathyroid and adrenal scanning methods are also presented.

6 **The Respiratory System** 53
MOHAMMED YUNUS

Radionuclides for lung disease study are starting to resolve the clinical dilemma in diagnosis. Dr. Yunus deals with perfusion and ventilation lung scanning, covering the principles . . . safety . . . radiopharmaceuticals . . . patient preparation . . . procedures . . . and interpretation, for diagnosis of numerous respiratory ailments.

7 **The Gastrointestinal System** 63
FUAD S. ASHKAR AND AUGUST MIALE, JR.

Drs. Ashkar and Miale examine liver, spleen, and pancreas imaging, covering the principle . . . tracers used . . . instrumentation . . . results . . . and interpretation in normal and abnormal situations. They also point out sources of error.

8 **The Cardiovascular System** 80
STUART GOTTLIEB

Dr. Gottlieb presents dynamic radiotracer techniques and their interpretations in evaluating cardiovascular problems. Radionuclide angiocardiographic findings in normal pericardial effusion . . . ventricular aneurysm . . . . . . mass lesions . . . and valvular disease are discussed, and dymanic measurements are analyzed.

9 **The Skeletal System** 108
ALDO N. SERAFINI

Bone scanning techniques with better agents have revolutionized our understanding of skeletal disease. Dr. Serafini discusses the indications and uses of bone scanning, including neoplastic diseases . . . trauma . . . aseptic necrosis . . . inflammatory disease . . . differentiation of bone islands . . . and evaluation of metabolic disorder.

10 **The Reproductive System** 118
ALEX A. BEZJIAN

Dr. Bezjian's chapter deals with placental localization and the role of RIA in obstetrics and gynecology. The clinical use of HPL . . . HGG . . . estrogens . . . progesterones . . . and gonadotropins are discussed, as well as normal pregnancy . . . threatened abortion . . . toxemia . . . intrauterine growth retardation . . . signs of fetal demise . . . ovarian dysfunction . . . menstrual irregularities . . . amenorrhea . . . and infertility.

11 **The Renal System** 130
ALDO N. SERAFINI

The triple renal scintigraphic techniques and the more common radionuclides—radiochlormerodrin, radiohippuran, and radiopertechnetate—are discussed here. Indications for renal imaging are also presented, with reference to renal size and localization . . . evaluation of intra- or extrarenal space-occupying lesions . . . hypertension . . . renal outlet obstruction . . . detection of vesicoureteral reflux . . . and renal transplants.

12 **The Hematopoietic System** 141
MORTON B. WEINSTEIN

Dr. Weinstein's chapter deals with the in vitro hematological procedures . . . imaging of the bone marrow . . . spleen and lymph nodes . . . and immunohematology. Also discussed are the Schilling Test . . . blood volume . . . red cell survival . . . ferrokinetics . . . imaging of organs with reticuloendothelial cells . . . and the applications of radionuclides to red cell metabolism.

13 **Tumor Localization** 150
MORTON B. WEINSTEIN AND EUGENE B. ROSENBERG

Detecting neoplastic diseases with radiotracers has markedly improved the physician's capability to detect cancer. Drs. Weinstein and Rosenberg tell how the standard radiotracer is useful in localizing tumors . . . the methodology of study . . . clinical applications . . . and findings.

14 **Detection of Human Tumor-Associated Antigens** 160
EUGENE B. ROSENBERG, PATRICIA M. SMITH, AND MORTON B. WEINSTEIN

Tumor detection by radioimmunoassay is presented here, including methods of detection . . . RIA for carcinoembryonic antigen (CEA) . . . alpha fetoprotein . . . assays of cellular immunity which detect tumor antigens . . . lymphocyte transformation studies . . . and ^{51}chromium lymphocyte cytotoxicity assays.

15 **Radioimmunoassay** 168
FUAD S. ASHKAR AND ALBERT V. HEAL

Drs. Ashkar and Heal present the principle and applications of radioimmunoassay . . . the antigens . . . radiolabeling . . . antibody formation . . . assay separation of bound from free antigen . . . data derivation . . . and specific application.

16 **Radioisotope Therapy** 176
FUAD S. ASHKAR

Radioisotope therapy has had a major impact on thyroid disease therapy. Dr. Ashkar discusses the diagnosis of various types of hyperthyroidism, emphasizing isotope dose calculations and post-therapy hypothyroidism. The detection of thyroid carcinoma . . . the roles of surgery . . . and of radioiodine therapy are presented.

Glossary and Appendix Tables 182
SHARAD AMTEY

Definitions of terms commonly used in nuclear medicine are given. Tables of physical constants . . . units . . . and radiation doses associated with imaging procedures are included.

Self-Evaluation Section 199

Test your understanding in this comprehensive 200-question short-answer test.

Index 213

About the Editor

Fuad S. Ashkar, MD, is Assistant Professor of Radiology and Medicine at the University of Miami School of Medicine. He is also Director of the Nuclear Metabolic Section in the Division of Nuclear Medicine at Jackson Memorial Hospital in Miami and at Mount Sinai Medical Center in Miami Beach, as well as being Consultant in Endocrinology and Staff Physician at both hospitals.

A Fellow of the Royal Society of Health and a Diplomate of the American Board of Nuclear Medicine, Dr. Ashkar's memberships include the Alpha Omega Alpha Honor Medical Society, Society of Nuclear Medicine, American Association for the Advancement of Science, the American Thyroid Association, and American Diabetes Association.

The author or co-author of numerous original contributions to medical literature, Dr. Ashkar has helped edit two books and contributed to several others.

Contributors

Sharad Amtey, PhD, LLB
Associate Professor of Radiology
Department of Radiology
West Virginia University School of Medicine
Morgantown, West Virginia

Alex A. Bezjian, MD
Assistant Professor of Obstetrics-Gynecology and Radiology
Division of Nuclear Medicine
University of Miami School of Medicine

Albert J. Gilson, MD
Professor of Radiology
Division of Nuclear Medicine
University of Miami School of Medicine

Stuart Gottlieb, MD
Instructor in Radiology
Division of Nuclear Medicine
University of Miami School of Medicine

Albert V. Heal, PhD
Instructor in Radiology
Division of Nuclear Medicine
University of Miami School of Medicine

Homer B. Hupf, PhD
Assistant Professor of Radiology
Division of Nuclear Medicine
University of Miami School of Medicine and
Mount Sinai Medical Center

Peter J. Kenny, PhD
Associate Professor of Radiology
Division of Nuclear Medicine
University of Miami School of Medicine

August Miale, Jr., MD
Associate Professor of Radiology
Division of Nuclear Medicine
University of Miami School of Medicine

Eugene B. Rosenberg, MD
Assistant Professor of Radiology and Medicine
Division of Nuclear Medicine and Oncology
University of Miami School of Medicine

R. Roger Sankey, PhD
Instructor in Radiology
Division of Nuclear Medicine
University of Miami School of Medicine

Aldo N. Serafini, MD
Instructor in Radiology
Division of Nuclear Medicine
University of Miami School of Medicine

Patricia M. Smith, MS
Research Associate in Radiology
Division of Nuclear Medicine
University of Miami School of Medicine

William M. Smoak III, MD
Associate Professor of Radiology
Division of Nuclear Medicine
University of Miami School of Medicine

Morton B. Weinstein, MD
Assistant Professor of Radiology and Medicine
Division of Nuclear Medicine
University of Miami School of Medicine

Mohammed Yunus, MD
Fellow in Nuclear Medicine
Division of Nuclear Medicine
University of Miami School of Medicine

Introduction

The past two decades have witnessed the birth of nuclear medicine and its growth from a research and investigative tool into a major branch of medical science. The dramatic development of this field had a major impact on hospital and, to some degree, on office practice. The present rate of growth is estimated at 35% annually.

The availability of reliable, rapid, and safe nuclear diagnostic procedures has eliminated the need for other radical, invasive, and traumatic diagnostic tests. Precise, reproducible, and reliable in vitro tests in the areas of competitive protein-binding analysis and radioimmunoassay have shed new light on our understanding of thyroid diseases, anemias, diabetes mellitus, growth disorders, peptic ulcer disease, hypertension, adrenal abnormalities, drug therapy and addiction, and viral infections.

The great potential of nuclear medicine in the screening and staging of disease, in therapy planning and followup, and in treatment with radioactive isotopes is still to be explored.

This book outlines the present status of nuclear medicine as a practical diagnostic and therapeutic modality.

Fuad S. Ashkar, MD

Preface

This book fulfills two important purposes admirably. It makes available for the first time a self-instruction summary and defines the core of knowledge that should be mastered by anyone interested in nuclear medicine. More important, it accomplishes this increasingly difficult task in the most up-to-date way possible. Every other book covering nuclear medicine is almost of necessity out-of-date by the time it is published.

Another unique feature of this book is that it has been assembled by perhaps the only nuclear medicine division large enough and so well balanced that each system is covered with such authority. This group has previously demonstrated its balance and authority in teaching by conducting a unique series of annual nuclear medicine seminars in Miami, the last of which was a review course for the American Board of Nuclear Medicine.

As a result, all teachers of nuclear medicine—as well as learners—should be grateful to Dr. Ashkar and colleagues for this original and necessary contribution to our never-ending struggle to keep abreast of the rapid developments in nuclear medicine.

William H. Beierwaltes, MD
Physician-in-Charge
Division of Nuclear Medicine
University Hospital
Ann Arbor, Michigan

The moving rectilinear scanner and the stationary scintillation camera are the two types of imaging instruments. Both consist of a crystal detector, collimators, associated electronic circuitry, and a display mode.

1
Instruments for Imaging Procedures

Peter J. Kenny

The instruments used for imaging the distribution of an administered radionuclide in the body may be classified into two broad categories: moving rectilinear scanners and stationary scintillation cameras. In both types of instruments the detecting element is a crystal of sodium iodide which has the property of scintillating (emitting light) when gamma rays from a radionuclide interact in it. Each scintillation lasts approximately 1 μsec, and the light emitted is detected by one or more photomultiplier tubes and converted into a small electrical signal which is registered by the associated electronic circuitry.

> The detecting element is a crystal of sodium iodide which scintillates when gamma rays from a radionuclide interact in it.

The terminology of nuclear medicine and computerization is explained in the Glossary. Miscellaneous physical information appears in the Appendix.

Rectilinear Scanners

Many different types of rectilinear scanners are commercially available. The smaller models have a single detector capable of scanning an area 14 by 17 inches. Larger models have two detectors, one mounted

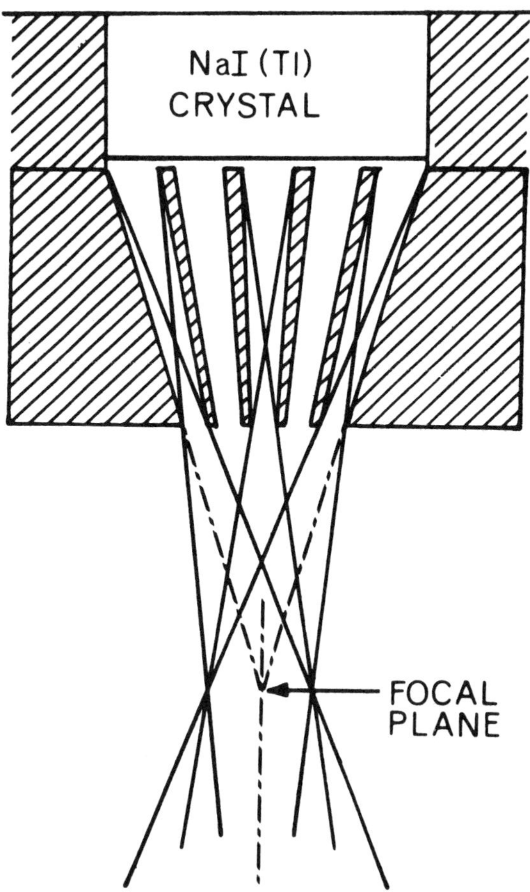

Figure 1-1 *Detecting element of rectilinear scanner. Sodium iodide crystal, usually 5 inches in diameter and 2 inches thick, is shielded with lead and fitted with a multihole focused collimator.*

above and one below the table on which the patient lies, and are capable of scanning the entire body. The most common detector is a crystal 5 inches in diameter and 2 inches thick, shielded with at least 2 inches of lead (Fig 1-1). Since gamma rays cannot be bent or focused to any useful extent (as can be done with light in the lens of a camera), the detector must be shielded and collimated so that it accepts radiation from only a narrow angle. The detector moves over the patient in a raster pattern (Fig 1-2). The count rate—the number of gamma rays interacting in the crystal per unit time—is registered at each position, and its variation over the area of the scan gives the relative distribution pattern of the radionuclide in the body.

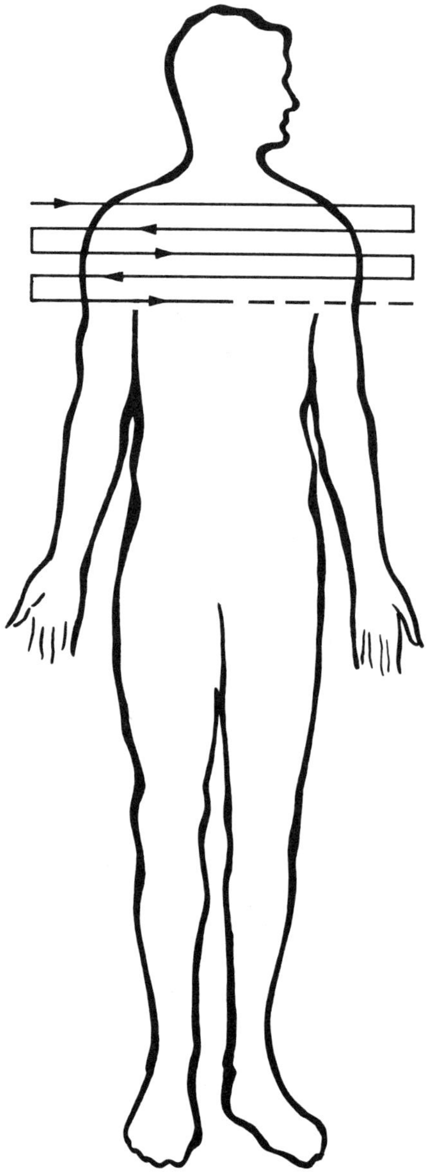

Figure 1-2 *Raster pattern of detector movement over patient.*

Collimators

The multihole focused collimator shown in Figure 1-1 is used to achieve a reasonable compromise between the conflicting requirements of sensitivity and spatial resolution. If no collimator were used, ie, if the full area of the crystal were exposed, more gamma rays could interact with the crystal and the counting rate at each point on the scan would be higher. However, the positional information regarding the direction of origin of each gamma ray would then be much less precise. Usually many different collimators are supplied with each scanner, and they can be interchanged depending on the particular application. For example, for scanning a small organ such as the thyroid gland, a fine-focus (high-resolution) collimator would be used to achieve the best definition and detail possible. For bone scanning a lower-resolution collimator would be used. For scanning large organs such as the liver or the lungs a collimator with a focal distance of approximately 5 inches would be appropriate.

Electronics

Figure 1-3 is a block diagram of the principal features of a scanner. The detector is moved by electric motors whose speed can

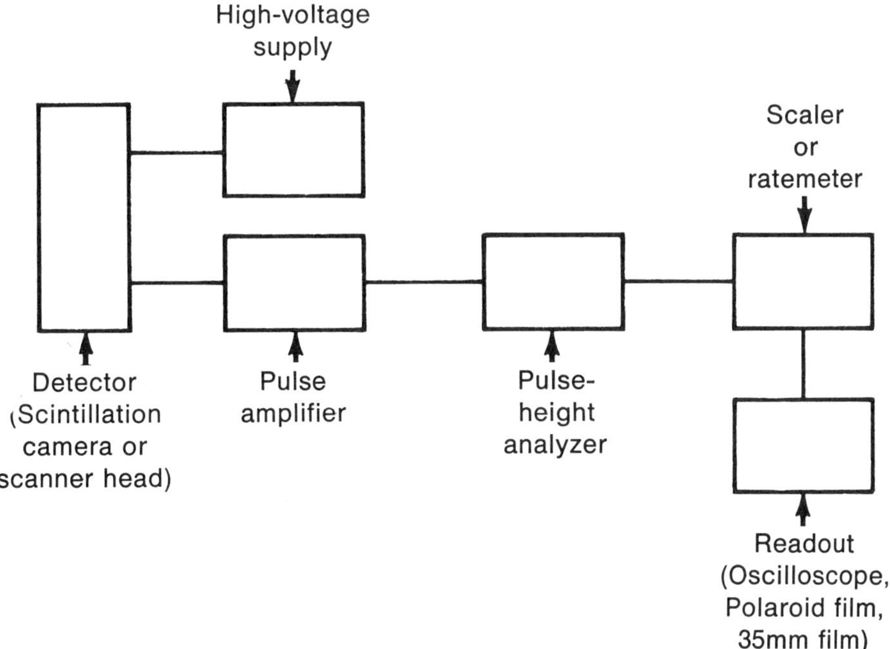

Figure 1-3 *Block diagram of imaging system.*

be adjusted by a dial setting. Speeds of up to 200 inches per minute are commonly available. The line spacing of the scan raster can also be selected, usually from a fine raster with successive lines 1/16 inch apart to coarser patterns with lines as much as 1 inch apart.

The function of the pulse-height analyzer is to ensure, as far as possible, that only gamma rays in the correct energy bracket are accepted. Each radionuclide used for scanning has its own distinctive gamma rays whose energies are specified in units of kiloelectron volts. For example, the principal gamma ray of technetium 99m is 140 kev; the principal gamma ray of iodine 131 is 364 kev. When gamma rays are scattered or deflected from their original direction of emission they lose some energy. These scattered gamma rays would degrade the quality of the image if they were counted. An energy channel or "window" can be set on the pulse-height analyzer which will accept only those pulses arising from gamma rays in a preselected range of energies.

Readouts

The final image of the radionuclide distribution in the body may be displayed in any of several ways. The so-called photoscan frequently takes the form of a 14- by 17-inch x-ray film on which each count registered places a small black dot by activating a light source which moves over the film in synchrony with the motion of the detector. Other forms of photoscan can be made on 35-mm, 70-mm, or Polaroid film which can be used to photograph the face of an oscilloscope on which each count accepted is briefly displayed in the correct positional relation. The display can also take the form of contour lines or can be made quantitative by the use of alphanumeric symbols from a typewriter or printer interfaced to the scanner.

Scintillation Cameras

In contrast to rectilinear scanners, the scintillation camera is a stationary device which views an entire organ at once. Several different models are now on the market with useful fields of view ranging from 10 to 15 inches in diameter. The detecting element is a large-diameter crystal of sodium iodide, 0.5 inch thick. The collimator may be a multiparallel-hole type (Fig 1-4) or a pinhole type (Fig 1-5). Organs larger than the useful diameter of the crystal may be viewed with the aid of a diverging collimator (Fig 1-6).

Gamma rays from the patient which interact in the crystal cause scintillations, just as in a rectilinear scanner. However, in the scintillation camera the crystal is viewed by 19 photomultiplier tubes whose outputs are connected to what is, in effect, an analog computer. The distribution of light among the 19 photomultipliers is sensed by the computer, which then determines where the scintillation occurred in the crystal. As with the scanner, a pulse-height analyzer is incorporated in the system to reject scattered gamma rays. Those scintillations corresponding to the interaction of unscattered gamma rays in the crystal are displayed briefly on an oscilloscope screen in the correct positional relation and are usually recorded on 35-mm, 70-mm, or Polaroid film. A unique advantage of the scintillation camera over the rectilinear scanner is its ability to perform rapid dynamic studies—for example,

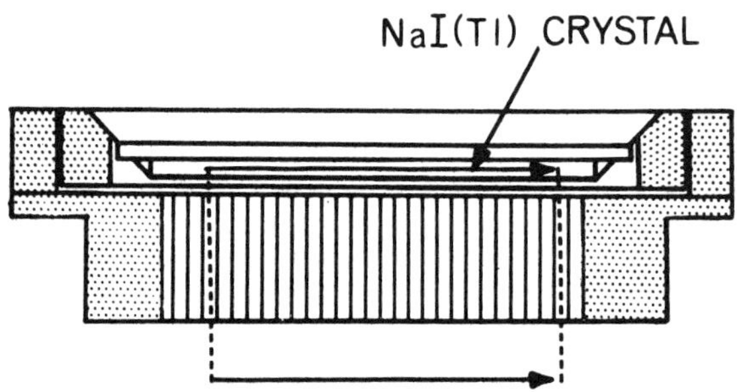

Figure 1-4 *Multiparallel-hole collimator for scintillation camera.*

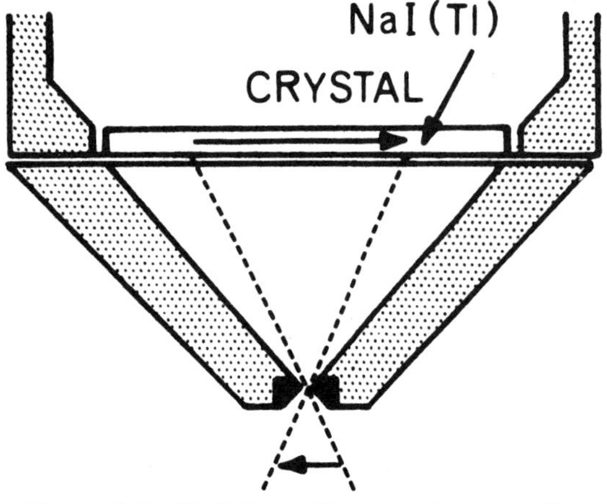

Figure 1-5 *Pinhole collimator for scintillation camera.*

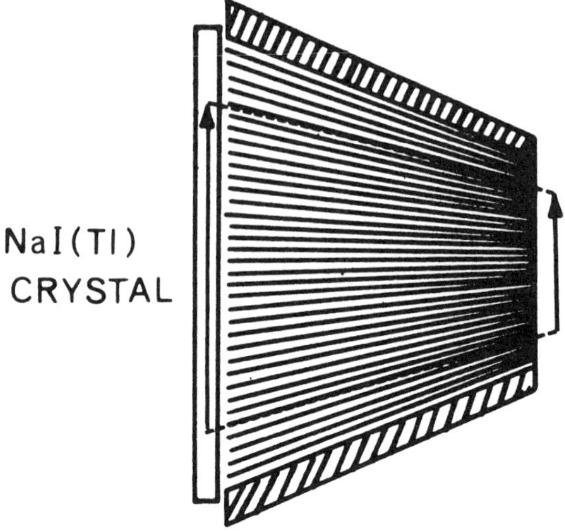

Figure 1-6 *Multidiverging-hole collimator for scintillation camera.*

An advantage of the scintillation camera over the rectilinear scanner is its ability to record rapid dynamic events, such as passage of radionuclide through the heart chambers.

---

to study the passage of a radionuclide through the chambers of the heart.

Because the camera crystal is only 0.5-inch compared with the 2-inch scanner crystal, the camera is best suited for use with radionuclides whose principal gamma ray energy is not much above 200 kev. With increasing energy, the efficiency of detection falls rapidly in the thin crystal. The autofluoroscope, a stationary camera-type imaging system, uses a large number of 1.5-inch thick crystals. It has therefore a higher efficiency than the scintillation camera but has a field of view limited to 6 by 9 inches.

Image Data Processing

Interfacing the scintillation camera to a small computer enables acquisition of quantitative data, especially from rapid dynamic studies, and permits such data-processing routines as correcting for nonuniformity of response across the large area of the crystal.

The most frequently used technique is to store the counts in a 64 by 64 matrix of image cells. Assuming a 10-inch useful crystal diameter, each image cell is then approximately 4 by 4 mm in size. The number of counts in each image cell per unit time (usually in the range 0.2 to 3.0 seconds, depending on the particular study) can be stored sequentially on a magnetic disc or tape, and time vs activity curves for various regions of interest in an organ can be displayed following completion of the study. Such systems add considerable flexibility to the options available with imaging systems, but they require the services of at least one individual to program and operate the computer.

So-called hard-wired systems—those which do not require programming, but rather provide a limited number of functions (eg, count integration over selected areas)—are also available commercially. These are simpler to operate but not as versatile as the minicomputer.

References

1. Anger HO: The instruments of nuclear medicine. *Hosp Practice* 7:45–54, 192.
2. Brookman VA, Bauer TJ: Collimator performance for scintillation camera systems. *J Nucl Med* 14:21, 1973.
3. Kenny PJ: What Is Quantitative Organ Visualization in Nuclear Medicine? In Kenny PJ, Smith EM (eds). *Quantitative Organ Visualization in Nuclear Medicine.* Coral Gables, Fla, University of Miami Press, 1971.
4. Sharma RR, Fowler JF: Threshold detection tests in radioisotope scanning. *Phys Med Biol* **15**:279, 1970.

Radiopharmaceuticals in the form of compounds, complexes, colloids, and generator-produced agents are used in nuclear medicine. Organ specificity is the goal of their design and the basis of their clinical value.

2 Radiopharmaceuticals for Clinical Use

Homer B. Hupf

Characteristics

With few exceptions, radiopharmaceuticals are categorized as diagnostic aids and are called *pharmaceuticals* because they must meet the same federal and state specifications as nonradioactive pharmaceuticals. The chemical concentration of the radioactive carrier substance is small and generally does not produce a pharmacologic effect. Appendix Tables 3, 4, 7, and 8 describe commonly used radionuclides.

Classification

Radiopharmaceuticals may be classified chemically as compounds, complexes, colloids, and generators.[11]

COMPOUNDS

In a compound, the radionuclide is firmly attached to the carrier substance by a true chemical bond. If the carrier compound normally contains atoms of the same species as the radionuclide, the compound is labeled isotopically. For instance, since chlormerodrin normally contains atoms of mercury, chlormerodrin Hg 197 is an isotopically labeled radioactive compound. On the other hand, methionine does not normally contain atoms of selenium, so selenomethionine Se 73 is a nonisotopically labeled radioactive compound.

COMPLEXES

Products such as polyphosphate Tc 99m, diethylenetriamine penta-acetic acid (DTPA), and citrate Ga 67 are complexes, and the radionuclide is associated with the carrier substance through secondary bonding (electron orbital overlap) which can be described by a stability constant. The radioactive species may separate from the carrier compound owing to a change in pH or the addition of a stronger complexing agent. The in vivo and in vitro stability of complexes is more precarious than the stability of compounds.

COLLOIDS

Colloids are products in the intermediate state between a solution and a suspension. The particle size of a colloid has no sharp limits, but a generally accepted size range is from 1 to 500 mu. These particles are much too small to be seen with the eye or even with an ordinary light microscope. A colorless colloid such as sulfur colloid Tc 99m should appear clear to partly cloudy depending upon the chemical concentration. No individual particles should be observed.

GENERATORS

The term *radioisotope cow* may be unscientific but accurately describes a radionuclide generator. A generator is a radioactive parent which decays to a radioactive daughter. The half-life of the parent is generally long enough to provide a useful product for at least several days (T½ = 67 hours for ^{99}Mo, 118 days for ^{113}Sn) and the half-life of the daughter is generally short (6 hours for ^{99m}Tc, 100 minutes for ^{113m}In). The useful daughter is periodically "milked" by means of a sterile eluting solution from the parent, which is firmly absorbed to an insoluble support.

Transport and Specificity

Injected radionuclides are rapidly distributed throughout the body in the blood stream. Depending upon its physical and chemical nature, the product may remain vascular, collect in pools or spaces, or be actively or inactively removed from the blood by specific organs or tumors. Specific mechanisms are discussed in subsequent paragraphs. The radiopharmaceutical does not reach necrotic or nonfunctioning areas, and these appear as holes in the image or scan.

Organ specificity is the goal in the design of radiopharmaceuticals, and it has proved an elusive one. Iodide uptake by the thyroid, colloid removal by the liver, physical filtration of labeled aggregates by the lung, and filtration and fixation of iodohippurate I 131 and chlormerodrin Hg 203, respectively, by the kidneys are fairly successful examples of organ specificity.

Physical Properties

The physical properties of some medically important radionuclides are shown in Table 2-1.

Table 2-1. Physical Properties of Some Common Radionuclides

Nuclide	T½	Principal gamma emissions (kev)	Abundance (%)
^{131}I	8.05 days	364	82
		637	6.8
^{123}I*	13.0 hr	159	83
		530	2
		380	1
^{124}I*	4.15 days	511	50
		605	67
		644	12
^{99m}Tc	6.05 hr	140	90
^{197}Hg	65.0 hr	68	100
		77	18
^{203}Hg	46.9 days	279	77
^{75}Se	120.0 days	136	57
		265	60
		280	25
^{18}F*	110.0 min	511	194
^{67}Ga*	77.9 hr	93	40
		184	24
		296	22
^{111}In*	2.81 days	173	89
		247	94
^{113m}In	99.8 min	393	64
^{87m}Sr *	2.83 hr	388	80
^{51}Cr	27.8 days	320	9

* Accelerator-produced.

Adapted from Lederer CM, Hollander JM, Perlman I. *Table of Isotopes*, 6th ed. New York, Wiley, 1968.

General Methods of Preparation

Inorganic Compounds

Inorganic compounds (NaI, NaF, $NaTcO_4$) generally have a high ionic character and are carried by the blood as plasma-protein complexes. They are prepared simply by dissolving the target from which they were produced in dilute acid or base, and then adjusting pH. If the radionuclide is accelerator-produced a chemical purification is usually required.

Organic Compounds

Organic compounds are produced by exchange (orthoiodohippurate I 131), substitution (iodinated albumin I 131), or synthesis (chlormerodrin Hg 197, methionine Se 75).[5,9] Iodinated compounds are prepared by converting iodide I^- ions to $I^{\alpha+} + I^{\alpha-}$ (the zero oxidation state) with an oxidizing agent such as chloramine T, iodine monochloride, or hydrogen peroxide. The subsequent exchange or substitution is rarely quantitative, and the unbound iodide is separated from the product using an ion-exchange resin. For best results, the reacting volumes should be kept small and iodide of high specific activity (millicuries per milligram of iodine) should be used. Synthesis generally involves several reactions, and the desired product must be purified of intermediate and initial reactants. Synthesis can rarely be accomplished with carrier-free radionuclides and the final product has a low specific activity (millicuries per milligram of final product). The chemical stability of a synthesized compound is usually good.

Complexes

Complexes are composed of a central ion (most often a metal ion, which is the radionuclide) surrounded by groups of two or more of the complexing agent called ligands. Under proper conditions of pH and concentration, the metal ion no longer exhibits its own chemical properties, but rather the chemical properties of the complexing agent. For example, gallium ions tend to form an insoluble hydroxide at pH 6 but remain in solution at pH 6 if citrate is present in the solution. In some cases, the oxidation state of the central ion must be altered to accomplish complexation. This appears to be the case for Tc^{+7}, which must be reduced to a lower oxidation state to form complexes with albumin, polyphosphate, or DTPA. Stannous chloride, ferrous sulfate, ascorbic acid, and hydrochloric acid, or combinations of the same, are used to effect complexation in these products. The stability of complexes depends upon the pH of the solution, the oxidation state of the central ion, and the absence of a stronger complexing agent (plasma proteins?).

Colloids

The preparation of colloids varies from simple adjustment of the pH of the solution to complicated chemical manipulations.[7] Ions of any element which form insoluble oxides or hydroxides can be made colloidal with proper control of concentration, agitation, and pH. Most colloidal particles tend to aggregate on standing. This tendency is greatly reduced or eliminated by the timely addition of a protective colloid such as albumin, gelatin, or mannitol.

Technetium-sulfur colloid is prepared by the formation of the highly insoluble sulfide, Tc_2S_7, in acid solution. Since the chemical concentration of Tc_2S_7 is very low (practically carrier-free Tc), the simultaneous formation of a sulfur colloid acts as an inert carrier of the Tc_2S_7. At pH 6.5 and higher, Tc_2S_7 tends to redissolve and form TcO_4^- so the final product is buffered at pH 6.

Clinical Applications

The following is a brief summary of the widely used clinical procedures in nuclear medicine. Emphasis is on the mechanism of uptake of the radiopharmaceutical, not on the clinical aspects. Appropriate texts should be consulted for more detailed clinical information.

Brain

Static images of the brain provide diagnostic information about the existence, size, and location of space-occupying lesions, cerebral vascular accidents, and intracranial injury.[3] Normal brain tissue is protected from chemical substances in the blood by a membranous blood-brain barrier or series of barriers impervious to many chemical substances. A space-occupying lesion breaks down the barrier in the area of the lesion and allows these chemicals to be absorbed there. Radiopharmaceuticals such as chlormerodrin Hg 203, albumin I 131, and pertechnetate Tc 99m are used to detect the lesions and aberrant blood flow.

Sodium pertechnetate Tc 99m sterile solution, either aseptically "milked" from a generator or supplied by a local distributor, is currently the agent of choice for these procedures. The unique physical properties of ^{99m}Tc permit administered activities of 10 to 20 mCi, which produce good target/background ratios on imaging and constitute an accepable radiation dose to the patient. This radiopharmaceutical also allows dynamic flow images to be taken every one to three seconds showing the initial passage of the bolus through the head and neck following intravenous injection. Minor drawbacks are slow vascular clearance (three to six hours) and scattering of the 140-kev photon by tissue and bone.

Drs. Smoak and Gilson discuss this further in Chapter 4.

Commonly Used Organ-Specific Radiopharmaceuticals

- Brain
  - Chlormerodrin Hg 203
  - Albumin I 131
  - Sodium pertechnetate Tc 99m
- Thyroid
  - Sodium iodide I 131
  - Sodium pertechnetate Tc 99m
- Liver
  - Sulfur colloid Tc 99m
  - Rose bengal I 131
- Lungs
  - Macroaggregated iodinated albumin I 131
  - Albumin microspheres Tc 99m
- Kidneys
  - Orthoiodohippuric acid I 131
  - Chlormerodrin Hg 197
  - Sodium pertechnetate Tc 99m
  - DTPA Tc 99m

Thyroid

Sodium iodide I 131 (orally or by injection) and sodium pertechnetate Tc 99m assist in the diagnosis of a variety of thyroid malfunctions. Functional disorders are related to the ability of the gland to trap, organify, and store circulating iodide I-131. The mechanism of uptake is active removal of approximately 25% of the circulating blood pool of iodide daily by the gland for conversion to thyroxine and triiodothyronine.

The thyroid gland also traps pertechnetate ions (TcO_4^-), but without organification or storage. Transit time of a bolus of pertechnetate Tc 99m from the carotid artery to the thyroid has been used as a test of thyroid function. The chief use of ^{99m}Tc in thyroid disorders is to depict the gland. The image allows differentiation of functioning from nonfunctioning tissue and location of "hot," "warm," or "cold" nodules.

Sodium pertechnetate Tc 99m has the advantages of short half-life, low radiation dose to the patient, and an easily collimated photon for better resolution; it lacks the organification and storage properties of iodide. Sodium iodide I 131 provides a relatively high radiation dose to the thyroid, and, if used for imaging, the imaging is generally delayed 24 to 48 hours to allow blood pool clearance.

Thyroid evaluation procedures are described in Chapter 5.

Liver

Liver imaging is generally performed to evaluate the organ's size, shape, and position or to detect space-occupying lesions, hepatic cell dysfunction, and biliary obstruction.[4] The Kupffer cells of the reticuloendothelial system efficiently remove colloidal particles (20μ to 500μ in size) from the blood and this is the mechanism utilized by radiopharmaceuticals for liver imaging. Sulfur colloid Tc 99m, prepared in the hospital from commercially available kits, is currently the most widely used radiopharmaceutical for liver studies. A minor disadvantage is tissue scattering of the 140-kev photon by the relatively thick organ. Colloids of ^{113m}In and ^{111}In are being investigated as possible substitutes for ^{99m}Tc in liver imaging.

Liver function and biliary stasis can be evaluated with a radioiodinated fluorescein dye substance, rose bengal. The radiopharmaceutical is cleared from the blood (approximately 95%) by polygonal cells of the liver. In contrast to colloidal particles removed by the Kupffer cells, the dye does not remain in the polygonal cells but is secreted into the bile canaliculi and travels through the biliary tree to the duodenum. Rose bengal I 131 is not generally used to study liver morphology or space-occupying lesions. Danger of radiation overdose to the patient from the eight-day half-life nuclide limits the administered activity to 300 uCi, and this undoubtedly hinders its use. Future availability of the 159-kev, short-lived ^{123}I (half-life 13 hours) should regenerate interest in radioiodinated rose bengal studies.

Dr. Ashkar discusses liver scanning in Chapter 7.

Lungs

Lung imaging is performed to assist in the diagnosis of aberrant pulmonary artery perfusion and diminished perfusion in the peripheral capillary bed.[10] Radioactive particles, between 10u and 90u in size, are trapped in some of the 2.8×10^8 capillary segments of the lung (approximately 8u) following an intravenous injection. An area of the lung which has no or limited blood flow appears as a hole or defect in the resulting image. Techniques are discussed by Dr. Yunus in Chapter 6.

The mechanism of uptake of the radiopharmaceutical is physical occlusion of biologically degradable particles. Albumin can be aggregated to particles in the proper size range under carefully controlled conditions of heat, agitation, and pH. Macroaggregated iodinated albumin I 131, macroaggregated albumin Tc 99m, and albumin microspheres Tc 99m are the main products used.

The ^{131}I product is first tagged, then aggregated and shipped ready to use by the radiopharmaceutical companies. The quality assurance of the product is good, but it suffers the physical drawbacks of ^{131}I mentioned earlier in connection with liver scanning.

Sterile macroaggregated albumin particles are available from several companies in kit form. The user prepares the ^{99m}Tc product by adding sodium pertechnetate Tc 99m. A reliable product can be prepared from the kits, but the preparer should exercise some quality control measures—eg, examining a sample of the tagged particles on a hemocytometer placed under a microscope, and performing radiochromatography to estimate the amount of unbound pertechnetate.

A sterile albumin microspheres kit is also available commercially with instructions for preparing the ^{99m}Tc product. The tagging procedure is more complex and the tag is somewhat more labile than the above product, but the average size of the particles is well controlled by the manufacturer before shipment.

Kidneys

Nuclear medicine procedures to assist in the diagnosis of various renal disorders include renal imaging, renography, voiding studies, clearance measurements, and vascular studies.[8] The radiopharmaceuticals commonly used are orthoiodohippuric acid I-131, chlormerodrin Hg-197, and pertechnetate Tc-99m or DTPA Tc 99m. Each radiopharmaceutical is handled somewhat differently biologically and the choice of agent depends upon the desired test. They are described by Dr. Serafini in Chapter 11.

With normal blood supply and adequate tubular function, 80% to 95% of the administered orthoiodohippuric acid I 131 is cleared by tubular cells and excreted in the urine. It is principally used for renography and flow studies.

Chlormerodrin Hg 197 is also cleared by the tubular cells, but is excreted very slowly. It is most often used for imaging the kidneys, but can be employed for the other tests. Tissue scattering of the low-energy x- and gamma rays from ^{197}Hg is a major disadvantage. Use of chlormerodrin Hg 203 has been limited because of the radiation dose to the kidneys (50 to 250 mrad/μCi).

Pertechnetate Tc 99m is used for blood flow studies and imaging. DTPA Tc 99m is cleared by the glomeruli and used for clearance measurements.

References

1. Basolo F, Johnson R: *Coordination Chemistry.* New York, Benjamin, 1964.
2. Freeman LM, Blaufox MD (eds): Diagnostic radionuclide studies of the thyroid gland. *Semin Nucl Med,* 1:3, 1971.
3. Gilson AJ, Smoak WM (eds): *Central Nervous System Investigations with Radionuclides.* Springfield, Ill, Thomas, 1971.
4. Gilson AJ, Smoak WM, Weinstein MB (eds): *Hematopoietic and Gastrointestinal Investigations with Radionuclides.* Springfield, Ill, Thomas, 1972.
5. Hunter WM: Iodination of Protein Compounds. In Andrews G, Kniseley R, Wagner H Jr (eds). *Radioactive Pharmaceuticals.* USAEC Conf 651111. Springfield, Va, Clearing house for Scientific Information, 1966, pp 245–264.
6. Lederer CM, Hollander JM, Perlman I: *Table of Isotopes,* 6th ed. New York, Wiley, 1968.
7. Reber LA: Colloidal Dispersions. In *Remington's Pharmaceutical Sciences,* 14th ed. Easton, Pa, Mack, 1970, pp 319–329.
8. Timmermans L, Merchie G (eds): *Radioisotopes in the Diagnosis of Diseases of the Kidneys and the Urinary Tract.* Proceedings, First International Symposium, Liege. Amsterdam, Excerpta Medica, 1969.
9. Tubis, M: Special Iodinated Compounds for Biology and Medicine. In Andrews G, Kniseley R, Wagner H Jr (eds). *Radioactive Pharmaceuticals.* USAEC Conf 651111. Springfield, Va, Clearing house for Scientific Information, 1966, pp 281–304.
10. Wagner HN Jr, Holmes RA, Lopez-Majano V, et al: The Lung. In Wagner HN (ed). *Principles of Nuclear Medicine.* Philadelphia, Saunders, 1968, pp 472–530.
11. Wilson BJ: *The Radiochemical Manual,* 2nd ed. Amersham, England, Radiochemical Centre, 1966.

A computer consists of an input device, a storage device, a central processing unit, and an output device. A small computer interfaced to the imaging instrument facilitates data processing.

3 Data and the Computer

R. Roger Sankey

The Digital Computer

Definitions

A computer is a device which can perform a sequence of arithmetic operations upon data input to it and communicate the results of these operations to the outside world. It is a digital device and requires digital data input. Digital data are discrete and are presented in terms of a finite number of characters. The other form of data—analog data—is generally of a continuous nature, eg, voltage levels. If a digital computer is to operate on analog data, the data must be first digitized. The device that accomplishes this task is an analog-to-digital converter (ADC). The ADC is the link, or interface, between the computer and any device which may be a source of analog data.

It is important to recognize that a digital computer is incapable of performing any task until it is programmed to do so. At that time the computer attempts to carry out the program step by step to produce an answer. The correctness of that answer depends on the correctness of the executed program written by an individual.

A computer can perform only as it is programmed. The correctness of the answer it produces depends on the correctness of the man-made program.

Organization

Most electronic computers consist of four basic units: (1) the input device, (2) a storage device, (3) a central processing unit, and (4) an output device. The interaction of these units is shown in Figure 3-1.

INPUT/OUTPUT DEVICES

The function of the input/output (I/O) devices is communication with the outside world, and often one device serves both as input and as output. Data and programs can be input to the computer through a teletype keyboard, a punched-paper-tape reader, a punched-card reader, or a magnetic tape or disc system.

STORAGE DEVICES

Storage may be internal to the computer (core storage) or external to the computer (peripheral storage).

Core storage is magnetic. Each core consists of small individual rings of ferromagnetic material, and the cores are wired together as shown in Figure 3-2. A current passing through the wire sets up a mag-

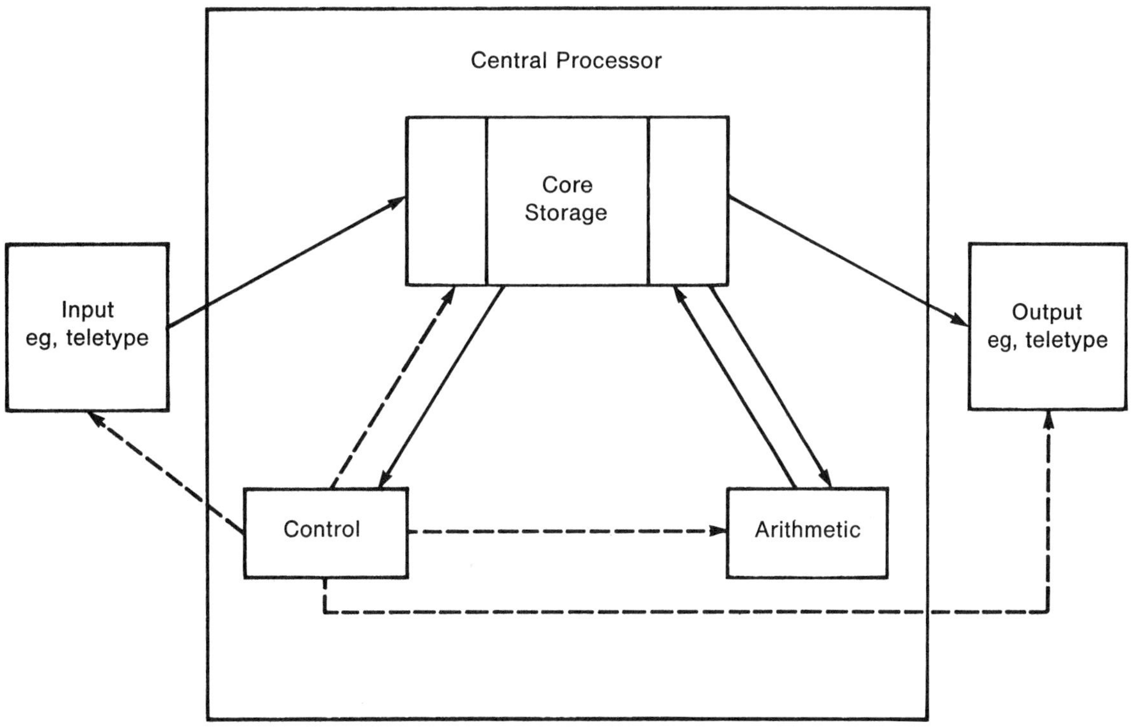

Figure 3-1 *Basic elements of digital computer system.*

netic field around the wire and induces a magnetic field in the ring. When the current is removed the ring remains magnetized. Depending on the direction of the current in the wire, the magnetic state of the ring has either a clockwise or a counterclockwise orientation. Current in one direction may be assigned the code number 1 and current in the opposite direction may be coded as zero. Therefore, a simple yes/no (binary) situation exists in the core of the computer and communication with the digital computer uses the binary number system which consists of 0 to 1. Detailed description of the binary and other numbering systems can be found in reference 2.

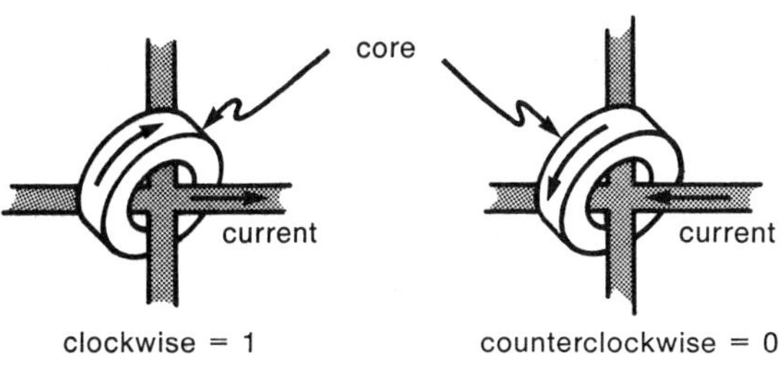

Figure 3-2 *Section of magnetic core.*

It is inefficient, and in most cases impossible, to use the core of a computer for long-term storage. Efficient *peripheral storage* on a magnetic tape or magnetic disc system is generally required.

A magnetic tape or disc consists of a large number of small sections, each of which can be magnetized in one direction or the opposite direction, forming a binary system completely compatible with the core storage of the computer. Speed is the basic difference between tape and disc. The tape is a sequential access system, ie, the computer must search a tape in a sequential fashion, record by record; the disc is a random access system, ie, any given record can be reached instantly. The disc, then, is the more rapid device and storage medium of choice.

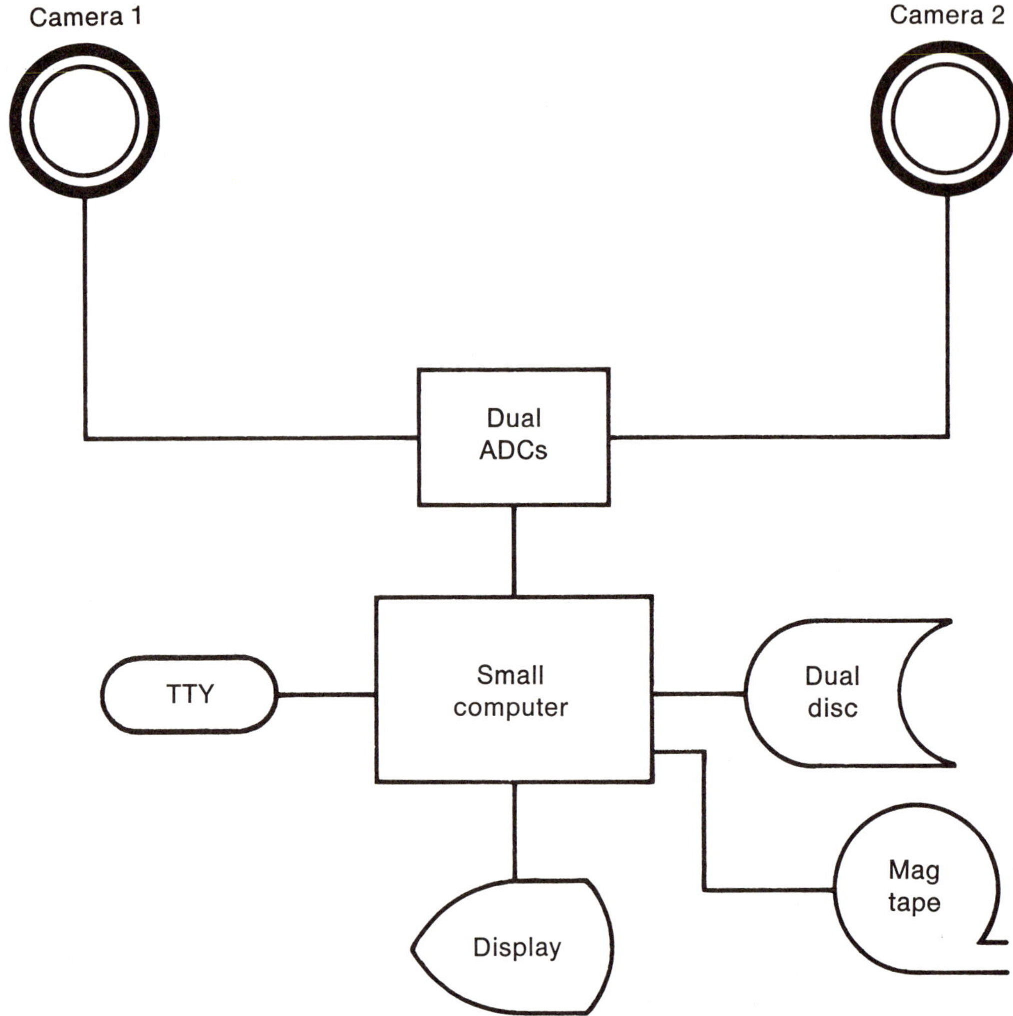

Figure 3-3 *Anger camera-computer system.*

CENTRAL PROCESSING UNIT

The central processing unit (CPU) consists of a control unit and an arithmetic unit. The control unit is the brain of the system. It is directly under human supervision. As shown in Figure 3-1, the control unit is in direct communication with all other components of the system. It interprets and forwards instructions to all the other components and ensures that all operations are carried out in the sequence prescribed by the stored program. The arithmetic unit is that part of the computer responsible for carrying out certain arithmetic operations.

The Computer and Nuclear Medicine

This discussion is limited to the Anger type gamma camera interfaced to a small digital computer. The reader should consult the works listed in the reference section for information on computerization in other areas of nuclear medicine.

Camera-Computer Hardware System

The gamma camera outputs analog positional information in the form of analog X and Y voltage signals which locate an event on the face of the crystal. (The operation of the camera is outlined in Chapter 1.)

The camera output, being analog, must be digitized before the image data can be interpreted and stored by the computer. This is usually accomplished with a succesive approximation ADC. This ADC is the interface between camera and computer and is under the influence of the control unit. Since the control unit is under human supervision, the decision to accept data and decisions about how it should be formatted, stored, etc, are made by the operator. Figure 3-3 presents the basic elements of a camera-computer system used in nuclear medicine. The I/O device for such a system is typically a teletype or high-speed thermal printer plus keyboard, the storage device is a magnetic tape or disc, the display device is a cathode ray tube, and the central processor is a minicomputer ("mini" because the storage capacity is limited in comparison with the large computer systems used in industry or universities). With these hardware elements various camera scans can be acquired, manipulated, and stored provided the appropriate programs are available.

Camera-Computer Software System

The software of the system is a compilation of all the programs that facilitate operation of the computer. The system software is in general unique for each application. Thus, the software required for acquisition and processing of camera studies is quite different in detail (though similar in concept and purpose) from the software necessary for scanner data acquisition and processing. Data acquisition from a camera consists of storing the positional X-Y information in an array in the core storage or memory of the computer. The array is typically 64 by 64 storage units in size. Each camera signal is used to increment one X-Y location in the 64 by 64 matrix (Fig 3-4). Each camera image consists of thousands of counts and each count is stored

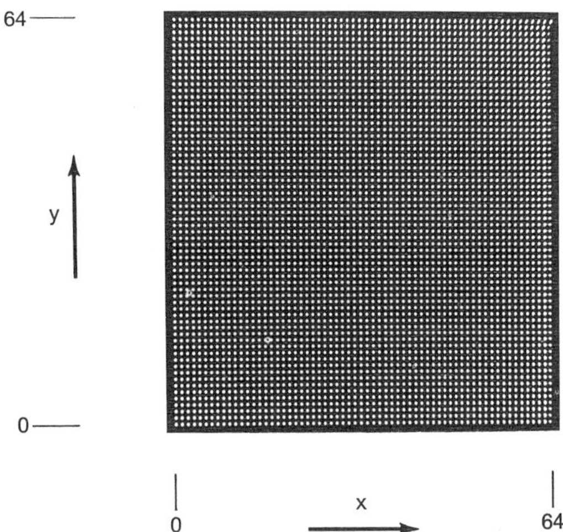

Figure 3-4 *Display matrix.*

in a given X-Y location of the matrix which corresponds to the position on the crystal at which it occurred. The final image displayed by the computer is a square 64 by 64 matrix of dots, each with an intensity determined by the number of counts received for that location. The image has a gray scale just as any photographic or x-ray image. The scan is then, by software command, stored on tape or disc or erased. The study may be static, consisting of a single image with a large number of counts, or dynamic, consisting of a number of sequential records, each collected for a prespecified number of seconds. The latter method of collecting data has proved useful in tracing the passage of a radioactive bolus through organs such as heart, liver, or kidney.

Described here are only those programs which the system operator utilizes in acquiring and processing a study. Software needed for storage, display of data, etc, are not discussed.

ACQUISITION SOFTWARE

Acquisition software may be considered in two categories: static study acquisition and dynamic study acquisition.

For accumulating a static image, the operator has the option of terminating the study by selecting either a preset time or a preset number of counts. In the former case the computer keeps track of the elapsed time and terminates at the requested time interval; in the latter case the computer integrates the number of counts and terminates acquisition when the desired number is reached. At the end of the study, storage may be either automatic to a preset disc record or commanded manually.

For a dynamic study the operator must furnish the computer with the number of frames to be collected, the time per frame, and a starting disc record. Each frame is stored on completion, the memory erased, and the next frame begun. The computer, upon receiving the start command, acquires the next frame, stores it in the starting record + 1, and so on until the study is completed.

The studies are available for instant recall and display so that photographs, enhancement maneuvers, etc, can be performed as required.

PROCESSING SOFTWARE

The purpose of processing software is to extract as much information as possible from a given study by allowing after-the-fact manipulations on the data not possible with a camera alone. Processing software is best considered by individual examination of the most common types of programs.

Uniformity Correction The sensitivity response across the face of the gamma camera is typically nonuniform by as much as 10%. This can be demonstrated by acquiring an image of a uniform flood source and observing the intensity pattern. If this image is digitized and stored in a 64 by 64 array, the computer can determine the correction factors necessary to make the image uniformly flat. These factors can be stored and applied to clinical images on a point-by-point basis to remove errors introduced by the nonuniform response. Figure 3-5 shows the flood data before and after correction.

Computer-Enabled Image Manipulations

- Uniformity correction
- Quality control
- Enhancement
- Region of interest assignment
- Smoothing
- Frame arithmetic
- Time-activity histograms

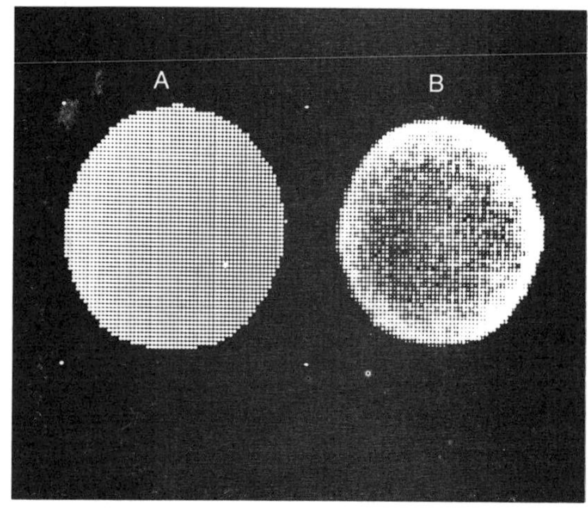

Figure 3-5 *Flood data displayed by computer before* (A) *and after* (B) *uniformity correction.*

Quality Control Because the camera can drift out of calibration and exceed the 10% nonuniformity limits, a rapid and simple check on day-to-day camera performance is useful. Figure 3-6 illustrates how the computer can be utilized to achieve this. Figure 3-6*A* shows a display of the raw flood source data; Figure 3-6*B* shows a display of all points 5% less than the average value of all the points. Figure 3-6*C* shows a display of all points 5% greater than the average; and Figure 3-6*D* shows a combination of *B* and *C*. This single image generated by the computer allows a

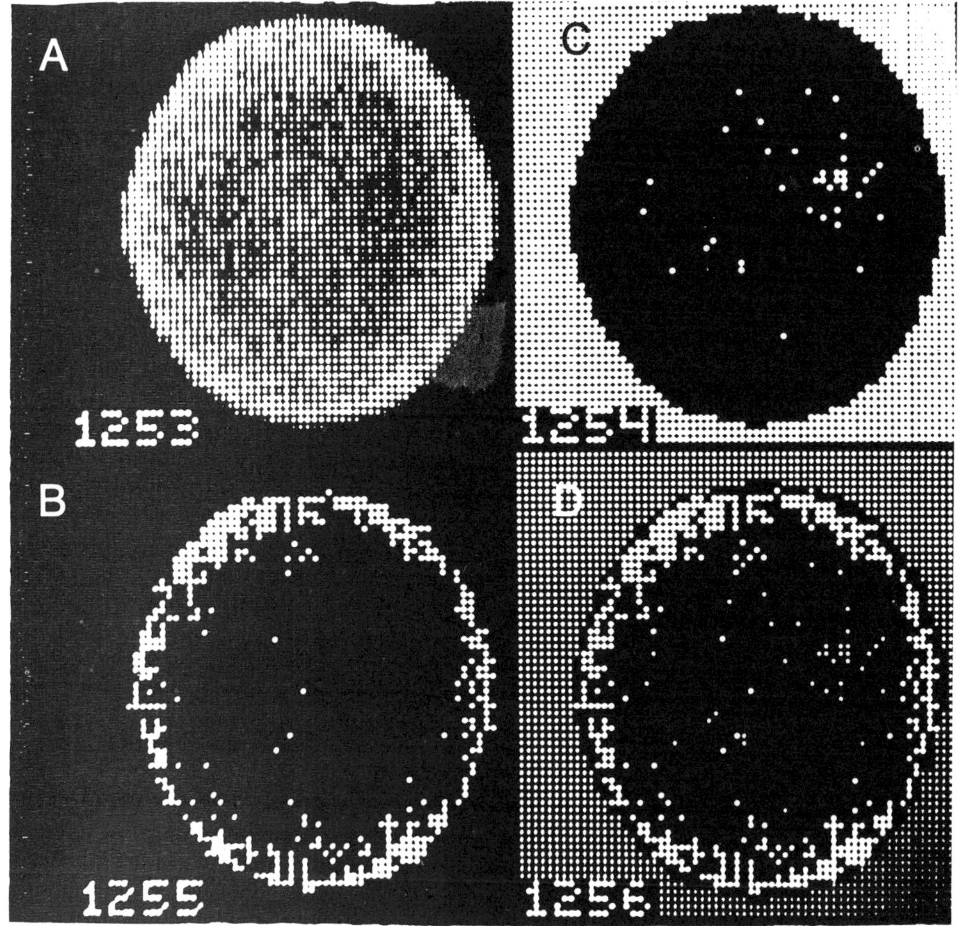

Figure 3-6 *Image quality control;* A, *raw flood image;* B, *display of all points 5% greater than average;* C, *display of all points 5% less than average;* D, *composite of* B *and* C.

quick visual assessment of a given camera's performance.

Enhancement Nuclear medicine images, like all other images, have a gray scale. The intensity of the image on the scope is usually set so that the highest-count-rate region in the image is at the top of the gray scale of the film used. This is not always desirable; often it is necessary to examine the low-count-rate areas which may be completely underexposed owing to a "hot spot" in the scan. A simple computer program allows the operator to adjust the gray scale (or color scale) by teletype commands. Figure 3-7 shows a liver scan that has been enhanced by adjusting the linear region of the gray scale. Figure 3-7*A* shows the usual image where the high-count-rate area is used to set the top of the scale with all other matrix elements in the image exposed proportionally. Figure 3-7*B* through *D* shows various alterations where high-count-rate areas are set to be exposed at the same level of saturation or simply deleted (blacked out) from the picture. The scheme utilized in making these pictures is shown in Figure 3-8. There are three variable parameters: (1) the cutoff level, (2) the background suppression, and (3) the saturation level. These parameters are expressed in percentages. The cutoff level

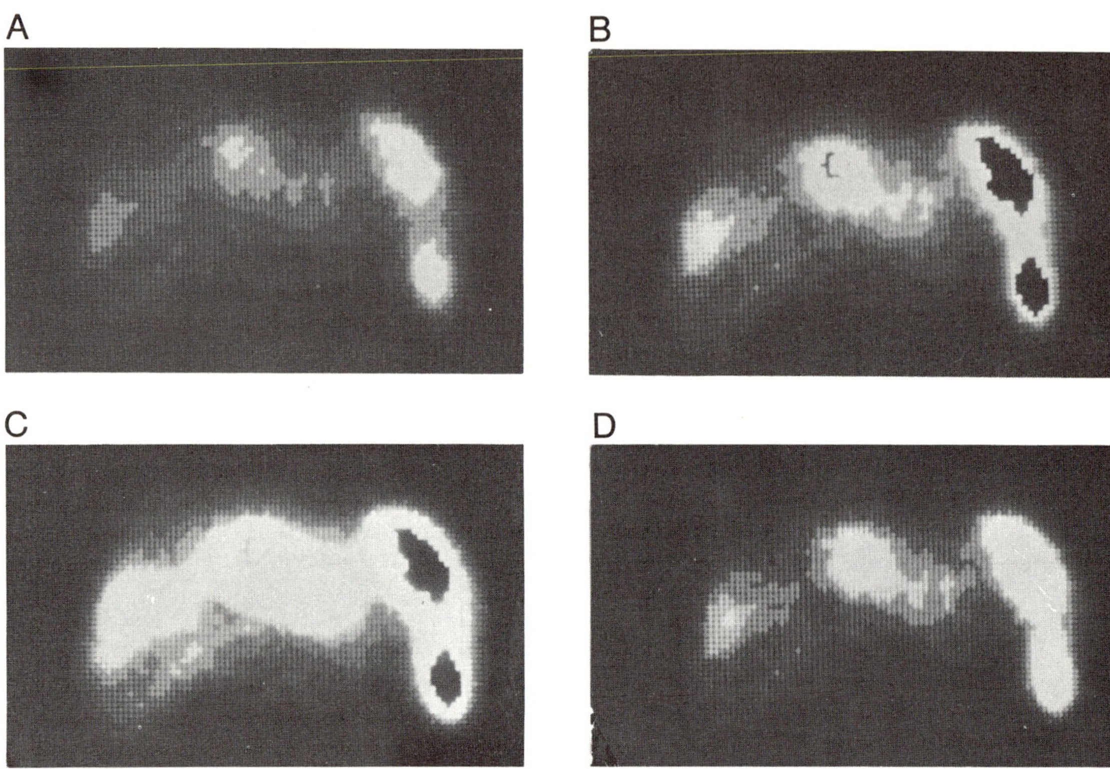

Figure 3-7 *Image enhancement of liver scan. Background suppression, saturation level, and cutoff level (in percents) are:* (A) *0, 100, 100;* (B) *10, 100, 80;* (C) *10, 80, 80;* (D) *10, 80, 100. (Images from Picker IES System.)*

is chosen as a percentage of the maximum count rate in the image. All points in the image having a larger number of counts than the percent cutoff level times the maximum count are blacked out. The product of the maximum count and the percent cutoff is the cut value. The background suppression is a percentage of the cut value. All points in the image containing fewer counts than the set percentage of the cut value are deleted. The saturation level is also a percentage of the cut value, and all points containing counts greater than this percentage and less than the cut value are set to the same intensity or color. All other shades of gray or colors are linearly distributed between the background level and the saturation level. The level percentages for the study shown in Figure 3-7 are indicated. The scheme described here is basically the one used on the Picker nuclear image enhancement system in conjunction with a Picker Dynacamera.

Region of Interest Assignment Any point or number of points in the image matrix can be selected by marking with a light pen or by typing in the X-Y coordinates of the desired region through the teletype. Once a point or region is flagged, the computer can compute and print out the number of flagged channels and the integrated count in the region. The flagged regions can be stored on a definite disc record for use later.

Smoothing The purpose of image smoothing is to create a smoothly varying

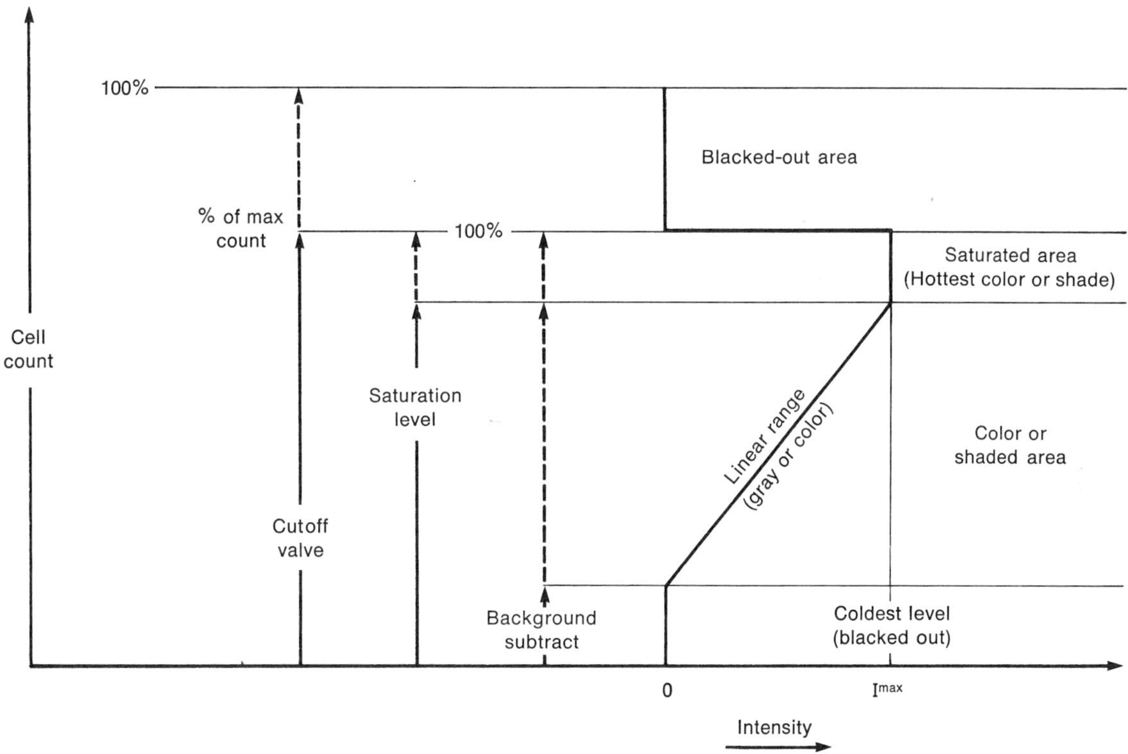

Figure 3-8 *Relation of cutoff level, saturation level, and background level to region of linear exposure. Enhancement scheme utilized on Picker IES System. (Reprint courtesy of Picker Nuclear, North Haven, Conn.)*

image by reducing statistical fluctuations. It is accomplished by averaging the matrix element of interest with adjacent elements. Consider nine elements of a given image numbered as follows.

7	8	9
6	1	2
5	4	3

Two common methods of smoothing this element of the image are five-point and nine-point. The five-point method involves a weighted average of the central point 1 with its closest neighbors—2, 4, 6, and 8. Nine-point smoothing involves a weighted average of the central point with all eight neighboring points. The process is carried out on each point in the image to obtain the final smoothed image. Smoothing of this type always degrades resolution to some degree.

Frame Arithmetic Dynamic studies consist of a number of timed frames which allow the assessment of blood flow to or through an organ as a function of time. The study is stored frame by frame on a disc in a fashion analogous to a movie film strip. The computer can be programmed to add frames to produce a composite or to subtract frames to reduce background. Figure 3-9 demonstrates the usefulness of frame addition. Figure 3-9*A* shows the right heart and pulmonary outflow of a dynamic heart study; it is a composite of selected frames from an early part of the study. Figure 3-9*B*, demonstrating the left heart and lung field, is constructed of se-

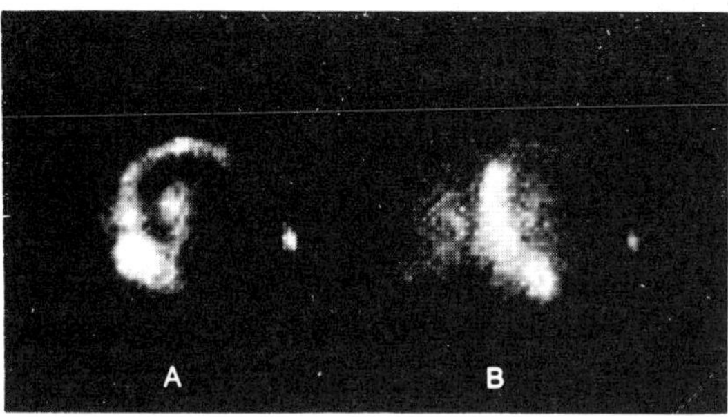

Figure 3-9 *Use of frame addition to create composite right heart image* (A) *and composite left heart image* (B). *Images generated with MDS Nuclear Medicine System on line to a Picker Dynacamera 2.*

lected frames later in the study.

Time-Activity Histograms A time-activity histogram is a plot of activity in a given region vs time. The application of the computer here is best described by means of an example of a cardiac blood flow study. A bolus of radioactive tracer is injected intravenously and the camera-computer system is started. The study is recorded at 0.5 second per frame for a total of 90 frames. A right and left heart image is formed as described in Figure 3-9. Regions in the right ventricle, right lung, and left ventricle are flagged with the light pen and displayed as intensified points in the image (Fig 3-10). The regions are stored and the study is played back frame by frame from the disc. As each frame is read from the disc, the total number of counts in each of the three stored regions is computed and stored sequentially. Upon completion, the generated points are displayed as curves on the cathode ray tube. Figure 3-11 presents the curves generated from the regions of Figure 3-9. Typically the curves are also printed out on the teletype, and with each point is printed the time elapsed from the start and the number of counts represented by the point. This figure clearly

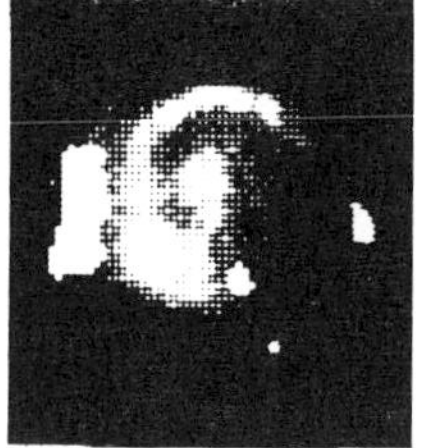

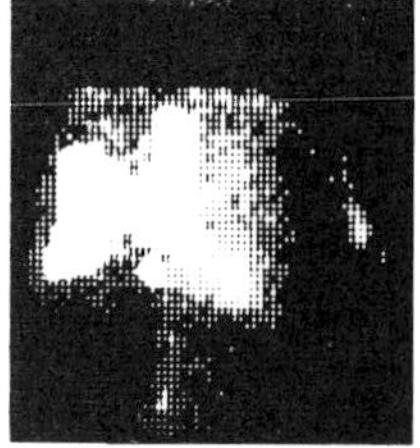

Figure 3-10 *Intensified regions over right and left heart demonstrate areas flagged for curve generation as applied to cardiac flow study.*

shows the passage of a tracer bolus through the right heart into the lungs and into the left heart. Transmit times, cardiac output, C_2/C_1 ratios, etc, can be calculated utilizing the information contained in the curve printout. Figure 3-12 is typical of the hardcopy (as opposed to photographic) output available.

A more detailed discussion of the dynamic computer-assisted cardiac blood flow study appears in Chapter 8. This type of analysis can be applied to liver blood flow, kidney blood flow, etc.

Conclusion

This chapter has dealt briefly with the organization of a small digital computer and how such a computer can be applied to problems in nuclear medicine. The use-

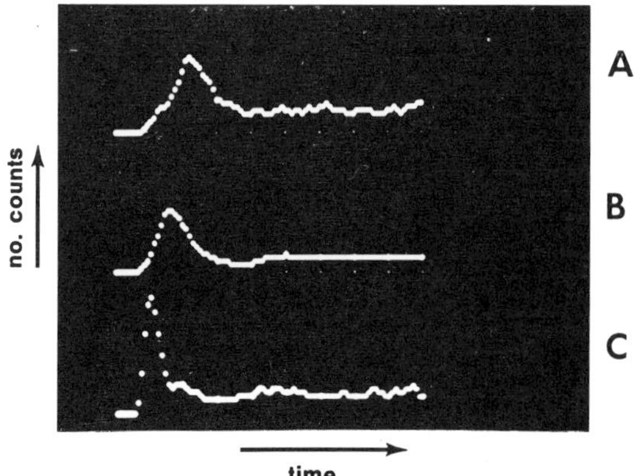

Figure 3-11 *Time-activity histogram.* A, *right ventricle curve;* B, *right lung curve;* C, *left ventricle curve.*

REGION 02

0.50	46	46
1.00	95	49
1.50	337	242
2.00	1019	682
2.50	1627	608
3.00	2088	461
3.50	2447	359
4.00	2706	259
4.50	2946	240
5.00	3111	165
5.50	3306	195
6.00	3452	146
6.50	3511	59
7.00	3622	111
7.50	3694	72
8.00	3811	117
8.50	3890	79
9.00	4001	111
9.50	4100	99
10.00	4176	76
10.50	4251	75
11.00	4339	88
11.50	4454	115
12.00	4581	127
12.50	4723	142
13.00	4883	160
13.50	5028	145
14.00	5195	167
14.50	5376	181
15.00	5581	205
15.50	5759	178
16.00	5956	197
16.50	6136	180
17.00	6301	165
17.50	6499	198
18.00	6676	177
18.50	6832	156
19.00	7002	170
19.50	7164	162
20.00	7323	159

Figure 3-12 *Hardcopy output of right ventricle curve showing time, counts per unit time, integrated with 30 characters per second thermal printer.*

fulness of a computer system (or nuclear medicine system) is becoming clearer with time. The literature attests to the success of the computer in the area of cardiac blood flow studies. Its potential in other dynamic studies has not been fully exploited.

The computer does not provide new information; it allows the extraction of more information from a given nuclear medicine procedure. Most importantly, it allows image manipulation after the fact, and spares the patient a reexamination.

References

1. Cole RW: *Introduction to Computing.* New York, McGraw-Hill, 1969.
2. *Introduction to Programming,* vol 1. Software Writing Group Programming Department, Digital Equipment Corporation, Maynard, Mass, 1970.
3. Kenny PJ, Smith EM (eds): *Quantitative Organ Visualization in Nuclear Medicine.* Coral Gables, Fla, University of Miami Press, 1971.
4. Krasnoff O: *Computers in Medicine.* Springfield, Ill, Thomas, 1967.
5. Lipkin SB, Rosenfeld A: *Picture Processing and Psychopictorics* New York, Academic Press, 1970.
6. *Proceedings, Symposium on Sharing of Computer Programs and Technology in Nuclear Medicine.* USAEC Conf–710425, Oak Ridge, Tenn, 1971.
7. *Proceedings, Second Symposium on Sharing of Computer Programs and Technology in Nuclear Medicine.* USAEC Conf–720430, Oak Ridge, Tenn, 1972.

Brain scanning is a safe, accurate procedure for detecting intracranial mass lesions and circulatory abnormalities. Complementary use of dynamic and static imaging gives the best results.

4 The Central Nervous System

William M. Smoak III and Albert J. Gilson

Procedure

Screening patients for central nervous system disease by radioactive isotope imaging techniques has proved one of the most useful functions of the nuclear medicine laboratory. The procedure, commonly referred to as brain scanning, is safe and accurate for detecting the presence or absence of most intracranial mass lesions. The study consists of two phases: dynamic scintigraphy and static scintigraphy. In the dynamic phase the radioactive material is injected as a bolus, and an Anger scintillation camera images its transit through the vascular system. Circulatory abnormalities can be identified by reviewing a tape recording or rapid-sequence filming of the transit. A dose of 10 to 15 mCi of technetium 99m in saline provides a low radiation exposure and high information yield. ^{99m}Tc has gained widespread acceptance as the radioactive isotope of choice for these studies. In the static phase, after the radioactive isotope bolus has equilibrated, alterations in the blood-brain barrier are recorded by scintillation camera or rectilinear scanner. These images are obtained one hour after the injection of the bolus. The static studies usually reveal the presence of an intracranial mass lesion and often demonstrate abnormalities of the skull and scalp. We consider these studies complementary in the same way that arteriography and plain skull roentgenography are complementary. This survey describes the spectrum of nervous system disease detectable by dynamic and static scintigraphy.

Advantages and Disadvantages

The majority of patients with *normal* dynamic and static scintigraphs are in fact free of major cranial vascular disease and of intracranial mass lesions. A normal scintigraphic study usually makes further diagnostic procedures, and their coexistent potential hazards to the patient, unnecessary. An *abnormal* scintigraphic survey demonstrating a mass lesion allows early use of a specific identifying procedure, expediting diagnosis and therapy.

> A normal scintigraphic study usually makes further diagnostic procedures unnecessary; an abnormal study allows early application of specific diagnostic tests.

The user of this nuclear medicine technique must, however, be aware of the intracranial diseases not readily detectable by brain scintigraphy. For example, vertebral-basilar artery stenosis can rarely be discerned. Small vessel occlusions and the punctate hemorrhages often seen in hypertensive patients are not identifiable. Metabolic diseases, degenerative diseases, and brain atrophy may be associated with normal brain scans. Small avascular tumors, such as the hematogenous spread of metastases from a breast or lung neoplasm, frequently go undetected. These apparent detractions from the value of this diagnostic study are more than offset by the procedures ability to detect potentially *curable* lesions such as partial carotid stenosis, meningioma, brain abscess, and subdural hematoma that are not obvious from the presenting clinical manifestations.

Interpretation

Interpretation of the brain scan involves two considerations: the phase of circulation (arterial, capillary, or venous) at which an abnormality appears during dynamic scintigraphy, and the relation between the dynamic and static survey findings. On the latter basis four types of scans can be described:

- Normal dynamic, normal static
- Abnormal dynamic, normal static
- Normal dynamic, abnormal static
- Abnormal dynamic, abnormal static

The discussion that follows explains the implications of each type of scan pair.

Normal Dynamic, Abnormal Static Scans

In a normal dynamic study the arterial, capillary, and venous phases of circulation can be distinctly identified (Fig 4-1). Carotid artery flow normally dominates the *arterial phase,* as the vertebral artery circulation is somewhat slower, represents only about 30% of the visualized radioactivity, and is posterior in location. At the region of the circle of Willis the flow divides into three parts representing the two middle cerebral groups and the anterior cerebral group. The *capillary phase* is identified by its diffuse pattern of activity. The normal *venous phase* is identified by the appearance of the superior sagittal sinus. Occasionally large superficial veins can be seen passing over the convexities. The washout may pass symmetrically down the cervical region or may pass through one dominant lateral sinus and give an asymmetrical pattern as depicted in the sketch.

Figure 4-1 (and subsequent similar figures) shows only the anterior view of the *static study,* although anterior, vertex, posterior, and both lateral projections are routinely recorded. The static views are obtained one hour after the dynamic study is performed. Prior to one hour, high blood levels of radioactivity may obscure delineation of intracranial lesions. If the static study is questionably abnormal, it is repeated at three hours (Fig 4-2).

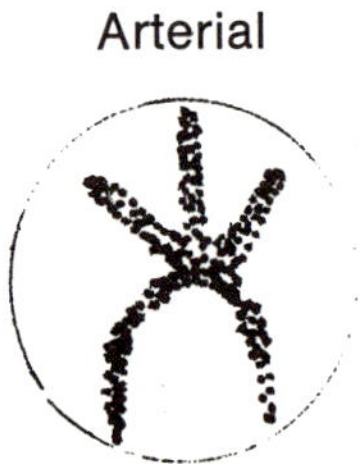

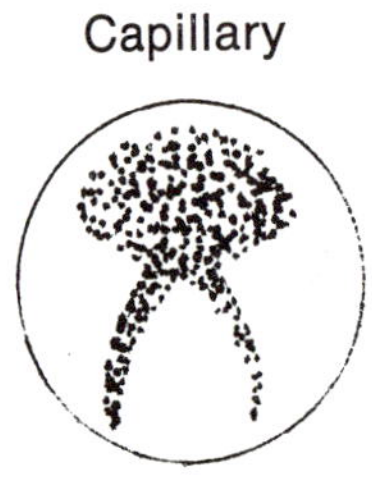

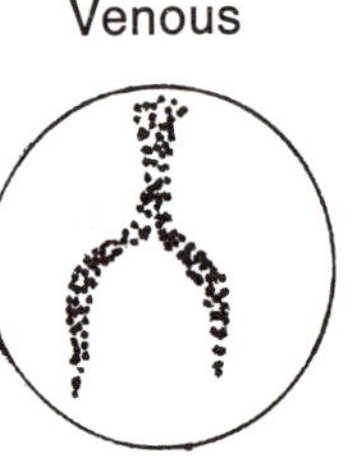

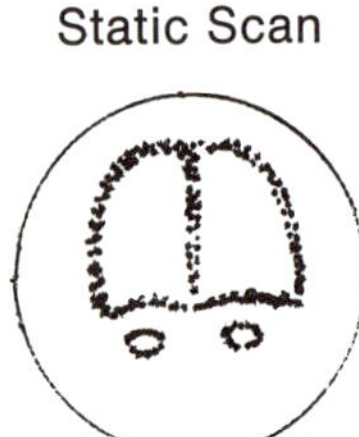

Figure 4-1 *Normal dynamic and static brain scans.*

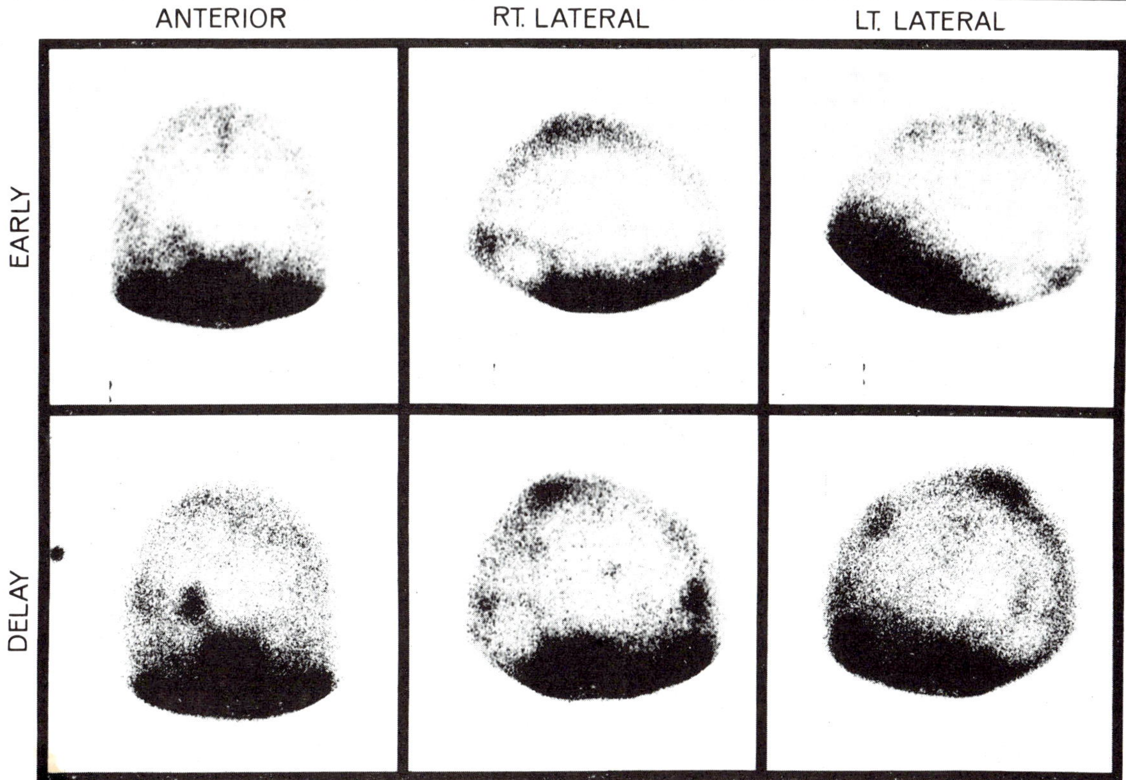

Figure 4-2 *One-hour and three-hour delayed static scintigraphs in patient with metastatic disease to brain and bone. When a questionable abnormality is identified on one-hour delayed static survey, further delayed static views usually show intensification of abnormality, while venous lakes tend to decrease with time. Here a suspicious area is seen over cranial vault and above right orbit at one hour. Views at three hours show intensification of radioactivity in abnormal areas compared with decreasing blood background radioactivity.*

Abnormal Dynamic, Normal Static Scans

UNILATERAL ABSENCE OF CAROTID ACTIVITY

The appearance of radioactivity in one carotid artery before the opposite fills (Fig 4-3) may be due to partial or total occlusion of a carotid artery or its internal or external branches. The most common site of obstruction is in the internal carotid artery just beyond the bifurcation. (This must not be confused with unilateral jugular reflux on the side of the injection. The latter is easily recognized by its appearance on the side of the injection and its failure to im-

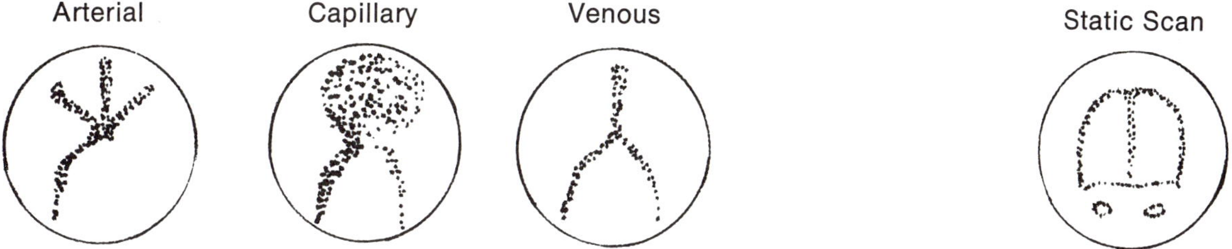

Figure 4-3 *Unilateral absence of carotid activity.*

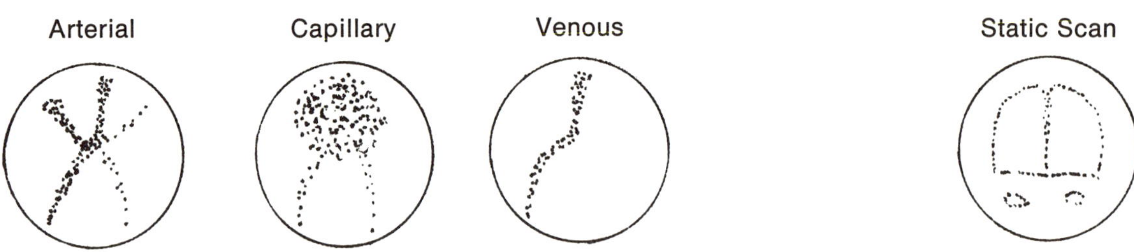

Figure 4-4 *Unilateral decrease of arterial activity.*

mediately perfuse the brain.) Even in the presence of total obstruction of an internal carotid artery, some radioactivity ultimately appears in the neck in arterial collaterals, in a vertebral artery, or in venous return. Therefore, the first scintigraph demonstrating absence of activity on one side in the carotid region is the most important.

A solitary defect in the column of radioactivity or bilateral defects in the column represent not a lesion but attenuation by mandible, gold fillings in the teeth, etc. To verify a lesion in this region, improved visualization of the carotid arteries can be obtained on a repeat study by slightly elevating the mandible. This is not done routinely as it obliterates the important intracranial component. Marked extension of the neck and shoulders may tamponade the incoming venous bolus and should be avoided.

In unilateral absence or reduction of carotid radioactivity, intracranial activity is primarily a function of the anatomic configuration of the circle of Willis and the adequacy of collateral development.

Vertebral and basilar artery stenosis is rarely if ever detected by dynamic scintigraphic studies. We have seen normal dynamic scans in patients with vertebral artery agenesis. However, an occasional cause of apparent asymmetry is filling of both anterior cerebral arteries from one internal carotid artery, causing more radioactivity to pass through the feeding carotid vessel.

UNILATERAL DECREASED ARTERIAL ACTIVITY

Decreased radioactivity throughout the distribution of carotid and middle cerebral arteries on one side (Fig 4-4) usually indi-

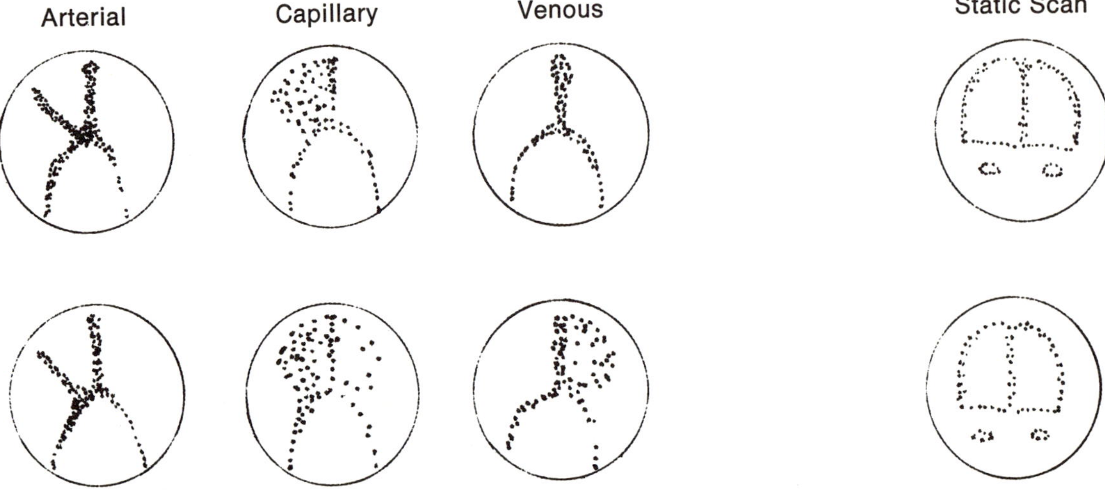

Figure 4-5 *Absent or decreased middle cerebral artery activity.*

cates partial occlusion on the affected side. The occlusion may be located anywhere along the course of the vessel. Following cerebral embolization or infarction, carotid flow as well as middle cerebral artery flow may be decreased.

Poor positioning of the patients may give a false appearance of asymmetrical flow. This rotation is easily identified by observing the superior sagittal sinus, seen in the venous phase, to appear as a curve rather than the usual straight line.

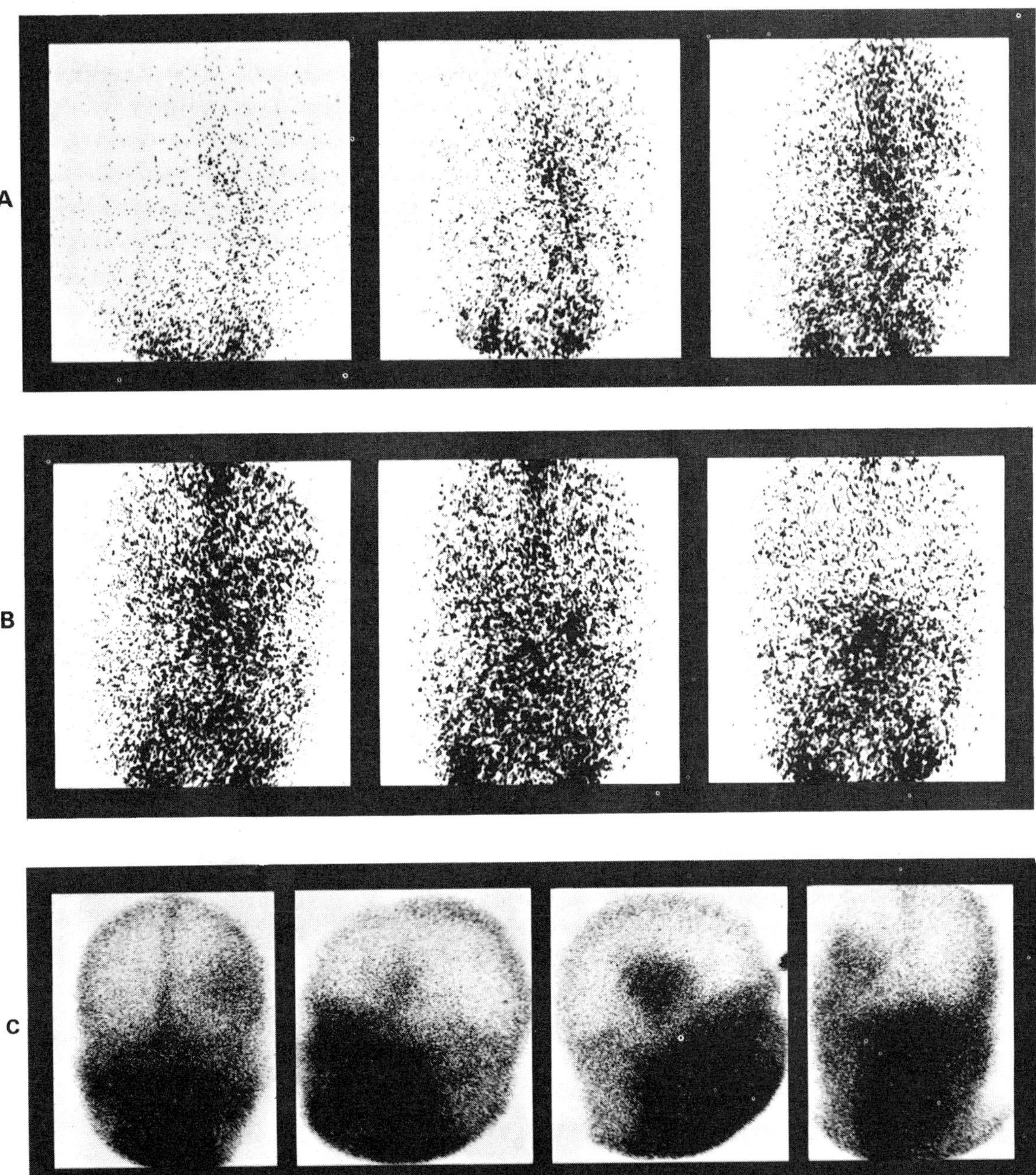

Figure 4-6 *Cerebral vascular accident ten days following onset. Decreased activity is seen in right carotid and right middle cerebral distribution in early frames of dynamic study (A). This has equilibrated during venous phase, and no abnormality is seen on washout (B). Static views (C) demonstrate lesion in distribution of right middle cerebral artery.*

ABSENT OR DECREASED MIDDLE CEREBRAL ARTERY ACTIVITY

This is one of the most common patterns seen in the first several days following onset of a cerebral vascular accident. The typical sequence of findings in uncomplicated stroke is as follows. For three or four days the dynamic study shows a decrease or absence of middle cerebral artery activity, but no abnormality is visible in the static views (Fig 4-5). (An abnormal static view at this early stage is highly suggestive of a preexisting tumor [metastasis or glioblastoma] that has undergone a recent hemorrhage.) One or two weeks following the stroke (Figs 4-6 and 4-7), the static study becomes abnormal, demonstrating the progressive changes in the blood-brain barrier. At this time, the dynamic study may revert to normal if there is revascularization, may demonstrate luxury perfusion (described in more detail later), or may continue to show total avascularity. This depends on the natural history of the disease in the particular patient. An additional finding occasionally identified on the dynamic study is displacement of vessels by a hematoma complicating a cerebral vascular accident. Over the next three to six weeks, the static brain images revert to normal. However, some patients with cerebral vascular accidents have completely normal dynamic and static studies throughout the course of the disease. This usually reflects areas of vascular damage too small for detection by the scintillation camera.

Minor asymmetries are commonly seen in the arterial phase of dynamic scintigraphs. These should be interpreted with caution. In our experience they are often not reproducible and result from statistical

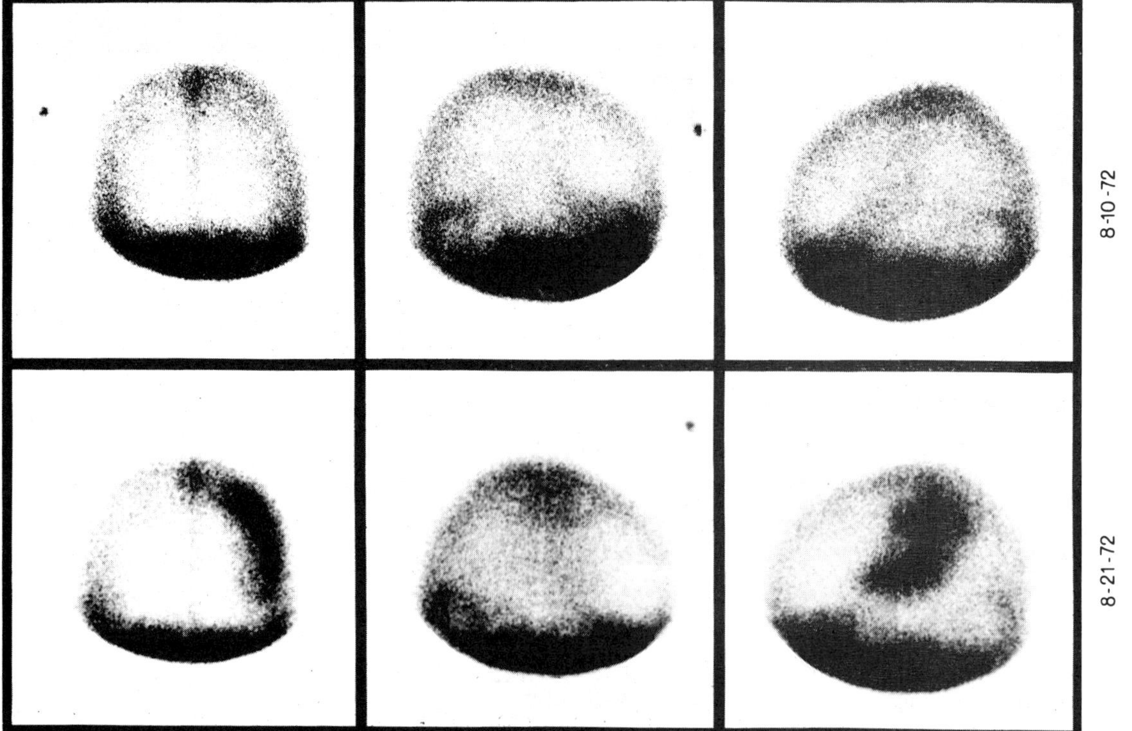

Figure 4-7 *Cerebral vascular accident on admission and 12 days later. Initial static scintiphotographs appear normal. Studies obtained 12 days later show typical configuration of left cerebral vascular accident involving several branches of middle cerebral artery.*

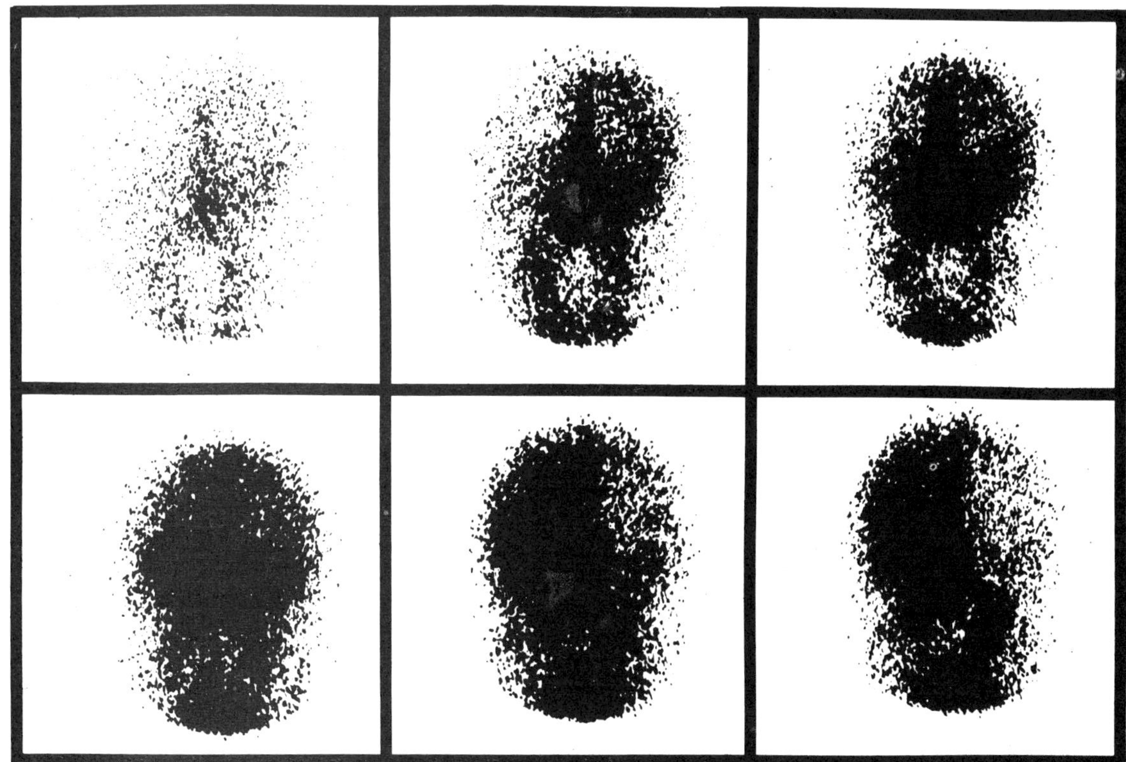

Figure 4-8 *Chronic occlusion of right middle cerebral artery with collateral filling of area from anterior cerebral and meningeal collaterals. Two-second dynamic scintigraphs demonstrate delayed appearance of radioactivity in right middle cerebral artery distribution. In subsequent images activity appears in this region and is retained while left side washes out.*

variations rather than disease. However, abnormality in the venous phase, in the form of retention of activity on the same side as delayed appearance in the arterial phase, confirms the presence of disease (Fig 4-8).

Lesions other than vascular occlusive disease are less common causes of absent or reduced radioactivity. Neurofibromas, cystic astrocytomas, and porencephalic cysts may appear as avascular areas without evidence of alteration of blood-brain barrier in the static views. In addition, following certain forms of intracranial surgery, an avascular region may result. The insertion of metal plates also attenuates the 140-kev photons of technetium 99m. A clue to the presence of this type of lesion is the finding of a void in the normal background activity seen in the static views.

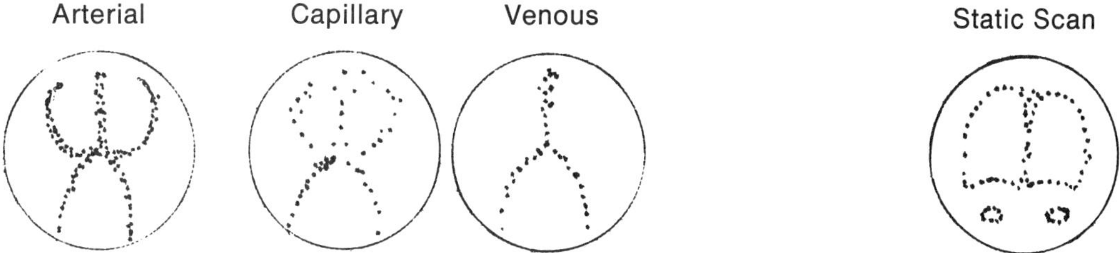

Figure 4-9 *Decreased central intracranial activity.*

DECREASED CENTRAL INTRACRANIAL ACTIVITY

The scintigraphic findings associated with enlarged ventricles range from normal to gross distortion of the images, depending on the extent of dilation and the age of the patient. The middle cerebral vessels may appear flattened laterally agains the convexities, leaving the central area relatively devoid of radioactivity in both the arterial and the capillary phases (Fig 4-9). If the foramen of Monro is obstructed on only one side, the abnormal pattern may be unilateral.

The static views are usually normal in an adult. A child may show the secondary characteristics of hydrocephalus, including enlargement of the head and low-lying position of the lateral sinuses.

Normal Dynamic, Abnormal Static Scans

SINGLE INTRACRANIAL LESION

A solitary lesion identified on a static study, without visible alteration of the vascular system on the dynamic scintigraphs (Fig 4-10), may be perplexing. Although its shape and location may suggest its nature, the lesion itself is usually nondescript. A linear lesion following a specific vascular distribution is usually an infarction. An infiltrating lesion crossing the midline is usually a glioblastoma. If the center of the lesion does not contain radioactivity—a so-called doughnut lesion—a cyst, hemorrhage, or necrosis may be the cause. At least one-half of such lesions are small avascular tumors (gliomas or metastases), abscesses, or cerebral infarctions.

MULTIPLE INTRACRANIAL LESIONS

Multiple small metastases, infarcts, and abscesses are frequently identified on static brain scans (Fig 4-11), without identifiable change on the dynamic study. Their differentiation from lesions involving the bony vault is sometimes difficult without skull roentgenograms or bone scans for additional information.

Abnormal Dynamic, Abnormal Static Scans

AVASCULAR INTRACRANIAL MASS

The presence of a region of intracranial avascularity with displacement of adjacent vessels away from the area suggests an avascular intracranial mass (Figs 4-12 and 4-13). Static images may offer a clue to the

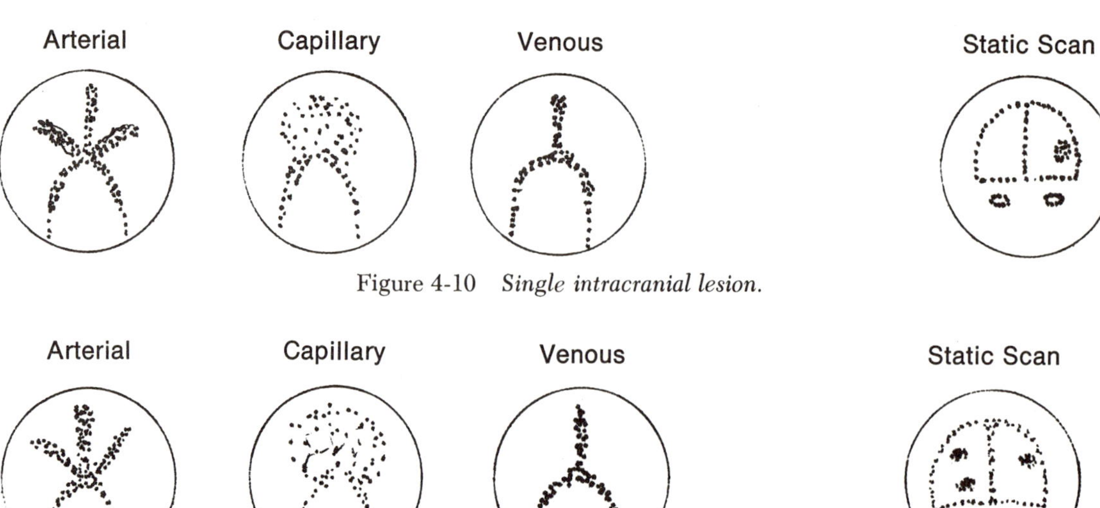

Figure 4-10 *Single intracranial lesion.*

Figure 4-11 *Multiple intracranial lesions.*

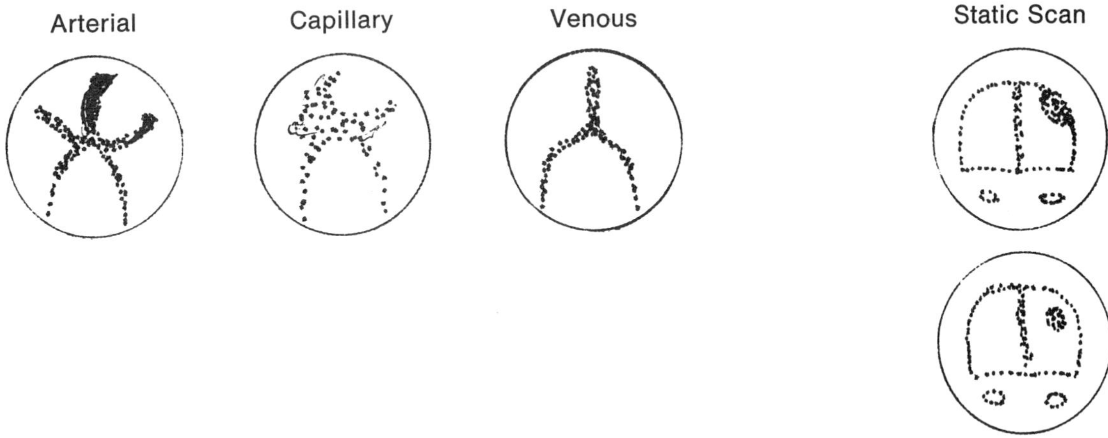

Figure 4-12 *Avascular intracranial mass.*

nature of the lesion. Meningiomas are frequently the cause of this configuration and usually are intensely active in the static views, have a flat base against a meningeal surface, and appear well circumscribed. This combination of findings is less often seen in astrocytomas, brain abscesses, and in solitary metastases. These lesions usually are not as intensely radioactive and tend to be deeper in the brain parenchyma.

VASCULAR INTRACRANIAL MASS APPEARING IN CAPILLARY PHASE

When the mass effect appears in the early arterial frames and radioactivity appears in the mass region in the capillary phase and persists through the venous washout, a "staining" meningioma is the likely cause (Fig 4-14). Over half of all meningiomas have this characteristic appearance.

INCREASED INTRACRANIAL ACTIVITY IN ARTERIAL PHASE WITH PARTIAL WASHOUT

This abnormality and the two that follow are somewhat similar and cannot always be clearly differentiated. Figure 4-15 shows the pattern typical of luxury perfusion, often identified 10 to 14 days following cerebral vascular accident. The abnormality is rarely asociated with increased carotid activity, appears in the arterial phase, tends to decrease during the venous washout, and follows a vascular distribution on the static images. In a patient with a history of recent stroke, a normal study on admission followed by this pattern two weeks later confirms the suspicion of a cerebral vascular accident with increased perfusion.

INCREASED CAROTID AND INTRACRANIAL ACTIVITY WITH RAPID VENOUS WASHOUT

Arteriovenous malformations may cause an increase in flow through the feeding carotid vesel and are easily identified by their sudden appearance and equally rapid washout in the dynamic scan (Fig 4-16 and 4-17). Static images further confirm the decreasing activity in the lesion as the pertechnetate clears from the blood pool.

INCREASED INTRACRANIAL ACTIVITY WITHOUT WASHOUT AND WITH NORMAL CAROTID ACTIVITY

When radioactivity in an intracranial lesion appears early and tends to remain in both the venous washout and static scans (Fig 4-18), intracranial malignancy is probably the cause. Although these lesions usually prove to be highly malignant gliomas, metastatic malignancy, particularly renal cell carcinoma, gives a similar pattern.

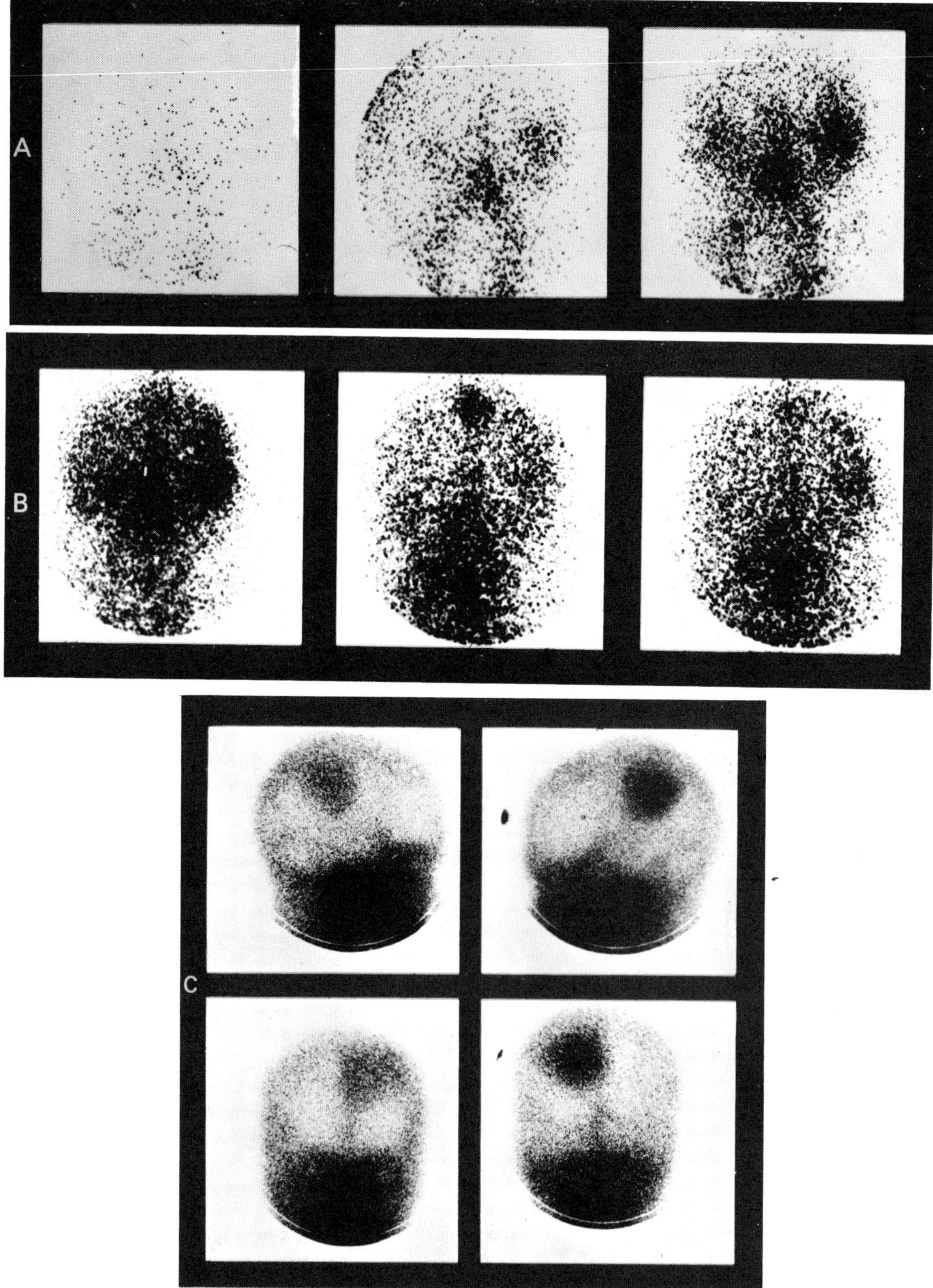

Figure 4-13 *Meningioma. Dynamic scintigraphy (A, arterial phase; B, venous phase) demonstrates progressive increase in radioactivity adjacent to right superior convexity. Static images (C) demonstrate peripheral flat-based lesion in this region.*

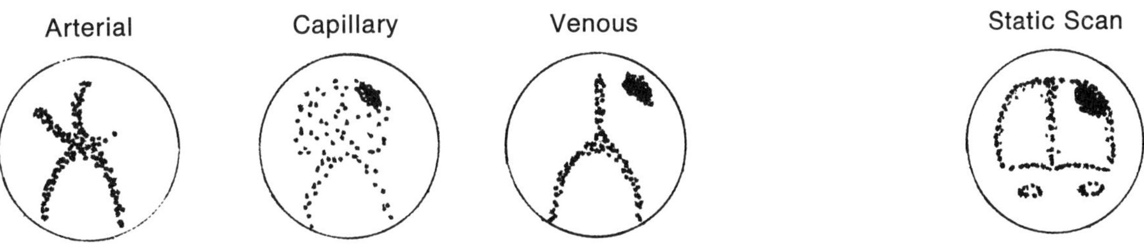

Figure 4-14 *Vascular intracranial mass appearing in capillary phase.*

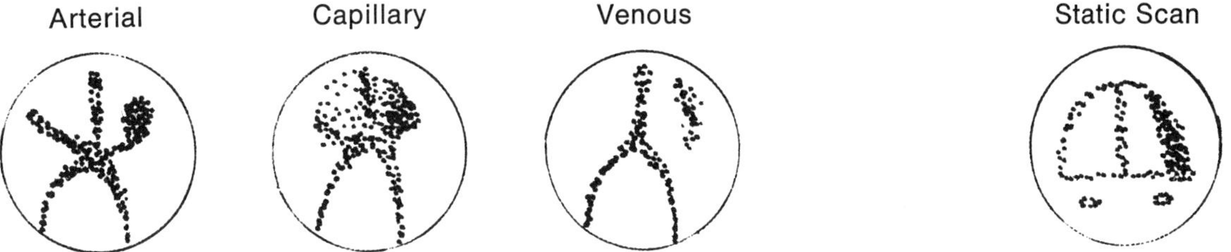

Figure 4-15 *Increased intracranial activity in arterial phase, with partial washout.*

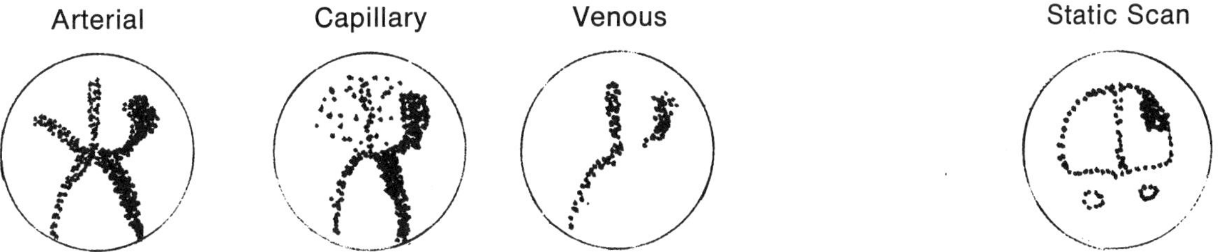

Figure 4-16 *Increased carotid and intracranial activity with rapid venous washout.*

Gliomas often have poorly defined borders on the static study, with vascular boundaries crossing at the midline.

INTRACRANIAL RIM

A concave intracranial distribution of radioactivity seen in the dynamic study (Fig 4-19) is the clue to epidural or subdural fluid accumulation. It is easily seen when the damage is of recent origin and there is hyperemia of the adjacent brain. In a patient with subdural hematoma the pattern is generally noted two weeks following the traumatic episode. Chronic subdural fluid collections may lose this configuration because of brain atrophy and loss of reaction to the accumulations. In these old lesions the hyperemic rim disappears, but the concave void persists. The static scans show a clearly discernible intracranial rim and thickening of skull convexity adjacent to it, forming an ellipse of increased radioactivity. These changes are often bilateral.

UNILATERAL EXTRACRANIAL INCREASED ACTIVITY

This common pattern of increased circulation over the cranial vault seen by dynamic scintigraphy (Fig 4-20) suggests scalp trauma or infection, metastases to skull and scalp, arteritis, sinusitis, early Paget's disease, or fibrous dysplasia. The dynamic scintigraphic findings are due to external carotid artery hyperemia and may mask intracranial abnormality.

The static scans are particularly helpful in suggesting the cause. A scalp hematoma

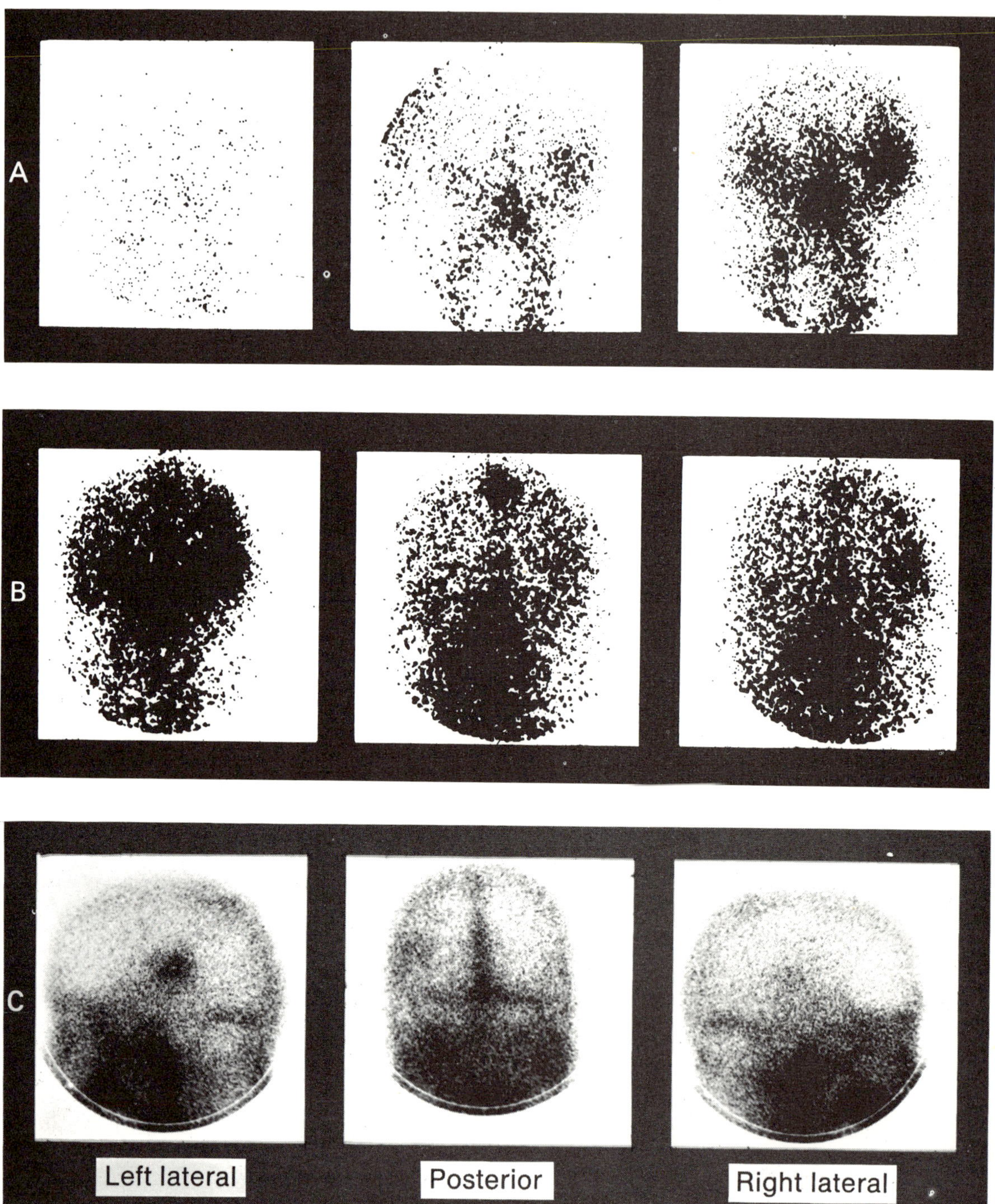

Figure 4-17 *Arteriovenous malformation. Dynamic study illustrates rapid appearance of activity in lesion in left middle cerebral distribution (A) that washes out in venous phase (B). Static scintiphotographs (C) demonstrate lesion in this region.*

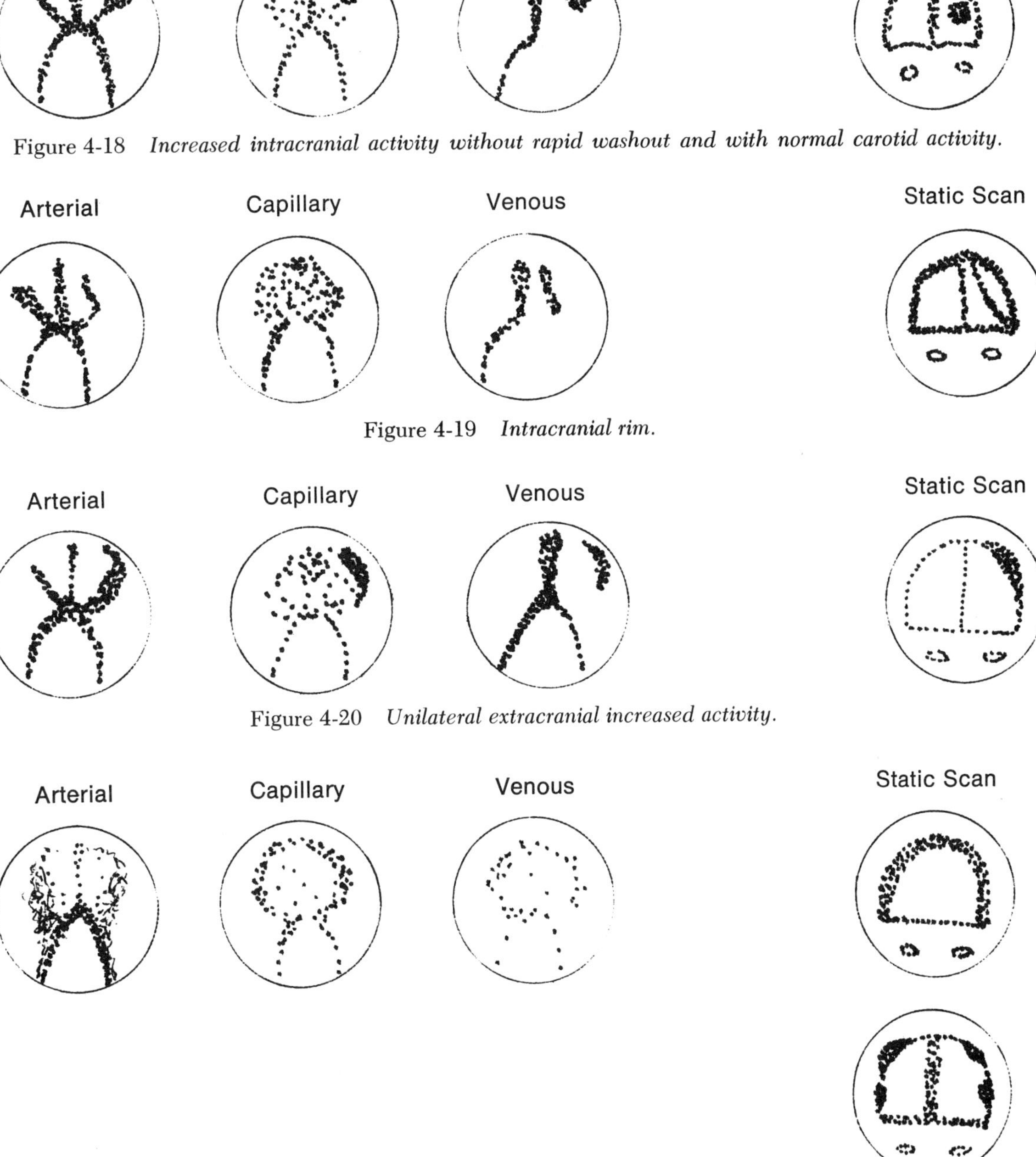

Figure 4-18 *Increased intracranial activity without rapid washout and with normal carotid activity.*

Figure 4-19 *Intracranial rim.*

Figure 4-20 *Unilateral extracranial increased activity.*

Figure 4-21 *Bilateral extracranial increased activity.*

tends to bulge outward from the cranial contours. Metastases are usually focal and are best seen three to four hours after injection on additional delayed views. Fibrous dysplasia usually avidly takes up the radioactive pertechnetate. Comparison of the scans with skull roentgenograms is generally of great assistance, the two studies usually yielding more information than either one alone.

BILATERAL EXTRACRANIAL INCREASED ACTIVITY

Paget's disease of bone in its advanced stages alters the external carotid circulation. This is visible in the early arterial phase as the radioactivity in the external circulation fills in the wedge normally seen between internal carotid and middle cerebral groups (Fig 4-21). Static images demonstrating a thickened cranial vault are easily identified as being due to this disease.

On occasion, numerous metastases and skull cause somewhat similar changes, but the skull has many discrete foci of increased activity in the static views. Patients with thickened skulls due to anemia usually have normal dynamic scintigraphs.

References

General

1. Bakay L: Blood-Brain Barrier Concept. In Gilson AJ, Smoak WM (eds). *Central Nervous System Investigation with Radionuclides.* Springfield, Ill, Thomas, 1971.
2. Cowan RJ, Maynard CD, Meschan I, Janeway R, Shigero K: Value of the routine use of the cerebral dynamic radioisotope study. *Radiology* **107**:111, 1973.
3. Gates GF, Dore EK, Taplin GV: Interval brain scanning with sodium pertechnetate Tc99m for tumor detectability. *JAMA* **215**:85, 1971.
4. O'Mara RE, McAfee JG, Chodes RB: "Doughnut" sign in cerebral radioisotopic images. *Radiology* **92**:581, 1969.
5. Watson DD, Nelson JP, Gottlieb S: Rapid bolus injection of radioisotopes. *Radiology* **106**:347, 1973.

Neoplasms

6. Baum S, Roghballer AB, Schiffman F Girolamo RF: Brain scanning in diagnosis of acoustic neuromas. *J Neurosurg* **36**:141, 1972.
7. James AE, Deland FH, Hodges FJ III, Wagner HN III: Radionuclide imaging in detection and differential diagnosis of craniopharyngiomas. *Am J Roentgenol Radium Ther Nucl Med* **109**:692, 1970.
8. Moody RA, Olsen JO, Gottschalk A, Hoffer PG: Brain scans of posterior fossa. *J Neurosurg* **36**:148, 1972.
9. Quinn JL III: Serial brain scans in glioblastoma multiforme. *Radiology* **101**:367, 1971.
10. Sheldon JJ, Smoak WM, Gargano FP, Watson DD: Dynamic scintigraphy in intracranial meningiomas. *Radiology* (to be published).
11. Smoak WM, Sheldon JJ, Gilson AJ: Characterization of intracranial neoplasms by dynamic radioisotope imaging. *J Fla Med Assoc* **59**:15, 1972.
12. Thompson RW, DeNardo GL, Kottra JJ: Diagnostic value of brain scanning in intracranial lymphomas. *Radiology* **103**:111, 1972.
13. Wickborn I: Angiographic determination of tumor pathology. *Acta Radiol (Diagn) (Stockh)* **50**:529, 1953.
14. Zachrisson L: Angiography of cerebral metastases. *Acta Radiol (Diagn) (Stockh)* **1**:521, 1963.

Ischemia and Infarction

15. Brinkman CA: Brain scanning as an aid to surgery for strokes. *Am J Surg* ***119***:453, 1970.
16. Glasgow JH, Currier RD, Goodrich JK, Tuton FT: Brain scans at varied intervals following CVA. *J Nucl Med* **6**:902, 1965.
17. Griep RJ, Wise G, Marty R: Detection of carotid artery obstruction by intravenous radionuclide angiography. *Radiology* **97**:311, 1970.
18. Taveras JM, Gilson JM, Davis DD, Kilgora B, Rumbaugh CL: Angiography in cerebral infarction. *Radiology* **93**:549, 1969.

Arteriovenous Malformations

19. Oldendorf WH, Kitano M: The free passage of 131-I antipyrine through brain as an indication of AV shunting. *Neurology* **14**:1078, 1964.
20. Rosenthall L: Radionuclide diagnosis of anteriovenous malformations with rapid sequence brain scans. *Radiology* **91**:1195, 1968.

Trauma and Subdural Hematomas

21. Cowan RJ, Maynard CD, Lassiter KR: 99m Technetium pertechnetate brain scans in detection of subdural hematomas: Study of age of lesion as related to development of positive scan. *J Neurosurg* **32**:30, 1970.

22. Gilson AJ, Gargano FP: Correlation of brain scans and angiography in intracranial trauma. *Am J Roentgenol Radium Ther Nucl Med* **94**:819, 1965.

23. Smoak WM, Gilson AJ: Scintillation visualization of a vascular rim in subdural hematoma. *J Nucl Med* **11**:695, 1970.

Inflammatory

24. Ferris EJ, Rudikoff JC, Shapiro JH: Cerebral angiography of bacterial infection. *Radiology* **90**:727, 1968.

25. Marion JC, Jones R, Mishkin FS: Tuberculosis meningitis diagnosed by brain scan. *Radiology* **104**:333, 1972.

26. Radcliffe WB, Gunto FC, Adcock DF, Krigman MR: Herpes simplex encephalitis: A radiologic-pathologic study of 4 cases. *Am J Roentgenol Radium Ther Nucl Med* **112**:263, 1971.

Pediatrics

27. Conway JJ: Radionuclide imaging of the central nervous system in children. *Radiol Clin North Am* **10**:271, 1972.

28. Fagan JH, Cowan RJ: Effect of potassium perchlorate on uptake of pertechnetate-99mTc in choroid plexus papillomas: A report of two cases. *J Nucl Med* **12**:312, 1971.

29. Ferry DJ Jr, Mylander K, Hardman J: Radiographic identification and surgical removal of teratoid tumor of roof of third ventricle. *J Neurosurg* **36**:231, 1972.

30. Hurley PJ, Wagner HN Jr: Diagnostic value of brain scanning in children. *JAMA* **221**:877, 1972.

31. Kuhl DE, Bevilaegra JE, Mishkin WM, Sanders, TP: Brain scan in Sturge-Weber syndrome. *Radiology* **103**:621, 1972.

32. Mishkin F, Truska J: Diagnosis of intracranial cysts by means of brain scan. *Radiology* **90**:740, 1968.

33. Van Houten FX, Holman LB, Treves S: Negative defect in an intracranial teratoma. *J Nucl Med* **13**:122, 1972.

Miscellaneous

34. Gize RW, Mishkin FS: Brain scans in multiple sclerosis. *Radiology* **97**:297, 1970.

35. Kieffer SA, Loken ME: Positive "brain" scans in fibrous dysplasia and other lesions of the skull. *Am J Roentgenol Radium Ther Nucl Med* **106**:731, 1969.

36. Vitye B, Ostiguy G, LeBel E: Abnormal 99mTc brain scan in cerebral sarcoidosis. *Can Med Assoc* J **101**:169, 1969.

Tumor Response to Therapy

37. Flipse RC, Vuksanavic M, Fonts EA: Sequential brain scanning in radiation therapy of malignant tumors of the brain. *Am J Roentgenol Radium Ther Nucl Med* **102**:92, 1968.

38. Handel SF, Powell MR, Wilson CB, Enot KJ: Scintiphotographic evaluation of response of brain neoplasms to systemic chemotherapy. *J Nucl Med* **12**:292, 1971.

Abnormalities of thyroid gland function and anatomy, as well as of the parathyroids and adrenals, can be identified by in vitro and in vivo tests using radioactive tracers and by scanning and imaging techniques.

5
The Thyroid, Parathyroids and Adrenals

Fuad S. Ashkar

The Thyroid

Radioactive isotopes have been used to study thyroid physiology and pathophysiology since 1940. They have proved highly valuable in assessing the gland's function and dysfunction, evaluating its size, and elucidating pathologic degenerations. The availability of isotopes of iodine with short and long half-lives have made possible the study of the thyroid, both in vivo and in vitro. The in vitro tests provide an accurate and reliable measure of thyroid hormone.

Radioactive iodine has revolutionized treatment of hyperthyroidism and thyroid carcinoma to the extent that nuclear medicine has virtually replaced surgery as treatment of choice.

Thyroid Physiology and the Iodine Cycle

Following ingestion of iodine into the body, the thyroid traps all that is present in the iodide form and concentrates it to levels sometimes as much as 500 times that in the plasma. Organification and storage follow. The iodine and the amino acid tyrosine are converted into thyroid hormone, which is bound to thyroglobulin and stored in the thyroid or released into the bloodstream according to need.

The trapping of iodine and the release of thyroid hormone are regulated by thyrotropin (TSH) from the pituitary gland through a balancing negative-feedback mechanism existing between the thyroid hormone level and a hypothalamic group of cells that secrete thyrotropin-releasing hormone (TRH). When the level of thyroid hormone in the bloodstream drops, TRH is released and TSH rises, resulting in increased iodine trapping and thyroid hormone release. When the level of thyroid hormone rises above normal, release of TRH and TSH stop until the hormone level drops again.

Because of the dynamic equilibrium in this system, measurement of any of these parameters reflects thyroid function.

In Vivo Thyroid Function Tests

24-HOUR RAIU

The 24-hour radioactive iodine uptake (RAIU) test measures the percentage of a small radioactive iodine tracer dose taken up by the patient's thyroid gland 24 hours following its ingestion. The uptake of radioactive iodine by the normal gland depends on the amount of iodine in the diet. Increased iodine ingestion produces a rise in the total-body iodine pool and overdilution

In vivo tests of thyroid function

- 24-hour radioactive iodine uptake
- TSH stimulation
- T_3 suppression
- Perchlorate discharge
- Dynamic study

of the tracer dose in it, resulting in a low uptake. Decreased iodine ingestion lowers the iodine pool, and uptake of the tracer dose is high.

Recent observations have shown that the normal range of RAIU is progressively declining because of increasing iodine pollution. The present normal national range, derived from averaging the data from numerous testing areas, is 5% to 35%. Table 5-1 summarizes the variation of RAIU associated with various clinical states and changes in the total-body iodine pool.

TSH STIMULATION, T_3 SUPPRESSION, PERCHLORATE DISCHARGE

The TSH stimulation, thyroid (T_3) suppression, and perchlorate discharge tests are variations of the RAIU designed to differentiate among types of hypothyroidism, to determine the presence or absence of hyperthyroidism or thyroiditis, and to detect enzyme deficiency in a nontoxic multinodular goiter.

The numerous pitfalls in these tests and the excessive time and cost of their performance limit their usefulness and confine their employment to those laboratories where the procedures can be standardized and the pitfalls avoided. Table 5-2 summarizes the indications, procedures, results, and pitfalls of these three tests.

DYNAMIC STUDY

A rapid, effective single-visit test for

Table 5-1. Radioactive Iodine Uptake in Various Conditions and Various States of Body Iodine Pool

	RAIU values		
Body iodine pool	**Increased (> 35%)**	**Normal (5%–35%)**	**Decreased (> 5%)**
Normal	Hyperthyroidism Recovering thyroiditis Antithyroid drug withdrawal rebound	Normal	Lingual thyroid Hypothyroidism Primary Secondary Tertiary Acute thyroiditis
High	Hyperthyroidism Chronic renal disease Congestive heart failure	Hyperthyroidism (with iodine contamination)	Hyperthyroidism Normal Hypothyroidism (with iodine contamination)
Low	Endemic goiter Prolonged use of diuretic	Normal	Hypothyroidism Primary Secondary Tertiary

Table 5-2. Characteristics of TSH Stimulation, T_3 Suppression, and Perchlorate Discharge Tests of Thyroid Function

Test	Indications	Procedure	Results	Pitfalls
TSH stimulation	Differentiation among primary, secondary, tertiary hypothyroidism	Obtain baseline RAIU Give TSH (10 U, IM, b.i.d.) Repeat RAIU	Normal and secondary or tertiary hypothyroidism RAIU value double or triple Primary hypothyroidism: no RAIU change	Unconfirmed hypothyroidism More TSH stimulation may be needed Iodine contamination limits test use
T_3 suppression	Differentiation between normal and hyperthyroid state Confirmation of active or early hyperthyroidism	Obtain baseline RAIU Give T_3 (100 ug/day for 7 days) Repeat RAIU on 7th day	Normal and nontoxic goiters: 20–40% of initial uptake suppressed Hyperthyroidism: less than 20% of initial uptake suppressed	Technical problems T_3 intake unreliable Iodine contamination limits test use
Perchlorate discharge	Investigation of multinodular gland (enzyme-deficiency goiter) with low RAIU value Suspicion of thyroiditis	Give tracer radioactive iodine Determine uptake slope Give 200 mg $KC10_4$ Determine change in uptake slope	Normal: slope remains above horizontal Thyroiditis or enzyme deficiency: slope drops below horizontal	Very low RAIU prevents test use Some antithyroid drugs cause positive result

evaluating thyroid function and anatomy employs pertechnetate Tc 99m and the scintillation camera. The test has the advantages of speed, accuracy, simplicity, low cost, and small radiation dose to the patient. The first transit of the radioactive tracer in the neck is recorded following its intravenous injection. Thyroid function is evaluated by recording the carotid-thyroid transit time (CTTT)—an index of trapping of the tracer, which is handled by the thyroid in a manner similar to iodine, except that it does not undergo organification.

A rapid, effective single-visit evaluation of thyroid function and anatomy employs sodium pertechnetate Tc 99m and the scintillation camera.

Since changes in the CTTT reflect changes in thyroid function, the dynamic

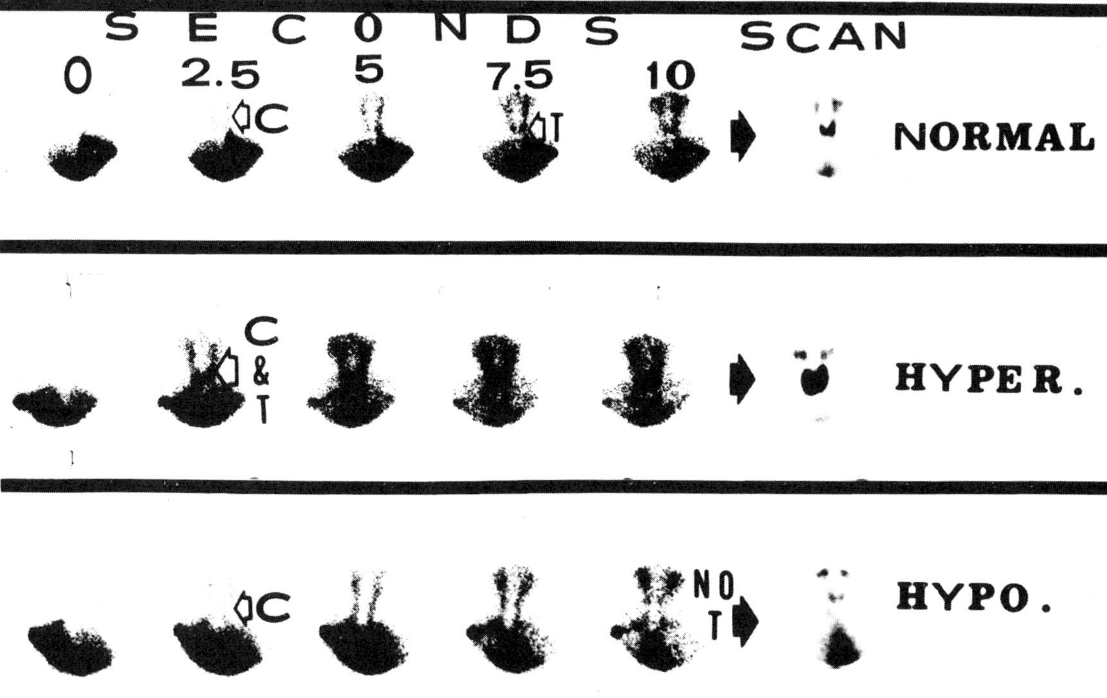

Figure 5-1 *Dynamic thyroid study.*

thyroid study is useful when employed in conjunction with stimulation or suppression tests, or as a follow-up to monitor the results of radioactive iodine therapy for hyperthyroidism. The following findings are present in the various thyroid functional states:

- Hyperthyroidism: CTTT rapid (zero to 2.5 seconds); thyroid image progressively darker due to increased trapping
- Normal: CTTT between 2.5 and 7.5 seconds; thyroid image constant
- Hypothyroidism: CTTT prolonged and undetermined; thyroid image not seen

At the end of the dynamic study a static scan is obtained with 300,000 counts. Figure 5-1 shows static scans typical of a normal gland, a diffuse toxic goiter, and an atrophic gland.

In Vitro Thyroid Function Tests

Murphy and Pattee have described a method of determining total serum thyroxine by using competitive protein-binding analysis (CPBA). Bound thyroixine is released from serum proteins by denaturation and precipitation with alcohol. The procedure leaves approximately 80% of the thyroxine in the alcoholic supernatant. After the supernatant is evaporated to dryness, a solution containing thyroxine binding globulin (TBG) fully saturated with radioactive thyroxine (T_4 I 125) is added to the thyroxine extract and to a series of thyroxine standards. This is followed by separating the protein-bound radioactive thyroxine from the free thyroxine. The thyroxine concentration of the unknown sample is then compared radiometrically with the standard and its value derived (Figure 5-2).

In vitro tests of thyroid function

- T_3 resin uptake
- T_4
- T_4N

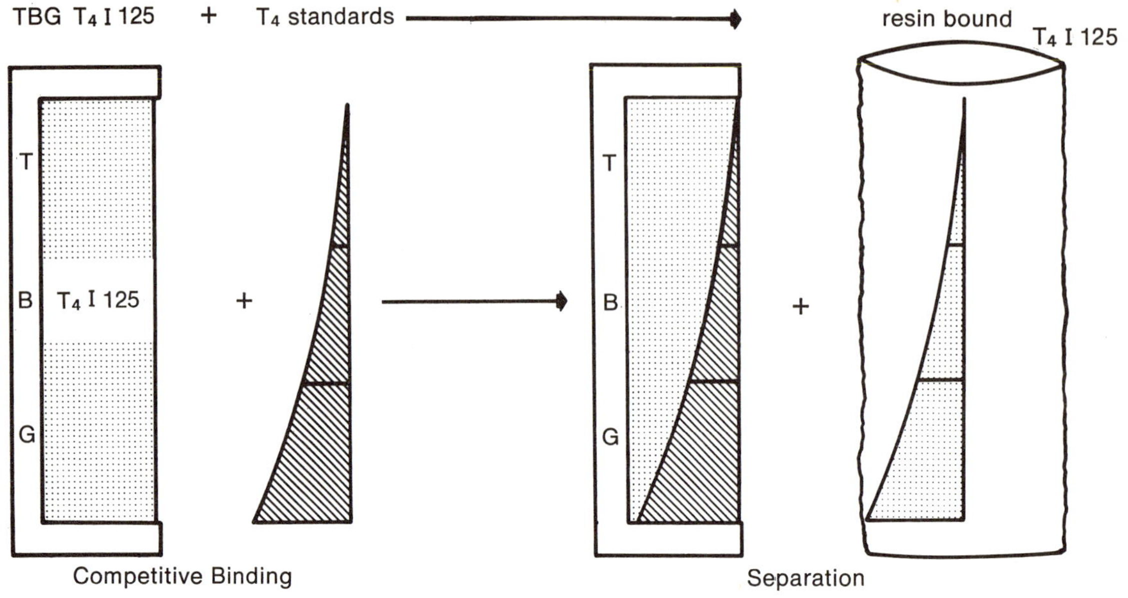

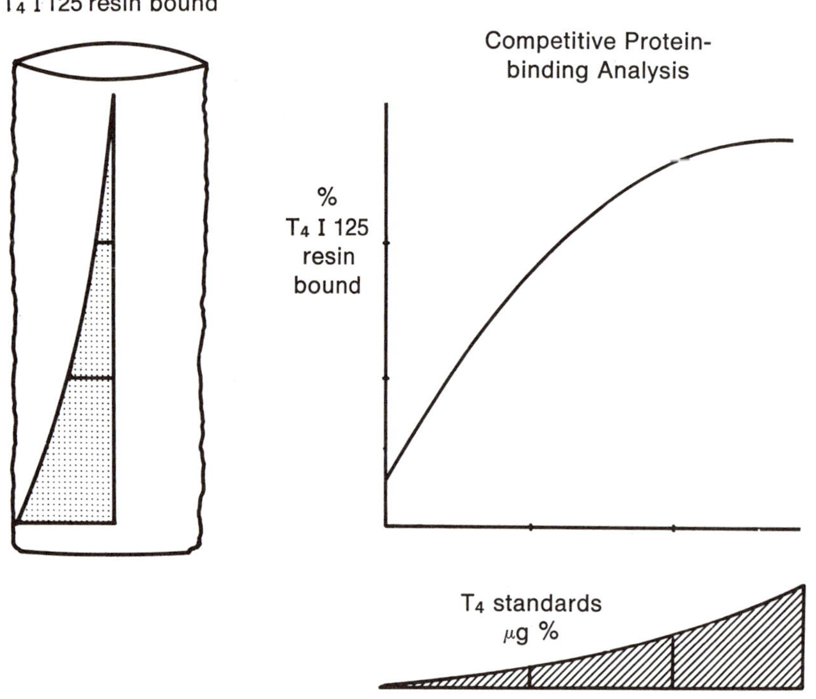

Figure 5-2 *Mechanism of competitive protein-binding analysis.*

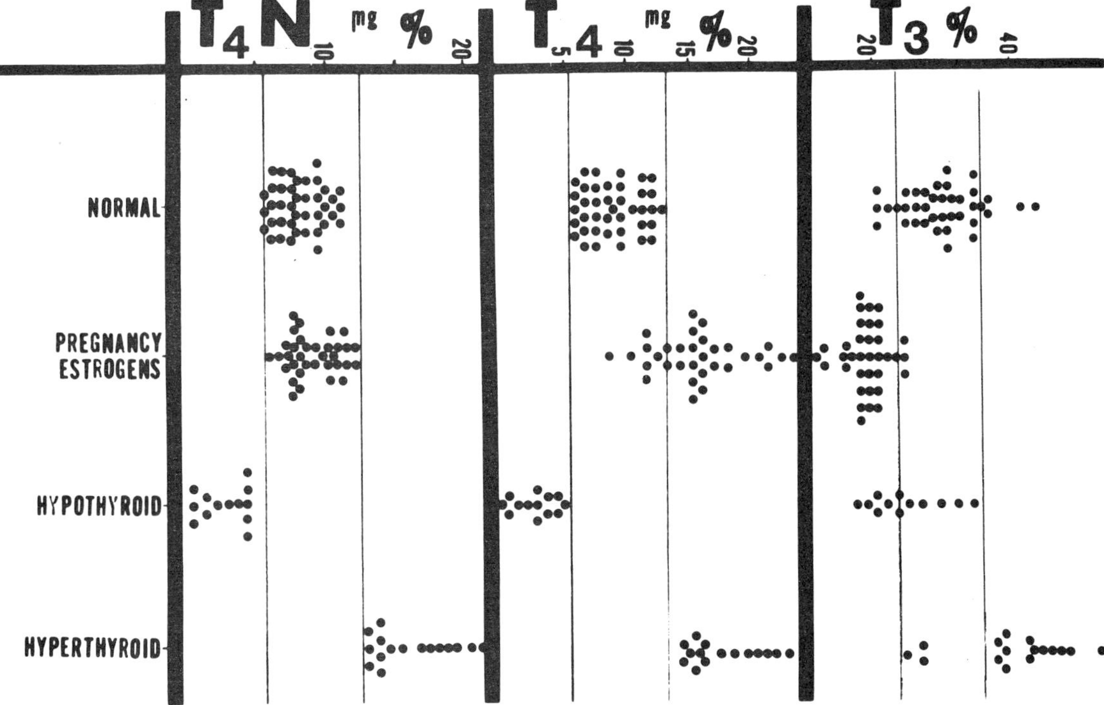

Figure 5-3 *Results of T_3, T_4, and T_4N tests of thyroid function in various conditions.*

T_3 RESIN UPTAKE

This test is the simplest adaptation of the CPBA principle applied to the measurement of thyroid function. When the patient's serum is mixed with a resin and a fixed amount of radioactive triiodothyronine, the radioactive tracer divides itself between the patient's serum and the resin, according to the available binding sites in the patient's serum. In hyperthyroidism the binding sites are saturated so the resin binds most of the tracer, resulting in a high value; in hypothyroidism the opposite occurs. The normal range is 24% to 36% (Fig 5-3).

In pregnant women and those undergoing estrogen therapy TBG increases, producing a falsely low T_3 uptake value in 88% of such patients.

T_4 TEST

The T_4 test measures total serum thyroxine by means of the CPBA. It is an accurate, sensitive method of assessing thyroid function. The normal range is 5.5 ug/100 ml to 12.5 ug/100 ml (Fig 5-3). The total serum thyroxine value is directly dependent on the TBG in the serum, which is altered by various physiologic states. In pregnancy, for example, increased TBG produces a falsely high test result in 77% of such patients.

T_4N TEST

Determination of normalized serum thyroxine (T_4N) values by dual CPBA overcomes the problem of false elevations or depressions in the T_4 test results by using the patient's serum at two stages in the test (Fig 5-4). The initial sample is used for thyroxine measurement; the second is used to correct any false alterations in the thyroxine level existing in the first sample. The standard curve is normalized by the addition of normal control serum to the

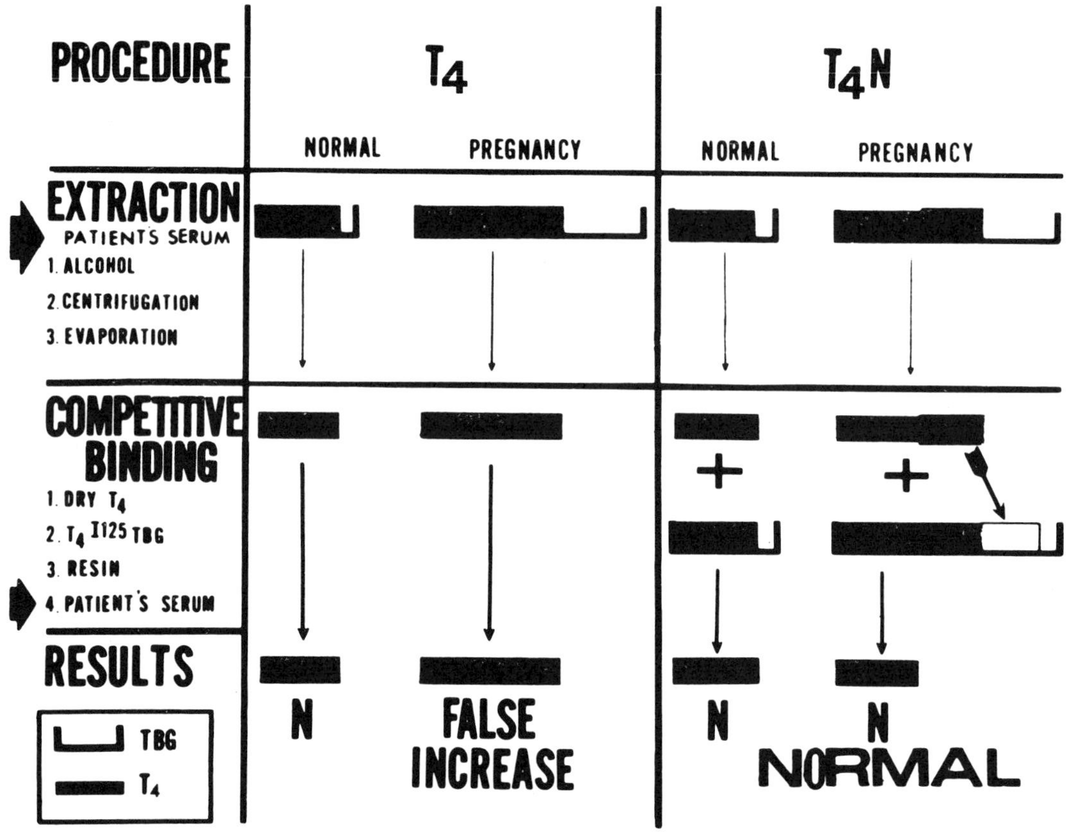

Figure 5-4 *Principle of T_4 and T_4N tests of thyroid function.*

thyroxine standards at the stage of competitive binding.

The ensuing drop in resin binding due to the dual competitive binding technique results in either proportional or disproportionate normalization. In proportional normalization the decline in the curve for normal and for pathologic thyroid states is equal and proportional; they cancel out and there is no appreciable change in thyroxine value. In dispropotionate normalization the decline in the normal curve is not equal to the decline in the value from an altered physiologic state associated with increased or decreased TBG binding, and these falsely abnormal thyroxine values are normalized.

Data obtained with this test correlate well in 94% of cases with the actual clinical state of the patient. This accuracy is superior to that of any other thyroid function test in use at the present time. The normal range is 5.5 ug/100 ml to 12.5 ug/100 ml. Normalization causes no change of thyroxine values in the normal and pathologic thyroid states, but physiologic states resulting in falsely high or low T_4 values, such as pregnancy, estrogen therapy, hypoproteinemia, androgen therapy, salicylate and drug therapy, are normalized and corrected (Fig 5-5).

Scanning and Imaging Techniques

The topographic, structural, and functional anatomy of the thyroid can be easily determined by scanning following the administration of a radioactive tracer (sodium iodide I 131, sodium pertechnetate Tc 99m, and selenomethionine Se 75) and the use of the scintillation camera. Thyroid imag-

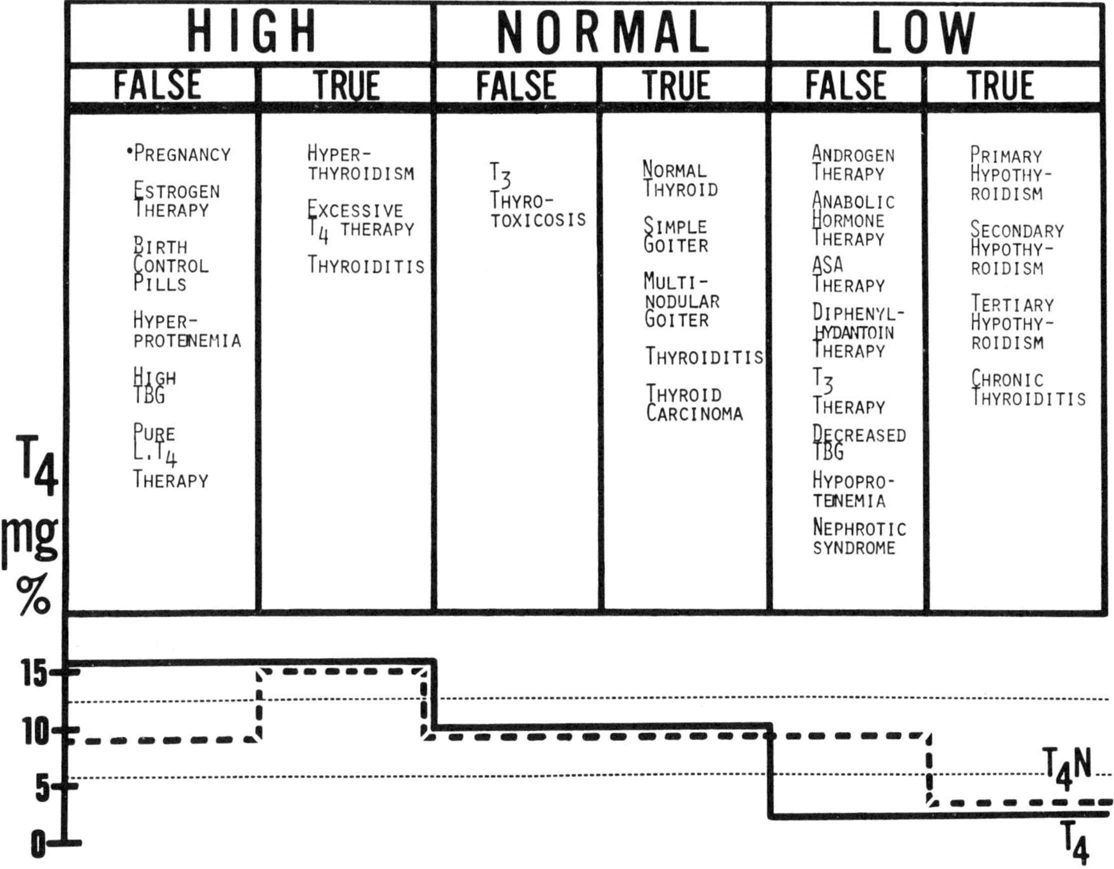

Figure 5-5 *T_4 and T_4N values in various clinical states.*

ing is started 24 hours following the ingestion or injection of 100 uCi of sodium iodide I 131 or 30 minutes following intravenous injection of 3 mCi of sodium pertechnetate Tc 99m or 250 uCi of selenomethionine Se 75.

The detector head of the scintillation camera with a pinhole collimator is centered over the neck of the supine patient. Thyroid images are recorded on Polaroid or 35-mm film from the oscilloscope of the camera.

EVALUATION OF THYROID REGULATION

Thyroid physiology and the maintenance of a normal thyroid hormone level are controlled by a negative-feedback mechanism involving the hypothalamus, anterior pituitary, and thyroid glands (Fig 5-6). TRH stimulates the secretion of TSH, which regulates thyroid hormone production and release.

Conditions Identifiable by Thyroid Scanning

- Abnormalities of thyroid regulation
- Goiter evolution
- Functioning thyroid nodule
- Nonfunctioning thyroid nodule

In thyrotoxicosis, an autonomous hyperfunctioning state associated with elevated thyroid hormone levels, TRH and TSH are low due to the normal feedback relation.

In the various types of hypothyroidism thyroid hormone level is low and the gland image is poor. In primary hypothyroidism

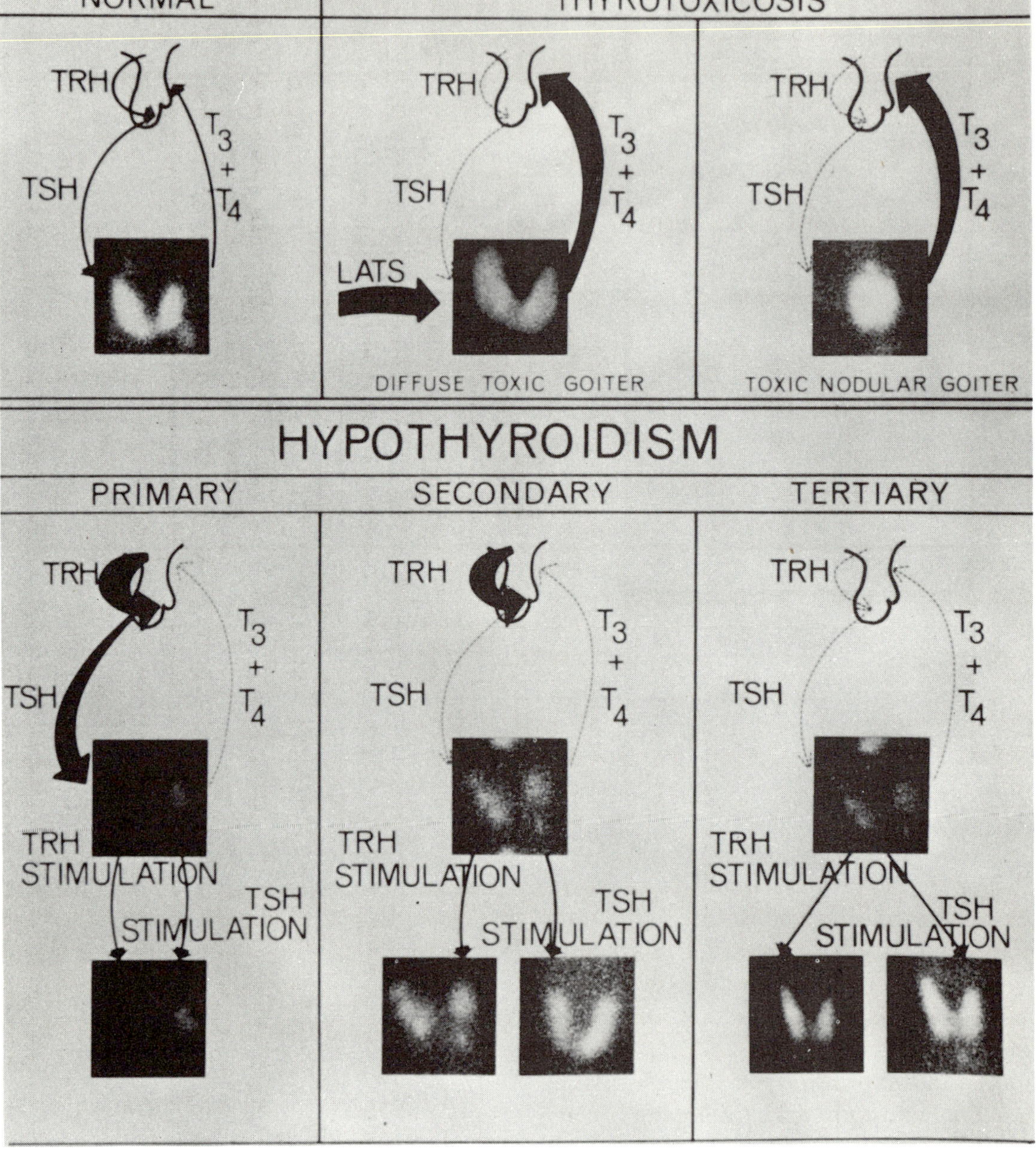

Figure 5-6 *Normal and abnormal thyroid regulation.*

due to thyroid gland disease, TRH and TSH are elevated and TRH or TSH stimulation cannot restore the normal thyroid image. In secondary hypothyroidism due to anterior pituitary disease, TRH is high but TSH is low; TSH stimulation, but not TRH stimulation, can restore the thyroid image to normal. In tertiary hypothyroidism due to hypothalamic disease, TRH and TSH are low and stimulation with either can restore the thyroid image to normal.

EVALUATION OF GOITER EVOLUTION

Abnormal stimuli acting on the thyroid

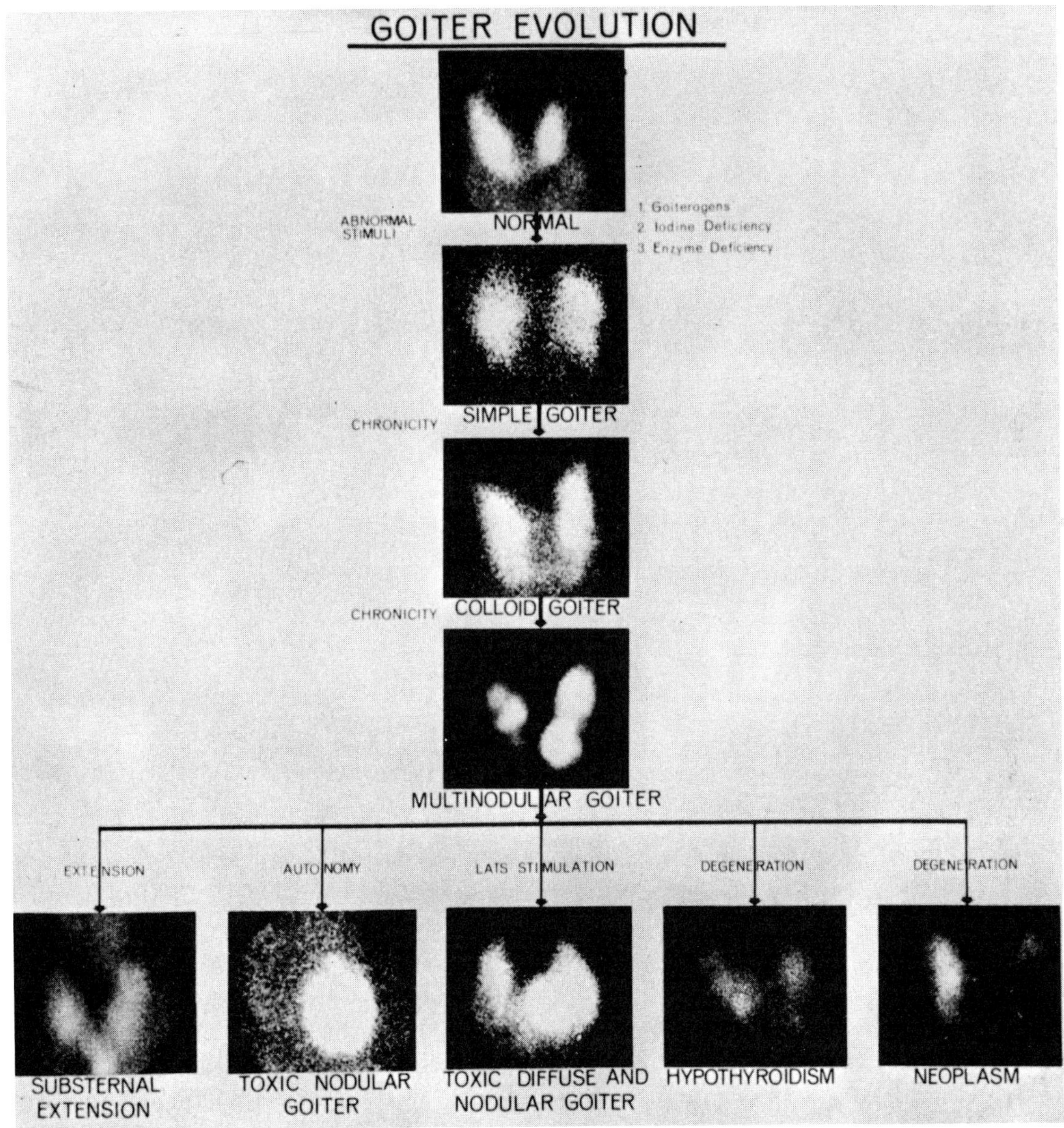

Figure 5-7 *Goiter evolution.*

produce pathologic changes in the gland that can be easily demonstrated by scanning. Use of the various radioactive isotopes of iodine, pertechnetate Tc 99m, and the scintillation camera has facilitated the diagnosis of various goiterous states. The distribution of the radioactive tracer in the gland demonstrates the changes induced by chronic overstimulation.

Various degenerative goitrous conditions can also be diagnosed. Examples are neoplasm, hypothyroid goiters, nontoxic nodular goiter, toxic diffuse and nodular goiters, and regional extensions (Fig 5-7).

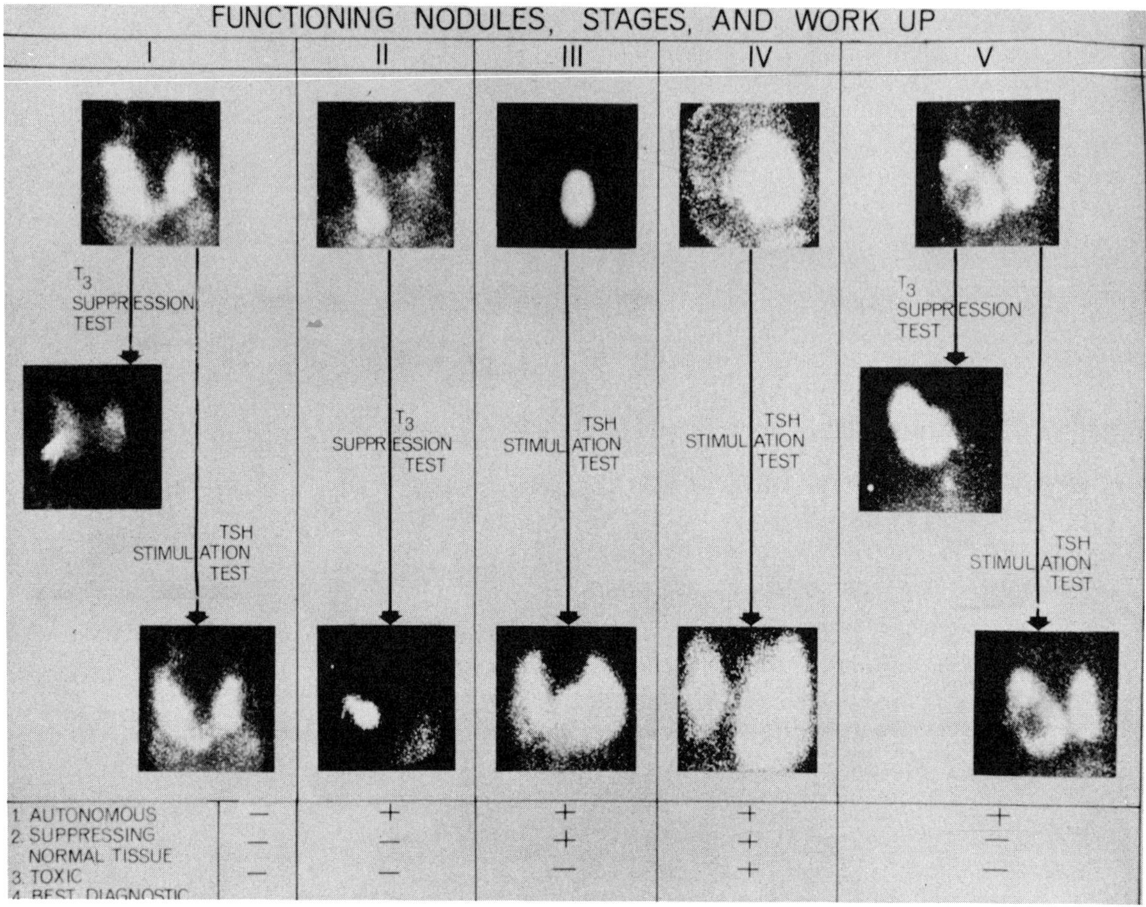

Figure 5-8 *Evaluation of functioning thyroid nodule.*

EVALUATION OF FUNCTIONING NODULE

The autonomous thyroid nodule evolves through various well-recognized stages (Fig 5-8). In addition, a cystic degenerative stage almost invariably occurs at some point in its natural history and can alter its functioning state and imaging appearance.

In 1972 we studied 447 patients with thyroid disorders. Of these, 25% had nodular thyroid disease; 8% were males and 92% were females, with a mean age of 54 years. The duration of the nodule ranged between 1 and 40 years, with a mean of 14 years. Of the patients with nodular thyroid disease, 72% had a single nodule, 24% had two nodules, and 4% had three nodules.

About 2% of the nodules were under TSH control; 24% were nontoxic and did not suppress the normal tissue; 29% were nontoxic but suppressed normal tissue; 12% were toxic and suppressed normal tissue; and 33% had reached the degenerative stage.

The cystic degenerative nodule was always clinically palpable, but was toxic in only 3% of cases. On scanning, it appeared as a nodule with a nonfunctioning center and hyperactive rim (owl's eye appearance) and did not concentrate selenomethionine Se 75. The contralateral lobe was normal in 80% of cases.

When cystic degeneration occurs in an autonomous nodule in a thyrotoxic patient, he may become euthyroid. The appearance

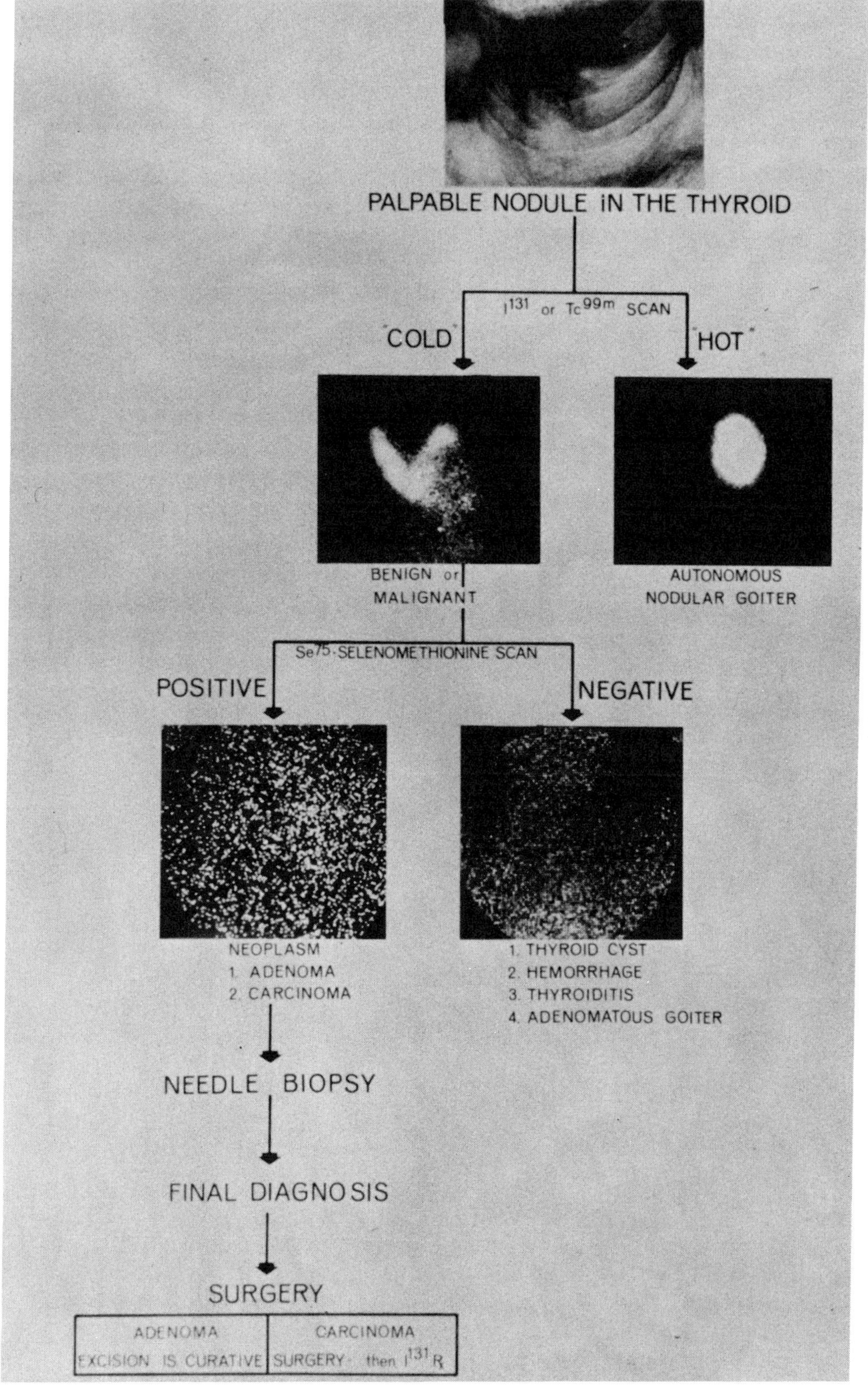

Figure 5-9 *Evaluation of nonfunctioning thyroid nodule.*

of the thyroid scan is so characteristic that it reliably distinguishes an autonomous degenerative nodule from a neoplasm.

EVALUATION OF NONFUNCTIONING NODULE

Thyroid scans performed with radioactive iodine or pertechnetate Tc 99m provide good in vivo assessment of the structure and function of the thyroid nodule (Fig 5-9).

Neoplastic lesions of the thyroid are unable to concentrate these tracers and appear "cold" in comparison with surrounding normal tissue. Since cyst, thyroiditis, and adenomatous goiter also produce "cold" areas on scans, differential diagnosis may be difficult. Neoplastic thyroid lesions can accumulate selenomethionine Se 75, an analog of the amino acid methionine, and use of this preparation allows their differentiation from nonneoplastic lesions.

In the well-defined lesion, needle biopsy is useful to distinguish benign from malignant lesions and is curative in cysts or hemorrhage of the thyroid. Once carcinoma is diagnosed a long-term therapy schedule should be planned for the patient in the form of surgery and ^{131}I ablation.

The Parathyroids

Diagnosis and localization of parathyroid adenomas or hyperplasia are challenging. Localization by the use of selenomethionine Se 75 and the scintillation camera, after thyroid gland suppression with stable iodine and perchlorate and parathyroid stimulation with glucagon, was successful in 80% of cases studied (Fig 5-10).

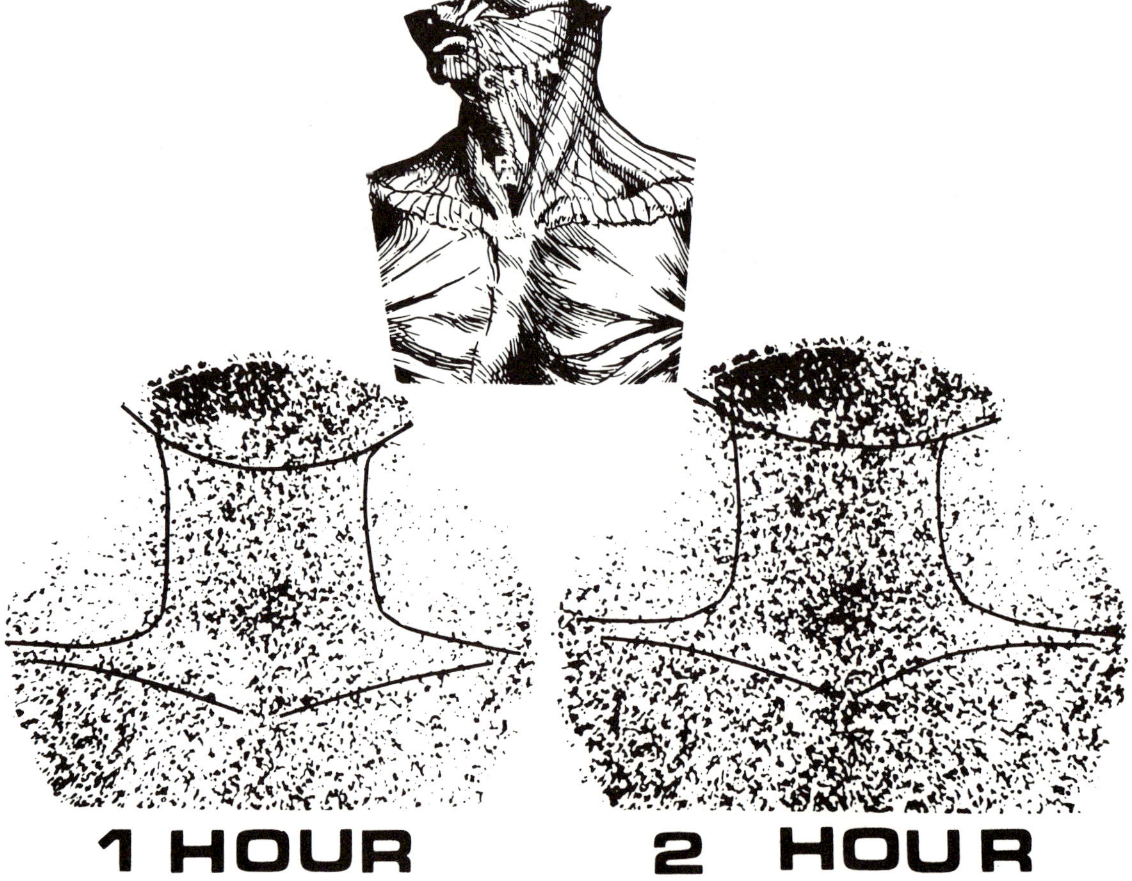

Figure 5-10 *Parathyroid adenoma.*

Table 5-3. Methods for Evaluating the Parathyroids and the Adrenals

	Scanning				Hormone Radioimmunoassay		
Gland	**Indications**	**Tracer**	**Precautions**	**Problems and pitfalls**	**Indications**	**Normal range**	**Problems**
Parathyroid	Hypercalcemia Parathyroid adenoma Parathyroid hyperlasia	Seleno-methionine Se 75 (250μCi; scan in 0.5, 1, 2 hours)	Thyroid suppression with SSKI (10 drops) $KClO_4$ (400 mg)	Lesion size is a limiting factor	Hyper-calcemia Hypo-calcemia	90–410 pg/ml	Normal and hyperpara-thyroid values overlap
Adrenal	Cushing's syndrome Adenoma Hyperplasia Postsurgical remnant Carcinoma	iodo-cholesterol I 131 (2 mCi; scan in 3, 6, 10 days)	Thyroid suppression with Lugol's solution (5 drops)	Long scanning time required	Cushing's syndrome Adrenal insufficiency Steroid therapy	10–80 pg/ml	Diurnal variations

Parathyroid hormone radioimmunoassay aids diagnosis of normal or abnormal parathyroid states. The normal range is between 90 and 410 pg/ml. Unfortunately, there is a considerable overlap between the normal and abnormal levels (Table 5-3).

The Adrenals

Adrenal tissue can be imaged successfully by the use of iodocholesterol I 131, an analog of cholesterol, the principal precursor of adrenal steroids (Fig 5-11). The

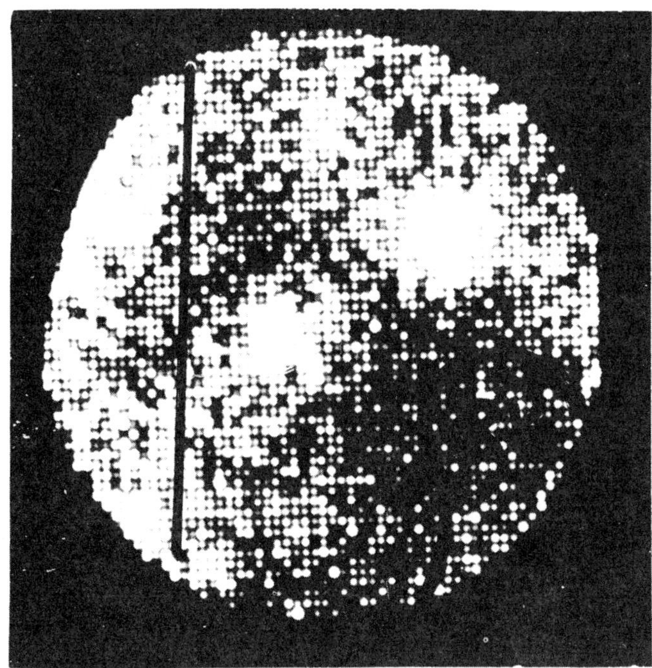

Figure 5-11 *Adrenal gland remnant.*

scan can establish the diagnosis of Cushing's syndrome and can differentiate among its causes.

Adrenal cortical stimulating hormone (ACTH) radioimmunoassay, available commercially, is useful in differentiating among the various adrenal functional states. The normal ACTH range is 10 to 80 pg/ml, and separation between the normal and abnormal states is good (Table 5-3).

References

1. Ashkar FS, Bezjian AA: Use of normalized serum thyroxine (T_4N). *JAMA* **221**:1483, 1972.
2. Ashkar FS, Naya JL, Smith EM: Parathyroid scanning with ^{75}Se-selenomethionine and glucagon stimulation. *J Nucl Med* **12**:751, 1971.
3. Ashkar FS, Smith EM: The dynamic thyroid study. *JAMA* **217**:441, 1971.
4. Beierwaltes WH, Lieberman LM, Ansari AN, et al: Visualization of human adrenal glands in vivo by scintillation scanning. *JAMA* **216**:275, 1971.
5. Bernard JD, McDonald RA, Nesmith JA: New normal ranges for radioiodine uptake study. *J Nucl Med* **12**:449, 1970.
6. Frohman LA: Clinical neuropharmacology of hypothalamic releasing factors: Medical progress. *N Eng J Med* **286**:1391, 1972.
7. Murphy BEP, Patte CJ: Determination of thyroxine utilizing the property of protein binding. *J Clin Endocrinol* **24**:187, 1964.
8. Weinstein MB, Ashkar FS, Caron CD: Se^{75} selenomethionine as a screening agent for the differential diagnosis of the cold thyroid nodule. *Semin Nucl Med* **1**:390, 1971.

Perfusion lung scanning provides information about blood flow; ventilation lung scanning, about gas exchange. Together they give a good picture of lung function and suggest possible causes of abnormalities.

6
The Respiratory System

Mohammed Yunus

Radionuclide Perfusion Study of the Lungs

Between 1962 and 1964 three groups of investigators described the use of labeled particles for determining the integrity of pulmonary blood flow. The use of these metabolizable macroaggregates of serum albumin labeled with I 131 has within a decade evolved into the now commonly performed perfusion lung scan—a safe, simple, and accurate means of evaluating pulmonary perfusion. Its major application today is as a screening test for pulmonary embolism.

The clinical dilemma in diagnosis of pulmonary embolism cannot be adequately discussed in this brief presentation. Several excellent reviews on the subject are available. Suffice it to say that although physicians are now more aware of the problem of pulmonary embolism, the majority of patients with the disease complain of such nonspecific symptoms as dyspnea, cough, and chest pain—all associated also with a wide variety of other cardiopulmonary disorders.

No specific laboratory tests are available; electrocardiography may be helpful but is not sensitive or specific. Chest roentgenograms may appear normal or may show a number of nonspecific changes. Pulmonary angiography, though more specific, cannot be used as a screening procedure because of its complexity and morbidity.

Radionuclide lung scanning, even though nonspecific, is a highly sensitive means of evaluating pulmonary perfusion. It is safe and simple; a normal lung scan virtually excludes the presence of angiographically demonstrable emboli.

Perfusion lung scanning is a safe, reliable screening test for pulmonary embolism. A normal scan virtually rules out angiographically demonstrable emboli.

Principle and Procedure

PRINCIPLE

The average pulmonary capillary diameter is about 8μ. Therefore, if larger particles (10μ to 50μ) are injected intravenously, approximately 90% of these particles is removed from the circulation during their first passage through the lung. They temporarily lodge in the terminal arterioles and capillaries as microemboli (Fig 6-1). The distribution of the labeled particles represents pulmonary blood flow which can be photographically displayed by external radiation detectors such as the Anger camera or the rectilinear scanner. While certain radioactive gases (Xenon 133), discussed

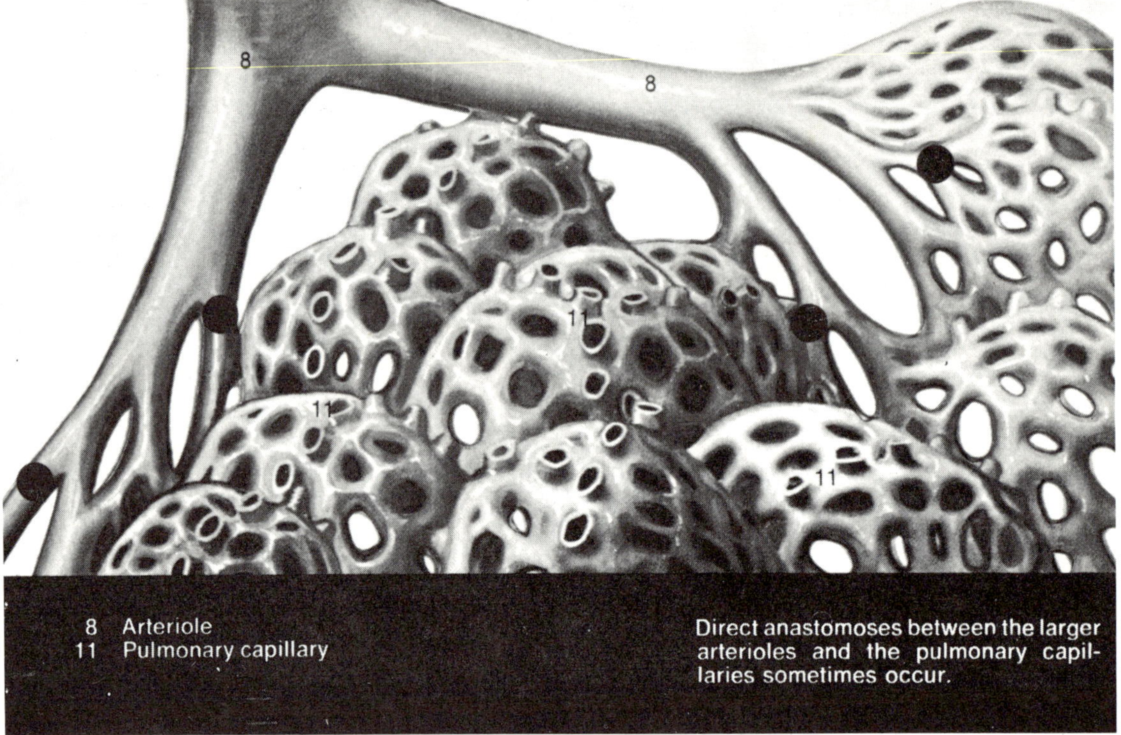

Figure 6-1 *Mechanism of perfusion lung scan. Radioactive particles are in pulmonary capillaries. Gamma rays emitted from these particles are detected by external radiation detectors. (From Roerig)*

later, can also be used to depict pulmonary blood flow, the particle method is more commonly employed because of several advantages:

- Multiple views can be obtained after single injection using a rectilinear scanner or Anger camera.
- This procedure is easier to perform even on sick patients.
- Commercial preparations are readily available and are less expensive.
- No additional equipment is necessary.

SAFETY

The transient iatrogenic microembolism produced to obtain a perfusion lung scan causes no ill effects, as the usual dose of macroaggregates for an adult occludes only 1 in 1000 of the total terminal vessels in the arteriolocapillary network; no alterations in pulmonary function or pulmonary artery pressure have been noted during the procedure. The amount of albumin used is too small to produce significant effects.

Even though a wide margin of safety exists, in patients with markedly compromised pulmonary vascular bed, eg, in severe pulmonary hypertension, it is wise to use a nonparticulate agent such as 133 Xe.

RADIOPHARMACEUTICALS

Several radionuclides have been used. The list includes macroaggregated albumin I 131, albumin microspheres Tc 99m, macroaggregated albumin Tc 99m, hydrated ferric oxide Tc 99m, and hydrated ferric oxide In 113m.

Macroaggregated albumin I 131 is still the most widely used radionuclide. Its advantages are:

- A shelf life of approximately two weeks that allows storage and makes the material readily available, especially in smaller laboratories

- Commercially available precalibrated, sterile solutions, ready for immediate use

Its disadvantages are:

- The need to prepare the patient with Lugol's solution to protect the thyroid gland
- A useless beta emission that limits administration to microcurie amounts

Newer agents such as macroaggregated albumin Tc 99m and albumin microspheres Tc 99m are gaining popularity. The short half-life (six hours) and lack of beta emission permits administration of larger doses and generally results in a better examination in a shorter time.

PREPARING PATIENT

Lugol's solution is given prior to the examination if macroaggregated albumin I 131 is used. No preparation is necessary with the other agents.

PROCEDURE

Lung scans of uniformly high quality are essential for proper interpretation. Strict adherence to standardized technique avoids production of artifacts.

- To eliminate the effect of gravity and ensure uniform particle distribution, injection should be made with the patient in the recumbent position.
- Imaging is started immediately and the anterior, posterior, right, and left lateral views are routinely obtained; the exception is the very sick patient.
- Chest roentgenography is performed immediately before or after the study.
- The total examination time is 10-30 minutes

Normal Lung

The normal scan (Fig 6-2) shows homogeneous distribution of radioactivity throughout the lungs. The cardiac outline is well delineated as an area of decreased activity more prominent toward the left side in the anterior view, and anteriorly in the left lateral view.

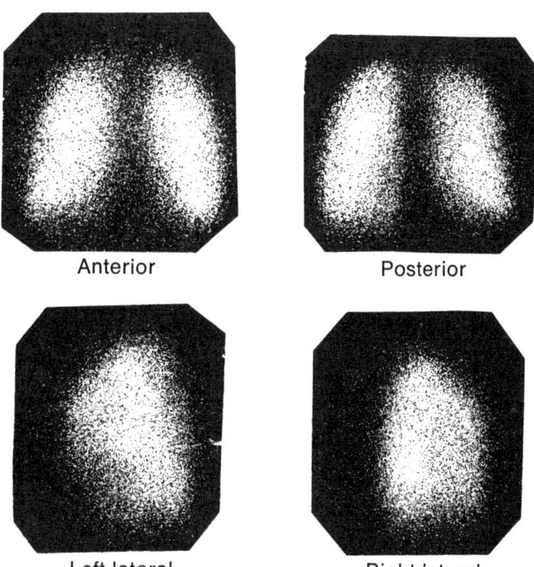

Figure 6-2 *Normal lung. Radioactivity is homogeneously distributed throughout lungs. Cardiac outline is well seen as area of decreased activity, more prominent in anterior and left lateral views.*

Pulmonary Embolism

The place of lung scanning in the diagnosis and management of a patient with suspected pulmonary embolism is outlined in Fig 6-3.

CHARACTERISTIC APPEARANCE

Pulmonary embolism with or without infarction produces areas of decreased perfusion on a lung scan. No appearance is specific for pulmonary embolism, but certain changes are consistently seen and are highly suggestive (Figs 6-4 and 6-5):

- Multiple, scattered, bilateral areas of decreased perfusion with areas of normal perfusion interspersed
- Peripheral perfusion defects with convex inner margins (toward the hilum)

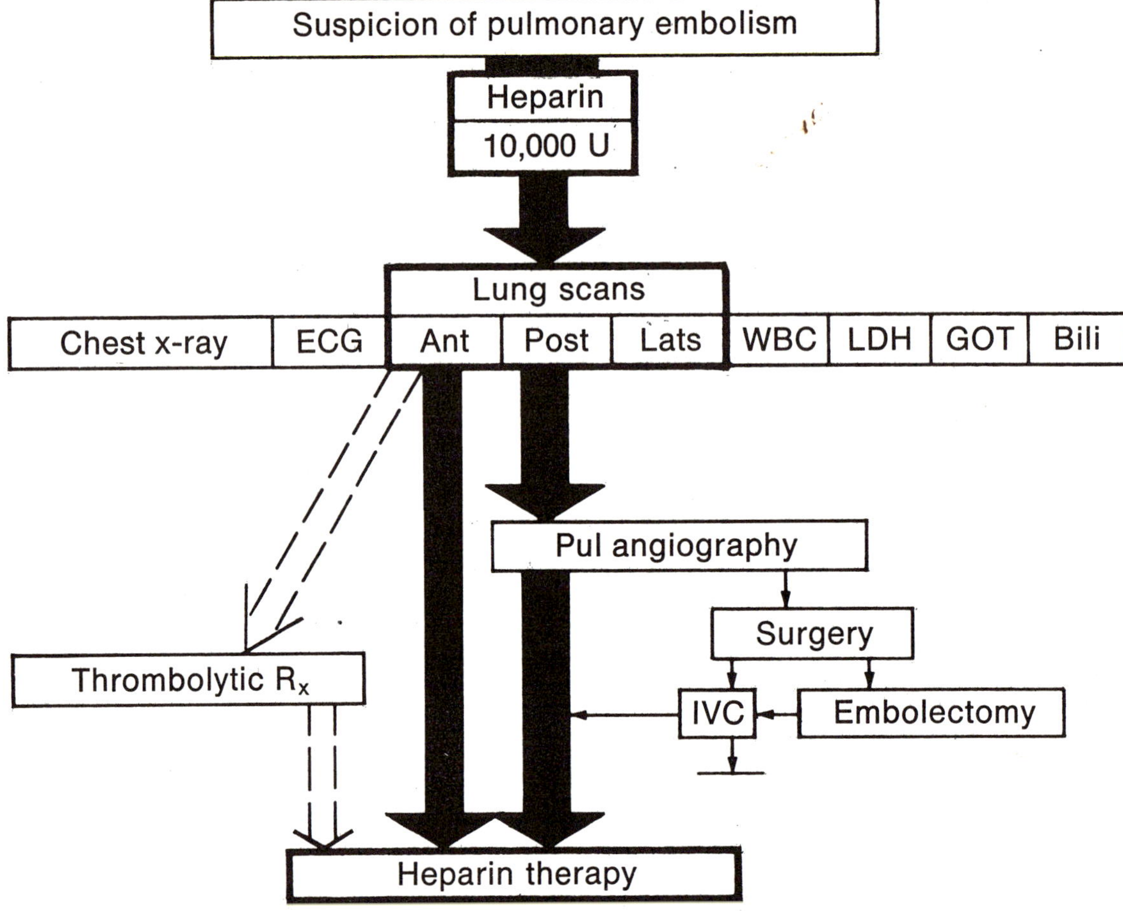

Figure 6-3 *Diagnostic and therapeutic approach to pulmonary embolism. On suspicion of pulmonary embolism, a single injection of heparin should be administered while diagnostic studies are completed. Although recommended pathway includes pulmonary angiography, lung scans in patients without previous cardiopulmonary disease may be sufficient to diagnose and treat embolism. However, when surgery is considered, particularly pulmonary embolectomy, angiography should be performed. Occasionally, in massive embolism, time may permit only pulmonary angiography. Ant, anterior; post, posterior; lats, laterals (right and left); WBC, white blood cell count; LDH, lactic dehydrogenase; GOT, glutamic oxalacetic transaminase; bili, bilirubin; IVC, inferior vena cava interruption; embolectomy, pulmonary embolectomy. (Reproduced from Sasahara, et al:* Cardiovascular Clin *1: 26, 1970.)*

Perfusion Scan Characteristics of Pulmonary Embolism

- Multiple, scattered bilateral areas of decreased perfusion with areas of normal perfusion interspersed
- Peripheral perfusion defects with convex inner margins
- Segmental perfusion defects without corresponding roentgenographic changes
- Hypoperfusion along the major fissure without demonstrable roentgenographic abnormality

- Segmental or lobar perfusion defects without corresponding roentgenographic changes
- Hypoperfusion along the major fissure without demonstrable roentgenographic abnormality (fissure sign)

These findings are not pathognomonic and may be seen in other diseases (Fig 6-6). A concurrent chest roentgenogram or ventilation study, and correlation with clinical findings, are necessary for correct interpretation.

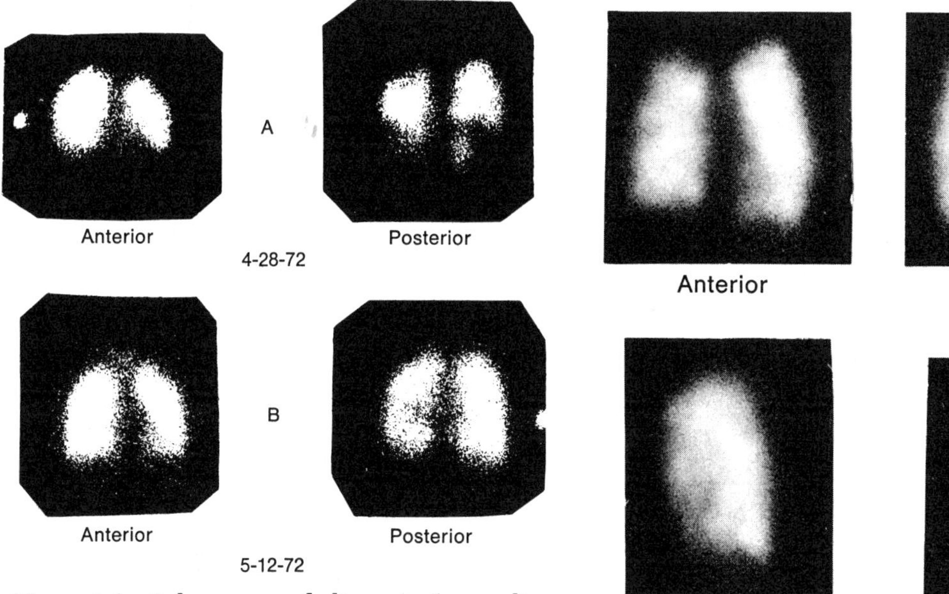

Figure 6-4 *Pulmonary embolism. A. Large discrete areas of perfusion defect without corresponding roentgenographic changes are highly suggestive of pulmonary emboli. B. Two weeks later perfusion is almost completely restored in affected areas.*

A single study is sometimes equivocal, but since acute pulmonary embolism shows a changing pattern, comparison with an earlier study or a repeat study in five to ten days may facilitate correct diagnosis.

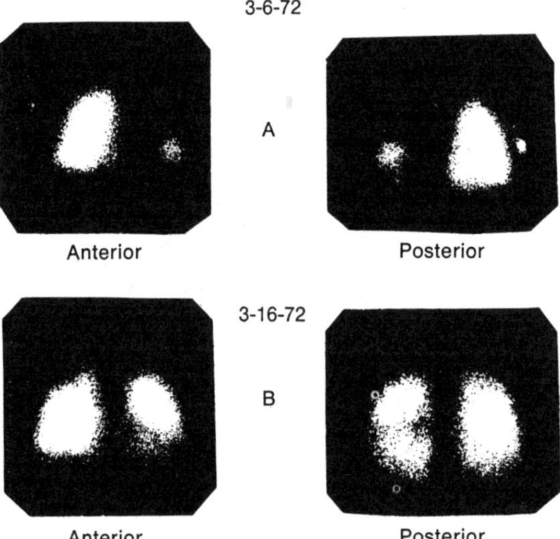

Figure 6-5 *Massive pulmonary embolism. A. Near absence of perfusion in left lung. No roentgenographic density was noted. B. Considerable improvement in perfusion of left lung ten days later.*

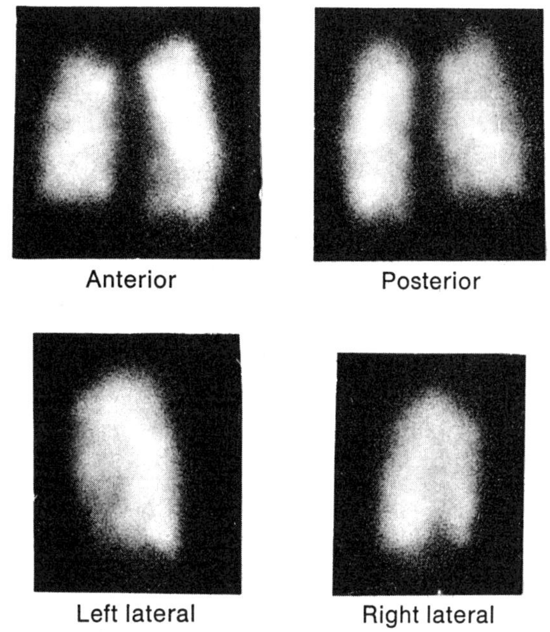

Anterior Posterior

Left lateral Right lateral

Figure 6-6 *Bronchial asthma. Perfusion is markedly abnormal. Patient, a young male, had a long history of bronchial asthma since childhood. Study, done during an acute episode, shows multiple perfusion defects.*

Lung scanning should be done as soon as possible after the onset of clinical symptoms since the characteristic changes may no longer be present after a few days.

USE IN PRESENCE OF ABNORMAL ROENTGENOGRAM

Lung scanning should be performed in patients with suspected pulmonary embolism even though chest roentgenography shows abnormal density. Demonstration of areas of perfusion deficit other than those ascertained by roentgenography establishes the diagnosis of pulmonary embolism with infarction.

DIFFERENTIAL DIAGNOSIS

Acute Bronchial Asthma Asthma can produce a lung scan indistinguishable from that characteristic of pulmonary embolism (Fig 6-6). Chest roentgenograms may also appear normal in these patients. The history and clinical manifestations differentiate the two diseases. Ventilation study may

Differential Diagnosis of Pulmonary Embolism

- Acute bronchial asthma
- Chronic obstructive pulmonary disease
- Pneumonia
- Pleural effusion
- Segmental or lobar atelectasis
- Congestive heart failure

be helpful, but is generally not necessary. A repeat lung scan 24 to 48 hours following successful treatment shows marked improvement or a return to normal in the asthmatic patient.

Chronic Obstructive Pulmonary Disease This may produce a markedly abnormal lung scan (Figs 6-7 and 6-8). Chest roentgenography and xenon ventilation abnor-

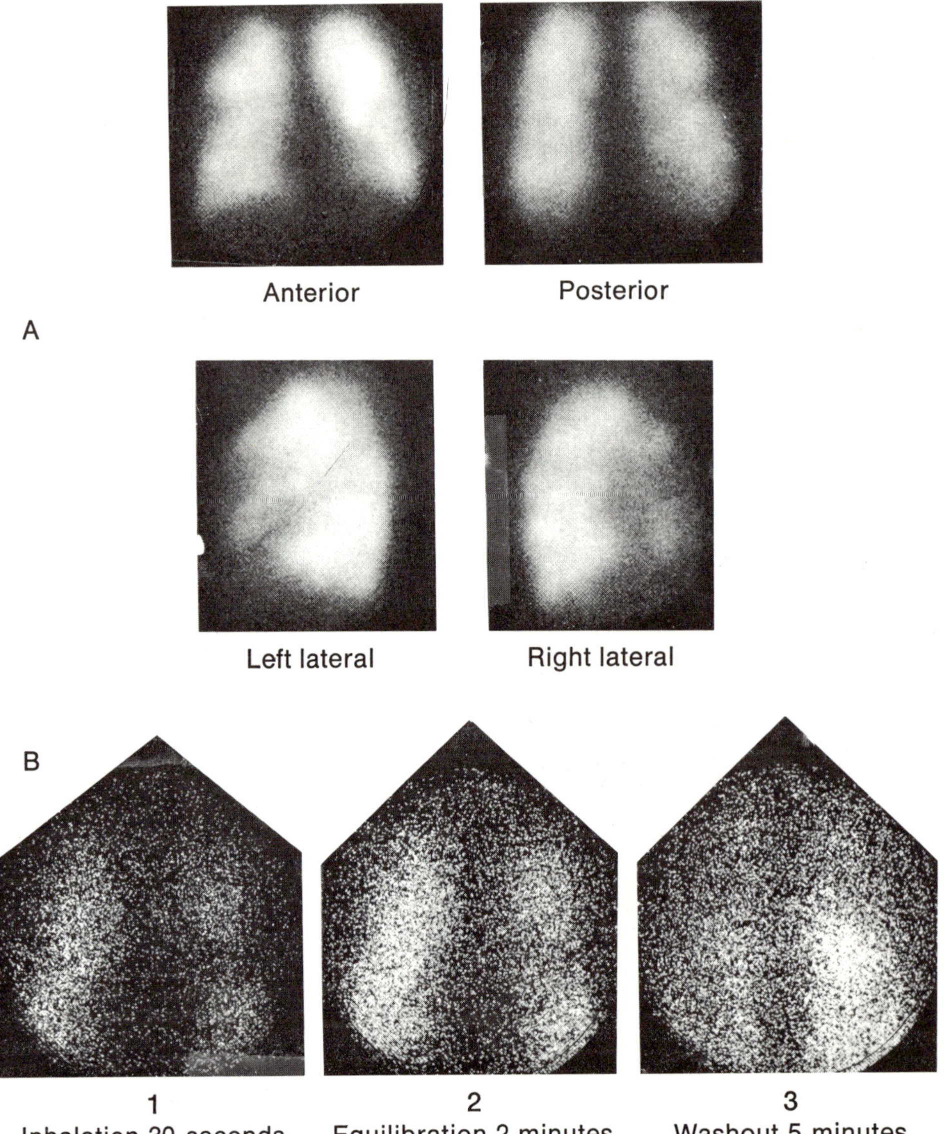

Figure 6-7 *Obstructive pulmonary disease. A. Perfusion study shows multiple perfusion abnormalities, most pronounced in region of right midline. B. Ventilation study shows decreased ventilation in this area and marked retention at five minutes.*

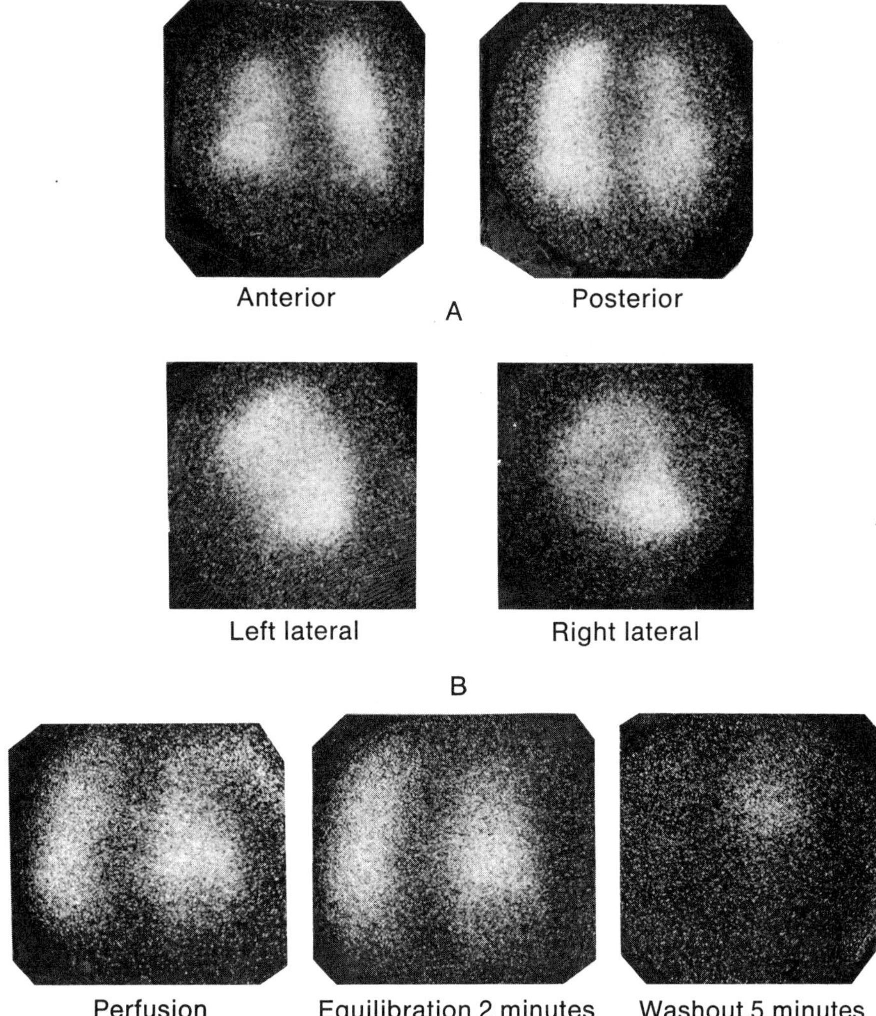

Figure 6-8 *Obstructive pulmonary disease. A. Perfusion study shows large area of decreased perfusion right upper lobe. B. Ventilation study shows large area of Xenon retention in washout phase.*

malities usually differentiate obstructive disease from pulmonary embolism. However, in some cases, especially when coexisting pulmonary embolism is suspected, pulmonary angiography may be necessary. A correct retrospective diagnosis can be established by a repeat lung scan in 10 to 14 days. The perfusion deficits of emphysema remain unchanged, whereas those of pulmonary embolism are somewhat altered.

Pneumonia The perfusion deficit in pneumonia corresponds solely to the area of roentgenographic density. Clinical manifestations and the absence of ventilation in the involved areas demonstrated by ^{133}Xe study confirm the diagnosis.

Pleural Effusion Localized pleural effusion may produce perfusion deficits suggestive of pulmonary embolism (fissure sign with interlobar fluid). Chest roentgenography with decubitus views enables differentiation.

Segmental or Lobar Atelectasis Perfusion defects correspond to distinct abnormalities seen on the chest roentgenogram. Dif-

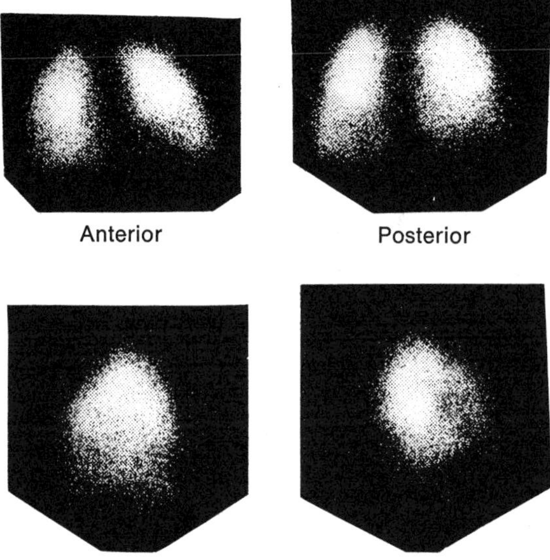

Figure 6-9 *Congestive heart failure. Perfusion study shows marked cardiac enlargement, redistribution of flow, and bilateral pleural effusion.*

ferentiation from pulmonary embolism is not difficult.

Congestive Heart Failure This produces a recognizable abnormality in the perfusion pattern (Fig 6-9). Pulmonary embolism cannot be excluded with certainty, and a repeat lung scan should be obtained following treatment of the acute episode.

Bronchogenic Carcinoma

Central lesions may produce a marked decrease in perfusion of the lungs even in the absence of roentgenographically demonstrable lesions. Several investigators have reported the use of lung scan in patients with suspected or proved bronchogenic carcinoma. This method may be useful in evaluating the resectability of the lesion and in following a patient during radiation or chemotherapy.

Chronic Obstructive Pulmonary Disease

Perfusion study combined with pulmonary function tests and radionuclide ventilation study has been used to determine the extent and severity of the disease process and to evaluate pulmonary perfusion prior to surgical removal of large bullae.

Characteristic perfusion abnormalities have been described in patients with alpha-1-antitrypsin deficiency.

Cystic Fibrosis

Perfusion and ventilation lung scanning, a more sensitive indicator of the presence of lung disease than either method alone, is being used to evaluate children with chronic lung disorders, especially cystic fibrosis.

Radionuclide Ventilation Study

The use of radioactive gases to determine regional pulmonary function dates back to the early 1950s. However, the method employed then required tracheobronchial catheterization and never gained popularity.

In the late 1950s, based on the knowledge that inhaled radioactive gases are distributed in the lungs similarly to air, a closed xenon system with external radiation detector was used to diagnose changes in ventilation with bronchial obstruction from bronchogenic carcinoma and other diseases.

The sensation created by the announcement of the availability of the labeled particles to diagnose pulmonary embolism overshadowed development of the ventilation study with radioactive gases. As described in the previous section, radionuclide perfusion study of the lung provides valuable data regarding the distribution of pulmonary blood flow, but offers insufficient information about the cause of the abnormality. Generally the cause of the abnormality detected by the perfusion lung scan is deduced on the basis of chest roentgenography, clinical manifestations, and pulmonary arteriography. Recent demonstrations of the value of ventilation studies in differential diagnosis of pulmonary embolism and the increased availability of a suitable imaging device (scintillation camera) have revived enthusiasm for the procedure.

Principle and Procedure

PRINCIPLE

Basic knowledge of the pulmonary physiology is essential to the interpretation of the ventilation study. Briefly, normal lung function (replacement of oxygen and removal of carbon dioxide) requires blood flow (perfusion) and gas exchange (ventilation). Diseases producing a change in one component will produce a corresponding change in the other.

Perfusion defects caused by acute or chronic parenchymal lung disease or bronchial obstruction (with atelectasis) are associated with abnormalities in the ventilation of the involved portions of the lung.

Pulmonary embolism without infarction classically produces marked perfusion abnormalities, but the involved areas show normal ventilation.

RADIOPHARMACEUTICALS

^{133}Xe, a reactor-produced and poorly soluble radionuclide, is at present the most widely used. Though its 5.3-day half-life is less than ideal, it allows for shipping and storage. It is also readily available commercially as a gas or dissolved in a saline solution. Clinically useful radionuclides of nitrogen, oxygen, and carbon are cyclotron-produced and have such short half-lives (minutes) that their routine clinical use is limited. Inhalation of small radioactive particles (0.5μ to 10.0μ) in size has been used to demonstrate pulmonary ventilation but has not proved totally satisfactory.

INSTRUMENTS

A rapid imaging device such as the Anger scintillation camera is necessary for the ventilation study. Special shielded spirometers and other required accessories are now commercially available, facilitating the routine use of radioactive gases.

PROCEDURE

No patient preparation is necessary. Several methods are currently in use, but only the two most commonly employed techniques will be discussed here. The intravenous method requires less cooperation from the patient and is therefore used in the very sick.

Intravenous Method After selection of the optimal view for the examination, as determined by the evaluation of the perfusion study, a solution of xenon and normal saline is injected intravenously during inspiration. This is the perfusion phase of the study. ^{133}Xe, being poorly soluble, rapidly diffuses from the pulmonary capillaries into the alveoli.

The subject is then instructed to rebreathe through a closed circuit equipped with a carbon dioxide trap. Two to five minutes of rebreathing in this manner results in uniform distribution of the gas. This is the equilibration phase. The subject then breathes in room air and breathes out the xenon. This is the washout phase.

Inspiratory Capacity Method The patient is connected to the spirometer circuit

Lung Scan Interpretation

- Pulmonary embolism
  - Decreased perfusion
  - Normal ventilation
- Pneumonia
  - Abnormal perfusion
  - Abnormal ventilation
- Emphysema
  - Decreased perfusion
  - Decreased ventilation
- Bronchial obstruction
  - Abnormal perfusion
  - Abnormal ventilation

containing ^{133}Xe during a maximal inspiratory effort. This is the ventilation phase. The equilibration and washout phases are executed as in the intravenous method. All phases of the study are constantly recorded.

INTERPRETATION

Normally the radionuclides are uniformly distributed in the ventilation and equilibration phases. Clearance is prompt, without focal retention.

An area of decreased activity during the ventilation phase or delay in clearance during the washout phase is abnormal.

Acute pulmonary embolism is characteristically associated with normal ventilation in areas of decreased perfusion. Pneumonia produces both ventilation and perfusion abnormalities, with the ventilation abnormality of greater magnitude. Pulmonary emphysema produces decreased ventilation and perfusion in the involved areas and may show abnormal retention of the radionuclide in affected areas during the washout phase (Figs 6-8 and 6-9). Bronchial obstruction from any cause produces marked abnormalities in perfusion and ventilation.

References

1. Dalen JE, Dexter L: Pulmonary embolism. *JAMA* **207**:1505, 1969.
2. DeNardo GL, Goodwin DA, Ravasini R, et al: The ventilatory lung scan in the diagnosis of pulmonary embolism. *N Eng J Med* **282**:1334, 1970.
3. Eaton SB, James AE, Potsaid MS, et al: Scintigraphic findings in pulmonary microembolism. *Am J Roentgenol Radium Ther Nucl Med* **105**:778, 1969.
4. Gilson AJ, Smoak WM (eds): *Pulmonary Investigation with Radionuclides.* Springfield, Ill, Thomas, 1970.
5. Gold WM, McCormack KR: Pulmonary-function response to radioisotope scanning of the lungs. JAMA **197**:146, 1966.
6. Henderson LL, Tauxe WN, Hyatt RE: Lung scanning of asthmatic patients with 131 I MAA. *South Med J* **60**:795, 1967.
7. Johnson P: The role of lung scanning in pulmonary embolism. *Semin Nuc Med* **1**:161–182, 1971.
8. Maynard CD, Cowan RJ: Role of the scan in bronchogenic carcinoma. *Semin Nucl Med* **1**:195–205, 1971.
9. Robinson AE, Goodrich JK, Spock A: Inhalation and perfusion radionuclide studies of pediatric chest disease. *Radiology* **93**:1123–1128, 1969.
10. Sasahara A, Belko J, McIntyre K: Problems in the diagnosis and management of pulmonary embolism. *Semin Nucl Med* **1**:122–130, 1971.
11. Smoak WM: Pulmonary Ventilation Studies with Radionuclides. In Maynard CD (ed): *Continuing Education Lectures.* Vol. II. Southeastern Chapter, Society of Nuclear Medicine, 1972.
12. Taplin GV, Dore EK, Johnson DE, et al: Colloidal Radioalbumin Aggregates for Organ Scanning. Exhibit at 1963 annual meeting, Society of Nuclear Medicine, Montreal, Canada.
13. Tow DE, Wagner HN Jr, Lopez-Majano V, et al: Validity of measuring regional pulmonary arterial blood flow with macroaggregates of human serum albumin. *Am J. Roentgenol Radium Ther Nucl Med* **96**:664, 1966.
14. Wagner HN Jr, Rhodes BA, Sasaki Y, et al: Studies of the circulation with radioactive microspheres. *Invest Radiol* **4**:314, 1969.
15. Wagner HN, Sabiston DC, Iio M, et al: Regional pulmonary blood flow in man by radioisotope scanning. *JAMA* **187**: 601–603, 1964.
16. Weibel ER: Morphometry of the Human Lungs. In Geometry and Dimension of the Alveolar Capillary Network. New York, Academic Press, 1963; chap 7.
17. Wellman HN, Mack JF, Romilt DW, et al: Evaluation of the relative efficacy of pulmonary scintigraphy and pulmony angiography in the diagnosis of pulmonary arterial obstructive disease. (Abstract.) *J Nucl Med* **10**:380, 1969.
18. Winebright JW, Gerdes AJ, Nelp WB: Restoration of blood flow after pulmonary embolism. *Arch Intern Med* **125**:241, 1970.

Radionuclide scanning of the liver, spleen, and pancreas supplies information about the size, shape, and functional integrity of these organs.

7
The Gastrointestinal System

Fuad S. Ashkar and August Miale, Jr.

Liver Scanning

In recent years, a new technique utilizing liver-seeking materials labeled with radioactive isotopes has been developed which provides additional highly accurate and useful diagnostic information about liver disorders. The size, shape, position, and integrity of the liver, and the patency of the biliary tract, can be evaluated by graphically recording the distribution of radioactivity in the liver.

Two practical photoscanning instruments for producing images of the distribution of radioactivity are now in use. One is a moving detector or rectilinear scanning device with a focusing collimator; the other is a stationary detector or scintillation camera with a multiaperture straight-bore collimator. The images are produced on x-ray film and Polaroid film, respectively. Moving detector (rectilinear photoscanning) instruments have long been available and were used for most of the initial work on the liver. In the past few years, use of the scintillation camera has increased because of certain advantages, including speed and versatility, not possessed by other commercially available instruments.

Principle

TRACERS

A labeled dye, rose bengal I 131, was the first material widely used for liver photoscanning. Although its rapid excretion from the liver through the biliary system produces undesirable variations in the distribution of activity, passage of this labeled compound into the gut provides an index of patency of the biliary tract.

Colloidal particles labeled with gold 198 or technetium 99m are at present the most widely used agents for liver photoscanning. These particles, less than 1μ in size, are removed from the blood by Kupffer cells in the liver or by reticuloendothelial cells in other organs, mainly spleen and bone marrow. About 80% appear in liver 30 to 60 minutes following injection. Once trapped, the particles remain fixed until all radioactivity has decayed. Newer radioactive labels for colloidal particles, particularly technetium 99m and indium 113m, have more favorable radiation characteristics than gold 198 and are more desirable for photoscanning.

INSTRUMENTATION

The scintillation camera designed and introduced by Anger (Nuclear-Chicago Pho/Gamma) provides an excellent method for photoscanning. The crystal detector, 11 inches in diameter, 0.5 inch thick, and backed by 19 photomultiplier tubes, has three degrees of freedom, allowing the detector face to be placed parallel to any plane. Thus, any area of the body can be viewed with the patient in a comfortable position. Since a complete scan of any projection of the liver can be done in from several seconds to four minutes, multiple views of the liver can be obtained from various angles for evaluation of anterior, lateral, and posterior aspects.

The amplified pulses from the photomultiplier tubes are displayed as dots on the face of an oscilloscope and are then accumulated on Polaroid film to produce an image display. Since no data are rejected as background cutoff or hidden in the density of overexposed areas of x-ray film, a relatively accurate estimation of the true distribution of activity is possible. The multichannel straight-bore collimator works well at the liver surface and almost as well at a depth of three inches, which is the same as the point of focus of the average focusing collimator. The high activities (in the order of 300,000 to 1 million counts per minute) obtainable when ^{99m}Tc-labeled compounds are used, do not overload the scintillation camera as they may other detectors designed with ratemeter circuits and smaller crystals. With count rates of this magnitude, a liver photoscan can be done in a few seconds, with the patient holding his breath to avoid marginal artifacts often produced by breathing motion.

Landmarks are easily added using lead markers or small radioactive sources located over the usual points on the patient. The high scanning speed possible with the camera and the ability to study patients in any position allow prompt and rapid evaluation of the liver in traumatized or acutely ill patients prior to surgery. As an alternative to speed, the high sensitivity of the camera can be utilized to reduce the radioactive isotope dose when liver scanning is needed in a child.

RESULTS

Interpretation of these scans depends on the differential uptake of radioactive material by normal and abnormal tissues. Abnormalities are indicated by a decrease in activity over a focal or diffuse area of the liver due to loss of normal vascular supply or of normally functioning hepatic cells. Labeled colloids are used when the diagnostic interest centers about the anatomic features of the liver. Since tumors, abcesses, cysts, hemorrhage, and fibriotic tissue do not concentrate these substances, corresponding areas devoid of radioactivity appear as "cold" areas on the scans (Figs 7-1 and 7-2).

> **Interpretation of the liver scan depends on differential uptake of radioactive material by normal and abnormal tissue, with abnormality indicated by decreased uptake.**

Liver scans using a radionuclide-labeled dye such as rose bengal I 131 can also reveal anatomic features of the liver. However, the dye is rapidly excreted in the bile and subsequently in the small intestine. Variability of excretion by liver cells may

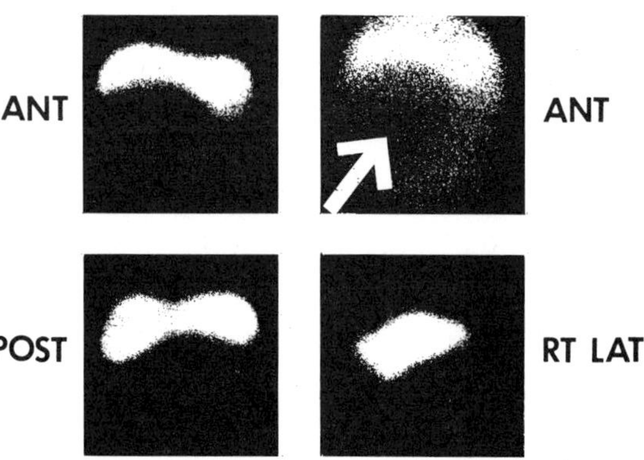

Figure 7-1 *Solitary intrahepatic cyst appearing as large "cold" area.*

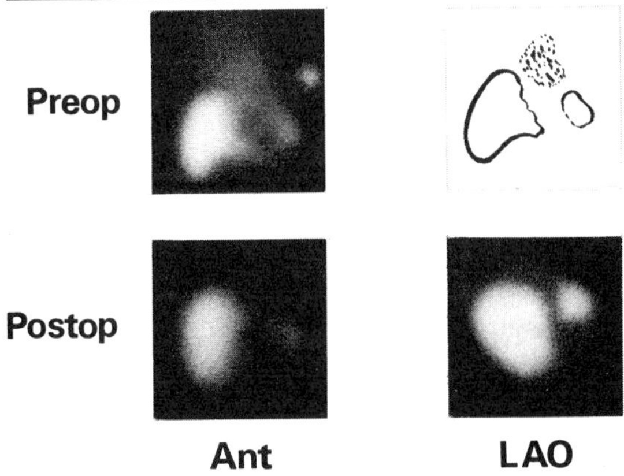

Figure 7-2 *Congenital hemangioma appearing as "cold" area.*

produce a nonohomogeneous distribution pattern of radioactivity within the liver which does not reflect a true anatomic defect. Rose bengal is more useful as a means of evaluating hepatobiliary patency, since demonstration of delayed or nonentry of dye into the small intestine indicates biliary obstruction.

Interpretation

NORMAL LIVER

Liver photoscans normally show minor variations from patient to patient, mainly with respect to shape; overall size is relatively constant. The thickest portion, usually representing the right lobe, appears as the area of highest density on the film. The

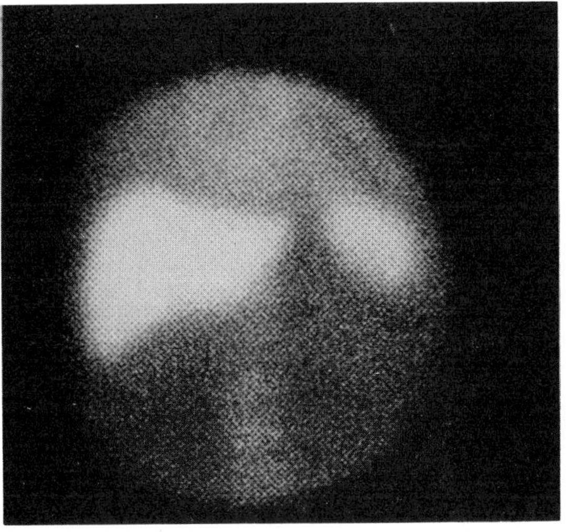

Figure 7-3 *Normal liver and spleen.*

liver dome curvature corresponds to the undersurface of the diaphragm; an indentation or concavity below the heart is a usual feature. The inferior portion of the right lobe is represented by a well-defined downward triangular projection reaching to about the costal margin. There is often some leftward projection of activity beyond the midline, but this is rarely prominent and often shows relatively less overall density (Fig 7-3).

Since liver size and shape vary in man, certain normal photoscan patterns should be recognized to avoid misinterpretation. The following normal variants have been described:

- Concavity of the inferior border
- Squareness of the liver
- Definite hilar indentation
- Exaggerated dome or inverted triangle with high diaphragm
- Globular liver
- Horn-shaped liver with concavity of the right lateral border due to indentation of the rib cage
- Downward extension of the right lobe (Riedel's lobe)
- Superior accessory lobe
- Inferior marginal indentation due to the right kidney
- Displacement due to interposition of the colon between the liver and the lateral abdominal wall

ABNORMAL LIVER

The most common abnormality detected is liver enlargement; its causes are listed in Table 7-1. The differential diagnosis of discrete filling defects is outlined in Table 7-2. Particular attention to defects in the area of the porta hepatis and left lobe will suggest other diagnostic possibilities listed in Tables 7-3 and 7-4.

The histologic character of the lesion or disease entity producing a defect cannot

Table 7-1. Abnormalities of Liver Size

Increase	Decrease
Malignancy	Normal variation
Laennec's cirrhosis	Artifactual
Fatty infiltration	Laennec's cirrhosis
Chronic passive congestion	Metastatic disease
Acute or subacute hepatitis	Cardiac cirrhosis
Distant inflammatory lesion	Biliary cirrhosis
Biliary cirrhosis	Collagen vascular disease
Chronic hemolytic anemia	Bilharziasis
Collagen vascular disease	Sarcoidosis
Hemochromatosis	
Amyloidosis	
Budd-Chiari snydrome	
Hydatid cyst	
Bilharziasis	

Table 7-2. Differential Diagnosis of Intrahepatic Filling Defects

Metastatic carcinoma and other malignancy
Hepatoma
Lymphoma
Abscess
  Pyogenic
  Tuberculous
  Amebic
Cyst
  Hydatid
  Simple
  Polycystic disease
Cavernous hemangioma
Hematoma and hematobilia
Amyloid mass
Cirrhosis
Extrinsic mass
Postsurgical defect

Table 7-3. Causes of Defects at Porta Hepatis

Normal variation
Metastatic malignancy
Direct invasion by malignancy of biliary tract, pancreas, or adjacent lymph nodes
Lymphoma
Hepatoma
Extrinsic pressure from emphysema or hydrops of gallbladder
Subhepatic abscess
Tuberculous abscess

Table 7-4. Causes of Apparent Absence or "Amputation" of Left Lobe of Liver

Congenital aplasia or neonatal atrophy
Hepatic metastasis occluding left portal vein
Hematoma
Hydatid cysts
Abscess
Hepatoma
Massive infarction
Extrinsic mass
Surgical removal
Radiation therapy

be identified from the scan alone (Fig 7-4). For example, a primary liver carcinoma cannot be differentiated from a metastatic lesion. Yet characteristic patterns do recur and are observed more commonly with certain entities. Multiple well-defined scattered defects frequently are caused by metastatic malignancy, but other forms of severe multifocal liver disease may produce a similar picture (Fig 7-5). Hepatomegaly with a diffusely mottled pattern of activity occurs frequently along with increased activity in spleen and bone marrow in advanced hepatic cirrhosis with or without fatty infiltration (Fig 7-6). A large well-defined right lateral marginal filling defect

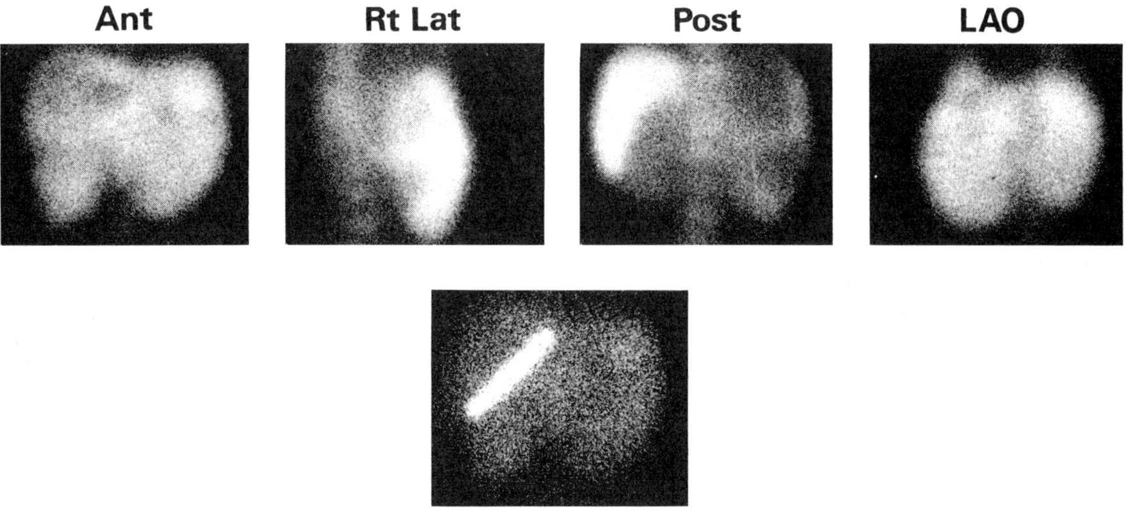

Figure 7-4 *Large defect in right lobe of liver, caused by primary hepatoma.*

suggests amebic or other abscess (Fig. 7-7). Massive left lobe enlargement with filling defects rarely is normal and frequently indicates malignancy. Discrepancy between the superior margin of the dome of the liver and the right diaphragm suggests a subdiaphragmatic lesion, usually an abscess. Scans of the liver and upper abdomen after injection of rose bengal I 131 are used to differentiate obstructive from nonobstructive jaundice. Normally, such scans reveal the presence of dye in the small intestine within 15 to 60 minutes after injection. This brisk passage of dye from the liver tends to introduce variations in the scanning image, particularly in a

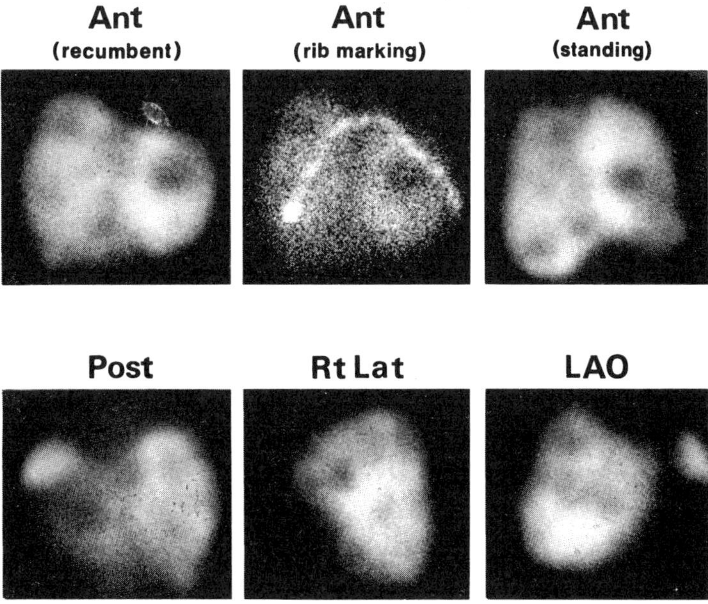

Figure 7-5 *Multiple well-defined scattered defects in liver, caused by metastatic carcinoma.*

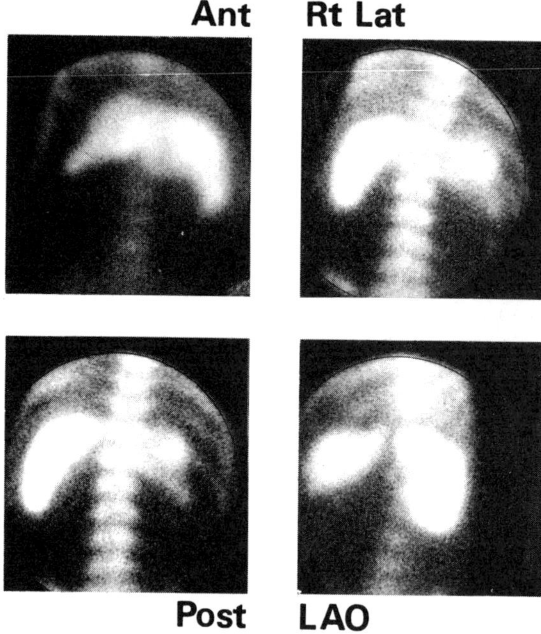

Figure 7-6 *Small contracted liver with splenomegaly and active bone marrow, characteristic of liver cirrhosis.*

diseased liver. Subsequent scans normally show rapid fading of radioactivity over the liver with concentration in the gallbladder and appearance in the small intestine more or less as a bolus. Usually by the end of two hours almost all the activity is in the bowel. When the common duct is obstructed, there is prolonged retention of radioactivity in the liver with little or none detected in the small intestine for several hours or as long as 24 hours after injection. The same pattern is observed with intrahepatic obstruction from cholestatic drugs, such as thorazine or testosterone; a history of their use should prevent misinterpretation.

Errors and Pitfalls

False-negative results may occur when lesions are smaller than the 2-cm resolving capacity of the scanning system or when they are deeply embedded in the liver or poorly differentiated from normal tissues. Occasionally, liver size is underestimated because abdominal obesity, ascites, or a marked increase in anteroposterior chest diameter with costal flaring increases the distance between the probe and the liver.

Information Obtainable

Useful information obtainable from a liver photoscan includes:

- Evaluation of size, shape, and position with respect to clinical findings
- Differentiation of liver mass from abdominal mass
- Detection of organ displacement or organomegaly
- Prebiopsy evaluation to determine optimal site
- Detection of space-occupying lesions
- Detection of biliary obstruction

Indications

Liver photoscans should be performed on patients who are candidates for surgery, chemotherapy, or radiation therapy in the presence of right upper quadrant pain, jaundice, abnormal liver function tests, and known primary malignancies of other sites. Further indications include the resolution of liver abscesses under chemotherapy (Fig 7-8), fevers of unknown etiology, and chronic ulcerative colitis. In all these situations, knowledge of the presence, location, and size of a diffuse or solitary lesion great-

Indications for Liver Scanning

- Right upper quadrant pain
- Jaundice
- Abnormal liver function tests
- Primary malignancy of other sites
- Chronic ulcerative colitis
- Fever of unknown cause
- Liver abscess under chemotherapy
- Intended biopsy

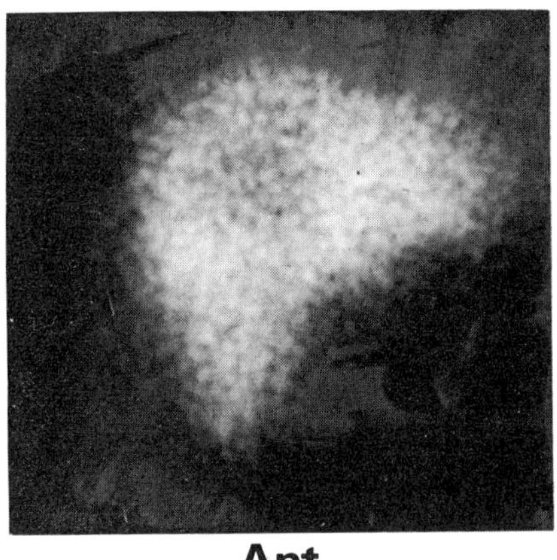
Ant

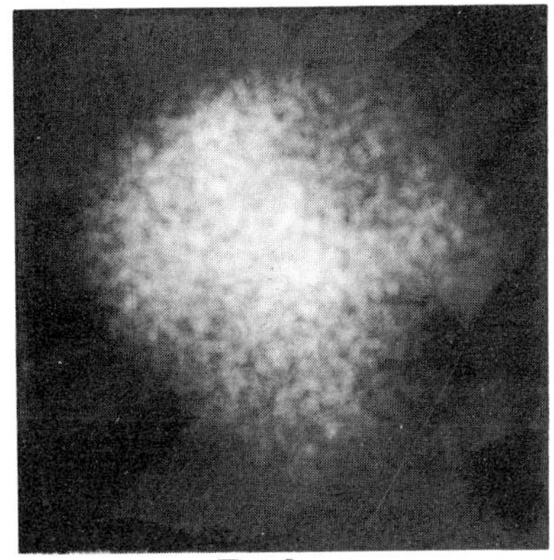
Rt Lat

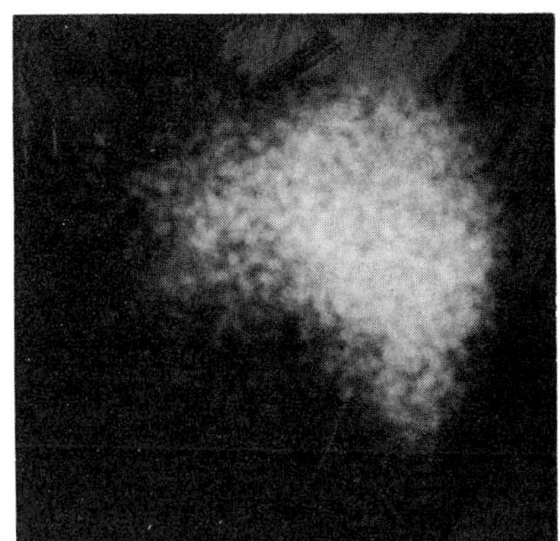
Post

Figure 7-7 *Large well-defined right lateral marginal filling defect in liver, caused by amebic abscess.*

ly facilitates the evaluation and management of each patient.

The most general indication is simply suspicion of liver disease based on clinical observations of the patient, even when liver chemistry determinations and liver biopsy are normal or only marginally disturbed. When liver biopsy is contemplated, the most effective biopsy site can be defined beforehand with the aid of a liver photoscan. This increases accuracy and avoids repeat biopsies. Even the initial biopsy or an exploratory laparotomy can sometimes be avoided when jaundice is thought to be due to multiple metastatic lesions. Demonstration of the multiple discrete filling defects typical of metastatic disease strongly militates against a single surgically corectable lesion in the common duct.

Diagnostic Accuracy

The diagnostic accuracy of the liver photoscan varies depending on the type of information the clinician expects to obtain. Hepatomegaly can be diagnosed with virtually 100% accuracy, while a deep-seated solitary tumor mass may be detected only

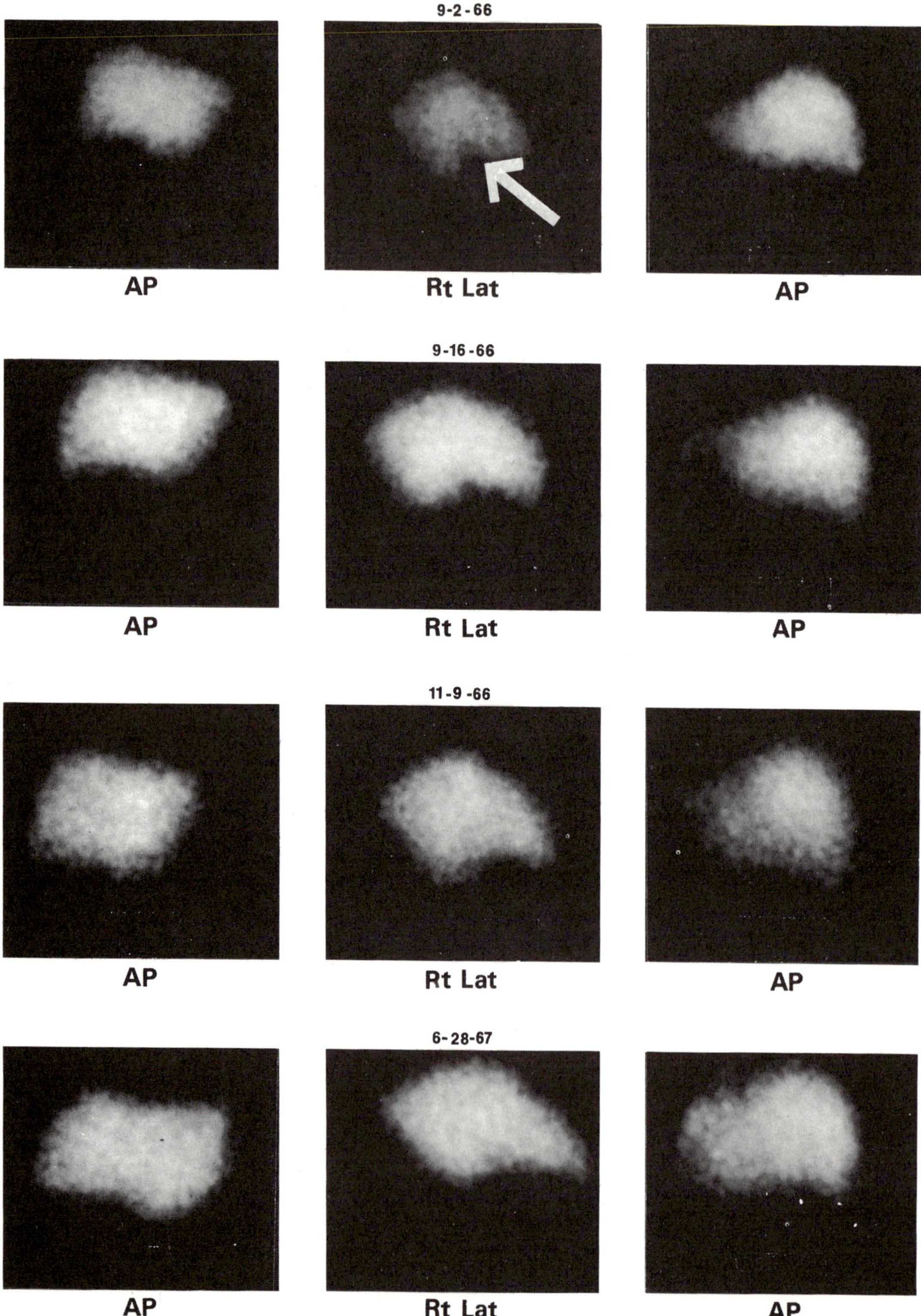

Figure 7-8 *Resolution of hepatic amebic abscess following chemotherapy.*

in about 60% to 70% of cases. Multiple metastatic lesions can be seen reliably in up to 83% of cases. However, the photoscan cannot diagnose the histologic identity of a given defect. In various reported series, the overall accuracy varies from 83% to 93%. False-positive diagnoses are made in about 5% of cases and false-negative reports or missed diagnoses, mostly of small or solitary defects, occur in about 10%.

Safety

Photoscanning poses essentially no risk to the patient. The newer short-half-life, generator-produced radioactive isotopes such as technetium 99m reduce radiation exposure to low levels. Toxic or allergic reactions to these radioactive pharmaceuticals are exceedingly rare—much rarer than reactions to the widely used Bromsulphalein dye.

> Toxic or allergic reactions to the radiopharmaceuticals used in liver scanning are much rarer than reactions to the Bromsulphalein used in liver function tests.

Spleen Imaging

The spleen in the normal adult is shaped like a coffee bean and lies in the left upper quadrant between the fundus of the stomach and left leaf of the diaphragm at the level of the 9th, 10th, and 11th ribs.

Tracers

The currently available colloids utilized in spleen imaging were initially developed for visualization of the liver. Phagocytosis of radioactive colloids by the reticuloendothelial cells of the liver, spleen, and bone marrow after the injection of short-lived radionuclides such as ^{99m}Tc and ^{113m}In allows excellent spleen visualization.

In the normal person, approximately 80% to 90% of the injected radioactive colloid enters the liver, 10% to 20% enters the spleen, and the remainder (representing a small amount seldom visualized in the normal person) enters the bone marrow and lung.

Particle size is important, since there is rapid blood clearance and maximum uptake in the liver and speen of particles 1 μ in size. Larger particles tend to lodge in the lung capillaries, while extremely small particles clear slowly and tend to be deposited in the bone marrow. Uniformity of particle size is also important for reproducibility and comparability of studies, but this has been practical only recently, following the development of albumin microspheres.

Of all the radioactive colloids presently available, colloid Tc 99m represents the ideal agent because of 140-kev energy, availability in commercial kits, rapid imaging, low radiation dose, and simultaneous visualization of the liver even though the liver may occasionally obscure parts of spleen or accessory splenic tissue. Colloid In 113m also is an excellent imaging agent but has not enjoyed the wide use of sulfur colloid Tc 99m (Fig 7-9).

Interpretation

SPLENIC RUPTURE

A ruptured spleen is usually secondary to acute trauma and is fairly common today. Occasionally, the spleen ruptures as a result of marked splenomegaly secondary to a systemic disease such as leukemia or infectious mononucleosis. Spleen imaging offers a safe, rapid, and fairly reliable method

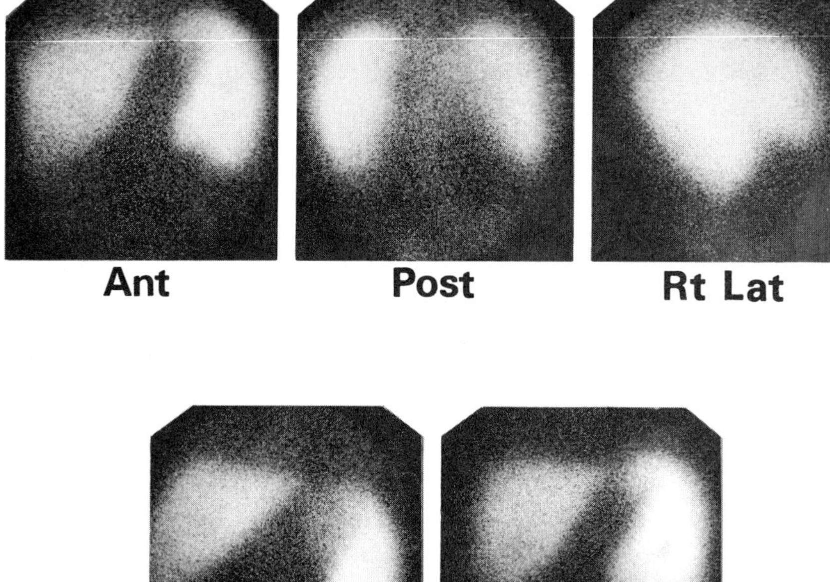

Figure 7-9 *Normal spleen. Artifact results from a coin in patient's pocket.*

> **Information Available from Spleen Scanning**
> - Splenic rupture
> - Spleen size
> - Absence of functioning spleen tissue
> - Accessory spleen
> - Splenosis

of determining if the spleen is ruptured (Fig 7-10).

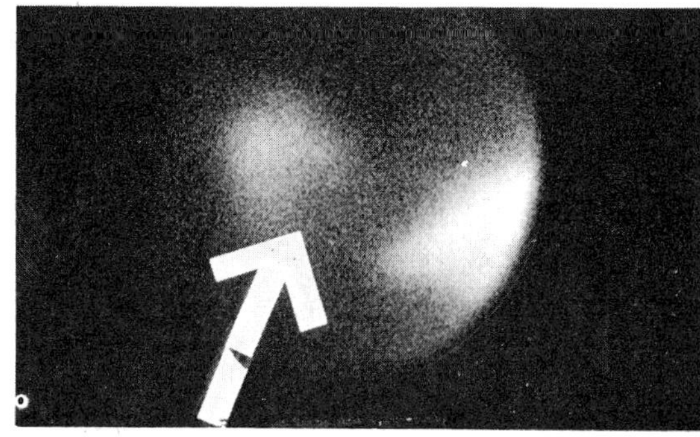

Figure 7-10 *Ruptured spleen with defect in superior border.*

SPLEEN SIZE

The simplest method of determining spleen size by imaging is to measure the posterior height. The normal spleen measures up to 14 cm. The weight can be derived fairly accurately from the equation:

$$W = 71.0L - 537$$

with W representing the spleen weight and L the length. Other methods for estimating the size and weight of the spleen are less simple and no more accurate (Fig 7-11).

ABSENCE OF FUNCTIONING SPLEEN TISSUE

Congenital absence of the spleen is rare and tends to be associated with severe congenital anomalies. Functional asplenia

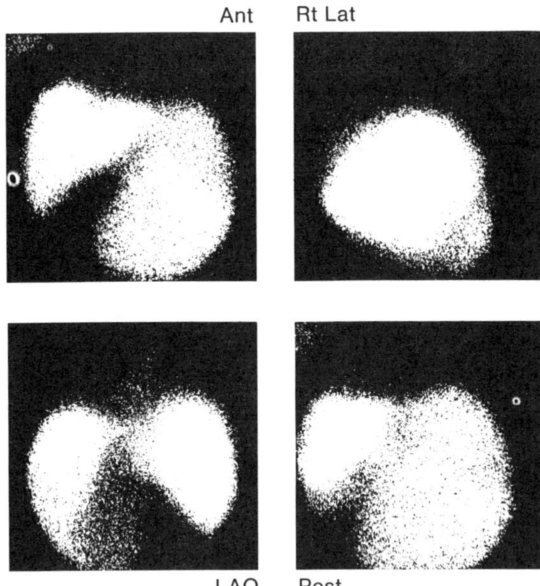

Figure 7-11 *Splenomegaly in lymphoma. Spleen is twice size of liver.*

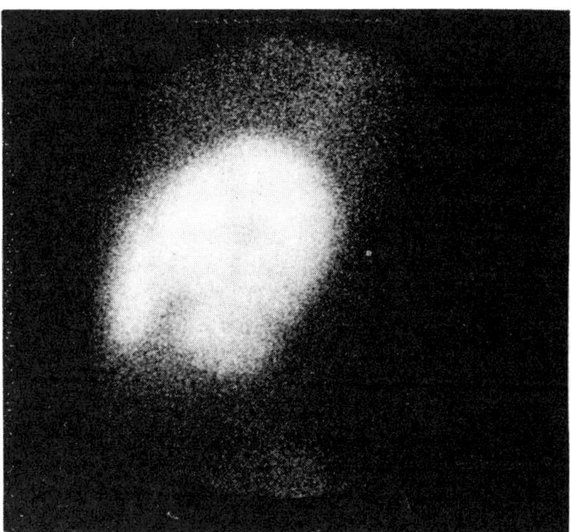

Figure 7-12 *Multiple splenic abscesses forming a left upper quadrant mass in patient with rheumatic heart disease and subacute bacterial endocarditis.*

refers to a palpable or roentgenographically visible spleen that cannot be imaged with injected sulfur colloid Tc 99m. It has been described with sickle cell disease, reticulum cell sarcoma involving the spleen, surgical transposition of the spleen, and persistent neutrophilic leukocytosis.

LEFT UPPER QUADRANT MASSES

Often it is difficult to differentiate between an enlarged spleen and a mass arising from another organ in the left upper quadrant. Spleen imaging offers a simple method of differentiation (Figs 7-12 and 7-13).

ACCESSORY SPLEEN AND SPLENOSIS

An accessory spleen has been found at one fifth to one third of all autopsies. Usually it is small and located in the gastrosplenic ligament or the tail of the pancreas, but it may be situated in the omentum or the mesentery of the intestines. The organ is best demonstrated when it sequesters altered red blood cells tagged with radionuclides, usually in a postsplenectomy patient. It can also be visualized adequately with radioactive colloids if overlap from the adjacent liver is not too great and if multiple views are obtained.

Splenosis occurs when the spleen is fractured and small fragments seed themselves in the peritoneal cavity and continue to grow. These minispleens are best visualized when they sequester altered red blood cells

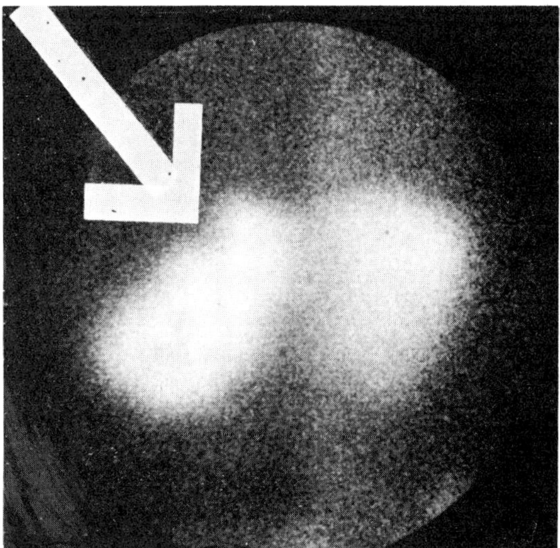

Figure 7-13 *Multiple splenic abscesses forming a left upper quadrant mass in a patient with subacute bacterial endocarditis and drug addiction.*

tagged with an appropriate radionuclide, and can also be demonstrated adequately with radioactive colloids.

LIVER-SPLEEN UPTAKE AND RETICULOENDOTHELIAL SYSTEM ASSESSMENT

The ratio of liver uptake to spleen uptake of radioactive colloids is fairly constant in a normal person. From 80% to 90% is trapped in the liver and from 10% to 20% in the spleen. One study has suggested that when this ratio is changed so that spleen uptake is decreased compared with liver uptake, systemic proliferative disease or hematopoietic neoplasm is likely to be present. If the spleen and bone marrow or bone marrow alone show increased uptake, the likelihood of cirrhosis or anemia is strong.

> **When spleen uptake of radioactivity is decreased compared with liver uptake, systemic proliferative disease or hematopoietic neoplasm is likely.**

> **When spleen and bone marrow uptake of radioactivity is increased compared with liver uptake, cirrhosis or anemia is likely.**

Pancreas Scanning

Detecting and evaluating pancreatic disease are important diagnostic challenges to the clinician, radiologist, and surgeon. Routine visualization of all pancreas utilizing selenomethionine Se 75 and the scintillation camera allows the identification of a normal pancreas in 95% of normal individuals. An abnormal pattern is found in 90% of patients with pancreatitis or pancreatic carcinoma.

Pancreas scanning appears most valuable in screening patients with suspected pancreatic diseases—particularly if performed early in the illness. Since the appearance of the radioactive tracer in the scan correlates well with the functional exocrine status of the pancreas, scanning is useful in evaluating pancreatic function.

Indications for Pancreas Scanning

- Chronic diarrhea
- Steatorrhea
- Malabsorption syndrome
- Recurrent abdominal pains
- Obstructive jaundice
- Epigastric mass
- Migratory thrombophlebitis
- Hard, nodular liver
- Hypoglycemia
- Diabetes
- Unexplained anorexia, melena, hematemesis, weight loss, ascites, fever, nausea, and vomiting
- Suspected pancreatitis, pancreatic tumor, pancreatic cyst, cystic fibrosis, islet-cell tumor

Indications and Contraindications

Pancreas scanning is indicated in all patients with chronic diarrhea, steatorrhea, malabsorption syndrome, recurrent abdominal pains, obstructive jaundice, epigastric mass, migratory thrombophlebitis, hard nodular liver, hypoglycemia, and some types of diabetes.

The procedure can aid diagnosis when the following conditions are unexplained:

anorexia, melena, hematemesis, weight loss, ascites, nausea and vomiting, and fever. It is also indicated when the following diseases are suspected: acute or chronic pancreatitis, benign pancreatic tumor, pancreatic carcinoma, cyst and pseudocyst of the pancreas, cystic fibrosis, and islet cell tumor.

The procedure is contraindicated in pregnancy, during lactation, and in patients allergic to selenomethione Se 75. Its use in the young should be weighed against its benefits.

Principle

For pancreas visualization, a considerable portion of the exocrine function must be intact. The organ must be able to synthesize digestive enzymes and trap from the blood enough selenomethionine Se 75 to allow visualization.

The exocrine pancreatic cells cannot differentiate between methionine, one of the basic amino acids in the enzymes secreted in the pancreatic juice, and the radioactive tracer selenomethionine Se 75. Therefore, the trapping of the tracer (localization process) begins immediately after injection of selenomethionine Se 75.

A test meal is simultaneously ingested, triggering a profuse output of enzymes from the pancreas. The incorporation of the tracer into the newly synthesized enzymes can then be recorded and observed on the serial exposures of the scintillation camera.

Instruments

Early pancreas scanning produced results that were variable and hard to reproduce —a reflection on the capabilities of the rectilinear scanner and its focused collimator. With the rectilinear scanner the organ was difficult to localize during the initial setup, the image formed slowly, correction for improper setting was impossible during the procedure, and overlap of liver and pancreas was common. Consequently, results were not always accurate.

The scintillation camera, however, has been used successfully to image the pancreas in both dynamic and static studies. Its advantages include:

- Easy location of the organ, since the image can be viewed immediately
- A freely adjustable detector angle that accommodates anatomic variations and reduces the frequency and degree of liver overlap
- Continuous data collection or uninterrupted scanning that allows functional or dynamic evaluation.

Procedure

Following an overnight fast to build up zymogen granulation in the pancreas, a liquid test meal is administered orally; 15 to 30 minutes later, after gastric emptying has occurred, 250μCi of selenomethionine Se 75 is injected intravenously.

The patient is supine on a stretcher with the scintillation camera detector head angled toward his right kidney or right costal margin. His left flank and shoulder are raised by a small pillow to improve separation of liver and pancreas images.

A parallel-hole collimator is used, and the camera spectrometer is set on the 269-kev photopeak with window width of 15% to 20%.

Immediately after tracer injection, six ten-minute serial exposures are started and are continued for an hour. This allows optimal visualization of the waxing and waning radioactivity in different portions of the pancreas. If visualization is poor, additional exposures may be obtained.

Interpretation

NORMAL PANCREAS

The pancreas consists of three parts: head, body, and tail. The common bile duct

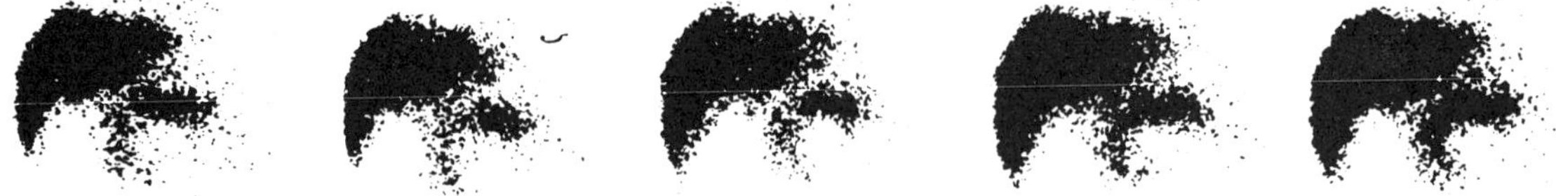

Figure 7-14 *Normal pancreas. Serial scans obtained ten minutes apart, showing lower border of liver and pancreas; all portions (head, body, and tail) are well visualized.*

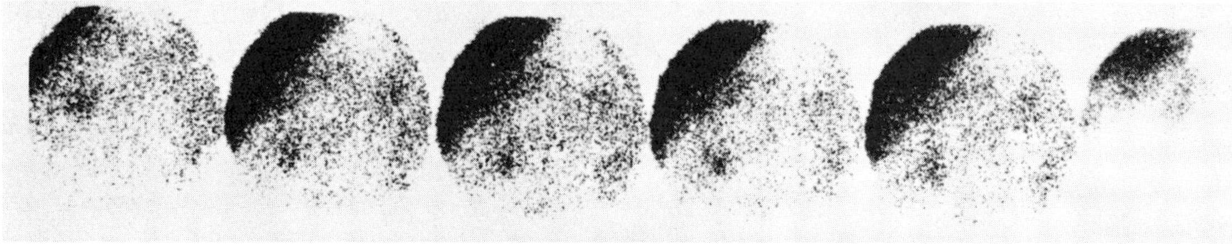

Figure 7-15 *Abnormal pancreas: Serial images obtained two minutes apart, revealing poor visualization of body and tail of pancreas.*

passes through the head of the pancreas; the aorta passes behind its body.

The shape of the normal pancreas varies. Pistol, horseshoe, sigmoid, and horizontal are the most common configurations.

Radioactivity appears in the normal pancreas within 20 minutes following the tracer injection (a range between 4 and 30 minutes is acceptable). All parts of the normal organ visualize well. If they do not, some

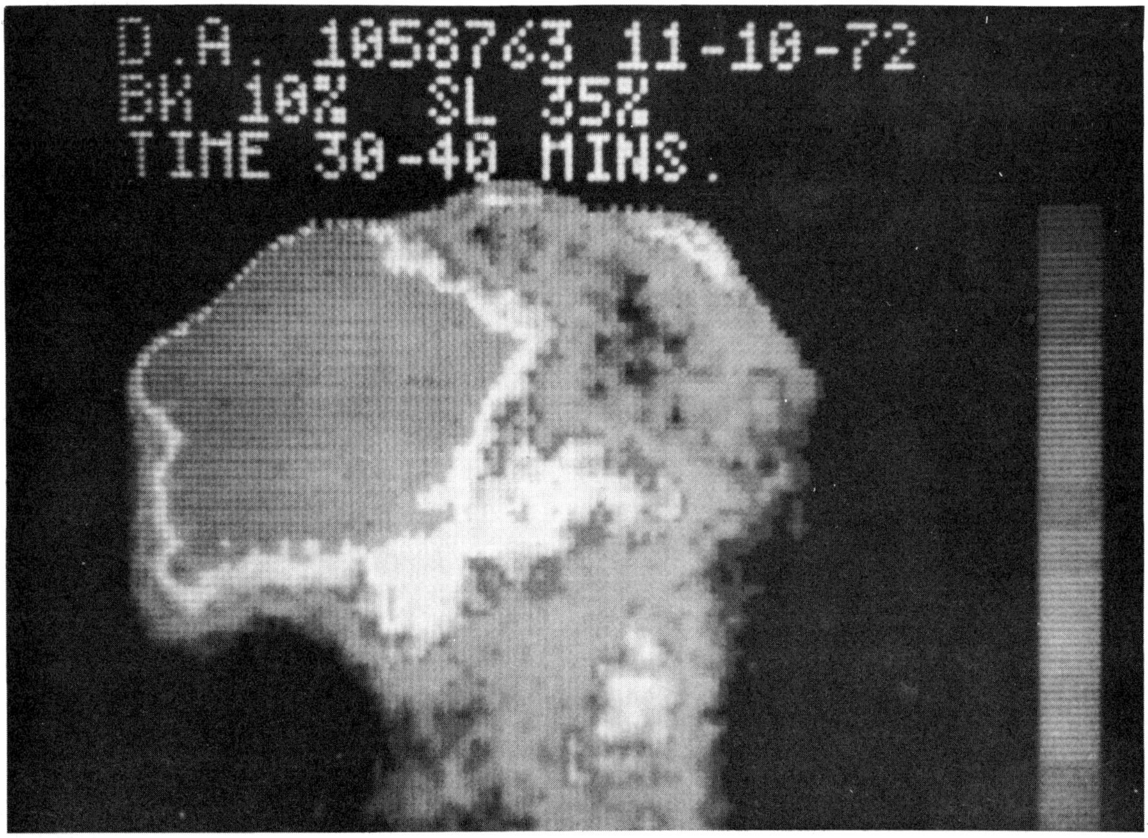

Figure 7-16 *Reduced visualization of the pancreas in acute pancreatitis.*

Disorders Suggested by Abnormal Pancreas Scan

- Acute hemorrhagic pancreatitis
- Chronic relapsing pancreatitis
- Cysts
- Carcinoma

type of abnormality is virtually certain. In two thirds of normal persons radioactivity tends to be more prominent in the tail of the pancreas than in the head (Fig 7-14).

ABNORMAL PANCREAS

Failure of the pancreas to visualize well in 20 to 30 minutes or imperfect visualization of some portion of the pancreas in the dynamic study constitutes evidence of abnormality (Fig 7-15). Three types of abnormal scans are recognized:

- Segmental visualization of the pancreas: part of the organ is well and promptly visualized, but one or two of the three parts cannot be seen.
- Reduced visualization of the pancreas: visualization is delayed or the image is poor.
- Nonvisualization of the pancreas: no radioactivity appears in the organ.

Reduced or nonvisualization does not always indicate pancreatic disease. The cause may be interference by other gastrointestinal diseases.

Acute Hemorrhagic Pancreatitis In 80% or more of patients with acute hemorrhagic pancreatitis scanning shows either reduced or nonvisualization of the pancreas. Generalized inflammation with edema and hemorrhage interfere with the normal concentration of the radioactive tracer, and this appears in the scan as reduced or nonvisualization of the organ (Fig 7-16).

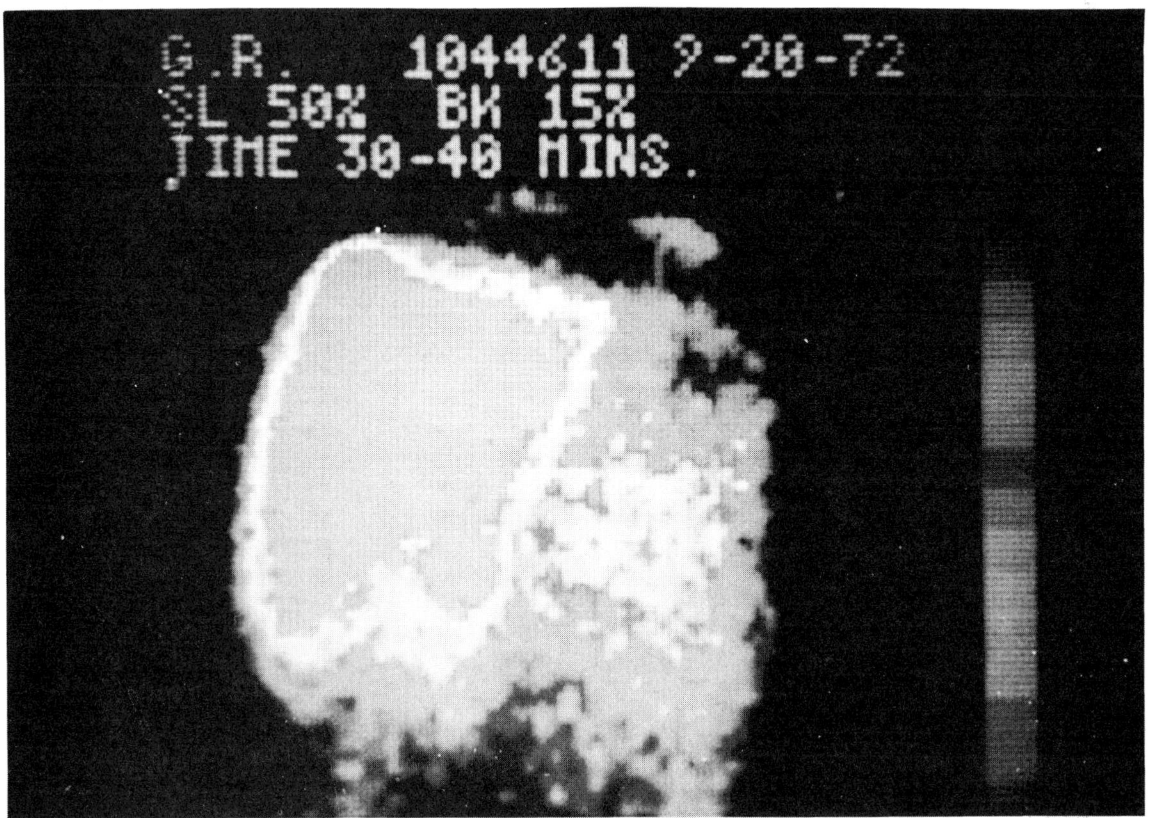

Figure 7-17 *Nonvisualization of pancreas in chronic pancreatitis.*

However, in some cases of mild, transient acute pancreatitis characterized by transient amylase elevations, the pancreas scan appears normal.

Chronic Relapsing Pancreatitis Extensive pathologic changes limit the ability of the pancreas to concentrate the radioactive tracer in certain areas or in general. In 96% of patients with chronic pancreatitis, scanning demonstrates reduced or nonvisualization of the organ (Fig 7-17).

Cysts Pancreatic cysts and pseudocysts appear on the scan as segmental defects.

Carcinoma Since the carcinoma is localized and the tumor concentrates the radioactive tracer at a different rate than does normal pancreatic tissue, the imaging abnormality produced is segmental and regional. In 95% of patients with pancreatic carcinoma, the scan shows a segmental area of nonvisualization (Fig 7-18). If a patient with suspected pancreatic carcinoma has a normal scan, detailed review of the original diagnostic premises is in order. In a patient thought to have carcinoma of the head of the pancreas, nonappearance of radioactivity over the head is strong presumptive evidence of cancer. Conversely, normal visualization of the head virtually rules out this diagnosis.

Cystic Fibrosis and Islet Cell Tumor Pancreas imaging in cystic fibrosis and islet cell tumor is nonspecific and allows only a general diagnosis of pancreatic abnormality.

Diagnostic Accuracy

The overall diagnostic accuracy of pancreatic scanning is 90%, with a 5% incidence

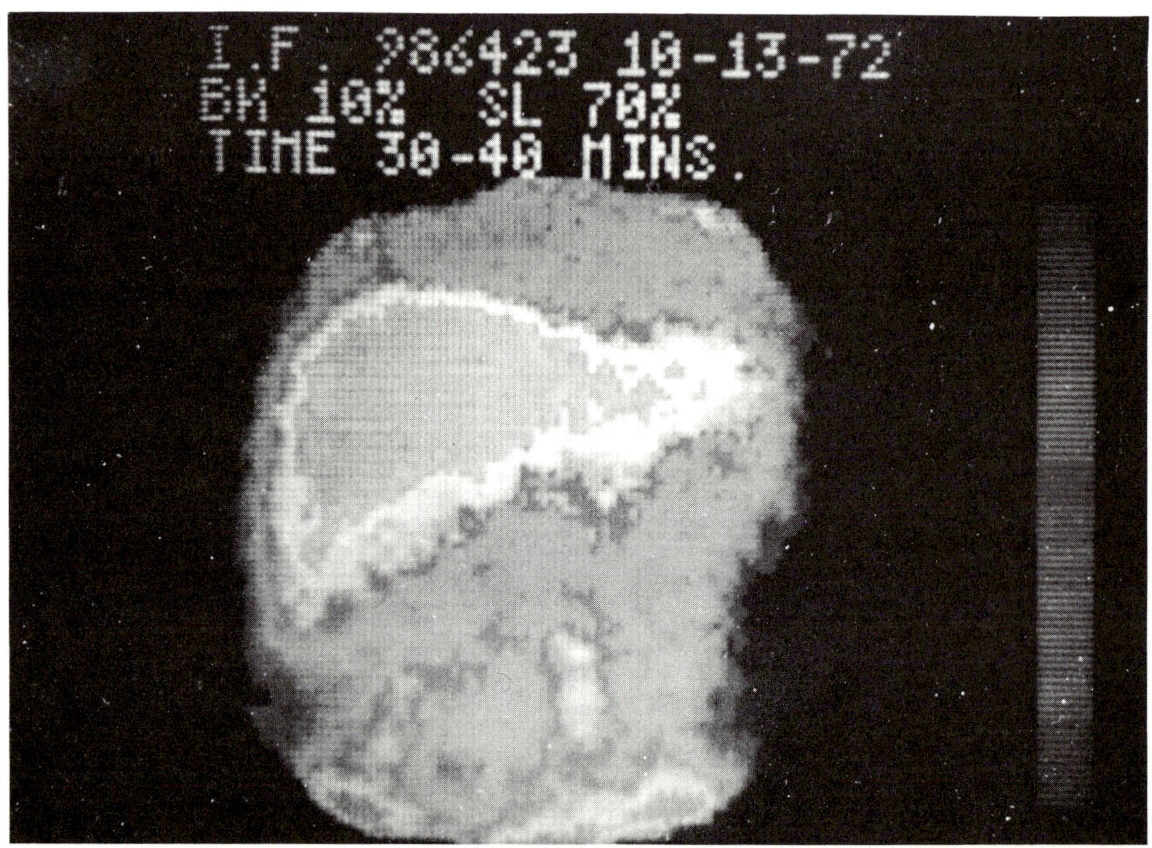

Figure 7-18 *Segmental defect in pancreas in carcinoma of that organ.*

of false-negative results and a 20% incidence of false-positive results. Other gastrointestinal diseases that interfere with pancreatic physiology and function are responsible for the high incidence of false-positive results.

When the patient exhibits no evidence of pancreatic disease, the likelihood of a normal scan is extremely high. In only 13 of a series of 225 patients was there an abnormal interpretation in a patient with a proved normal pancreas. Most patients with pancreatic carcinoma or established chronic pancreatitis have abnormal scans; in only 5 of 49 patients was the scan interpreted as normal.

References

1. Ashkar FS: The pancreatic scan: Easy index of function. *Consultant* **12**:8, 75–76, 1972.
2. Ashkar FS, Miale A Jr: *The Pancreatic Scan*. Medcom Famous Teachings in Modern Medicine. New York, Medcom, 1973.
3. Hewitt JC: Spleen Imaging. In Rohrer RH (ed). *Continuing Education Lectures*. Atlanta, Ga, Southeastern Chapter, Society of Nuclear Medicine, 1972.
4. Miale A Jr, Burke JS: Radioisotope Photoscanning of the Liver. In Sunderman FW, Sunderman FW Jr. (eds). *Laboratory Diagnosis of Liver Diseases*. St. Louis, Green, 1968, chap 34.

Radionuclide scanning of the heart, great vessels, and mediastinum is a noninvasive procedure for evaluation of various suspected cardiac defects.

8
The Cardiovascular System

Stuart Gottlieb

Rapid, noninvasive diagnostic techniques to aid in the cardiovascular workup are desirable because cardiac catheterization and contrast angiography pose a finite but significant risk to the patient and are costly in terms of money, time, and personnel. The morphologic detail provided by contrast angiography is not always necessary for clinically meaningful decisions. Particularly in the acutely ill patient, or when surgery is not planned, the lower resolution of the images provided by radionuclide angiography (RA) is frequently made up by the ease with which these studies can be performed and the wealth of physiologic data they provide. While it is unlikely in the foreseeable future that radioactive tracer techniques will replace more invasive procedures, they can allow more intelligent selection of those patients most likely to benefit from contrast angiography. Ideally, patients in whom no evidence of abnormality is found by noninvasive means may be spared the risk and cost attendant on catheterization. Since radionuclide studies can be repeated, clinical progress can be monitored over an extended time.

RAC aids selection of patients for contrast angiography. If RAC shows no evidence of abnormality, the patient may be spared catheterization.

Radioactive isotopes were first used to investigate cardiac function by Blumgart and Yens[2] more than 40 years ago. They employed radium C[1] and a modified cloud chamber. Prinzmetal et al[7] recorded the passage of an intravenous bolus of sodium 24 through the cardiac chambers and termed the resulting tracing a "radiocardiograph." Since the instrumentation utilized was cumbersome and the number of regions that could be reliably defined and monitored was limited, the technique found little general acceptance.

Development of static imaging devices, such as the Anger scintillation camera (Fig 8-1) and the digital autofluoroscope, which enable rapid sequential imaging of radionuclides during cardiopulmonary transit, and the availability of radionuclides possessing more nearly optimal imaging and counting characteristics, have revived interest in the application of radioactive tracer techniques to diagnosis of cardiac disease. Various data-processing accessories allow the retrospective construction of isotope-dilution curves or time-activity histograms, which describe passage of the radioactive bolus. While on-line computer facilities extend the applicability of the gamma camera, absence of such instrumentation does not preclude the performance of many clinically useful studies.

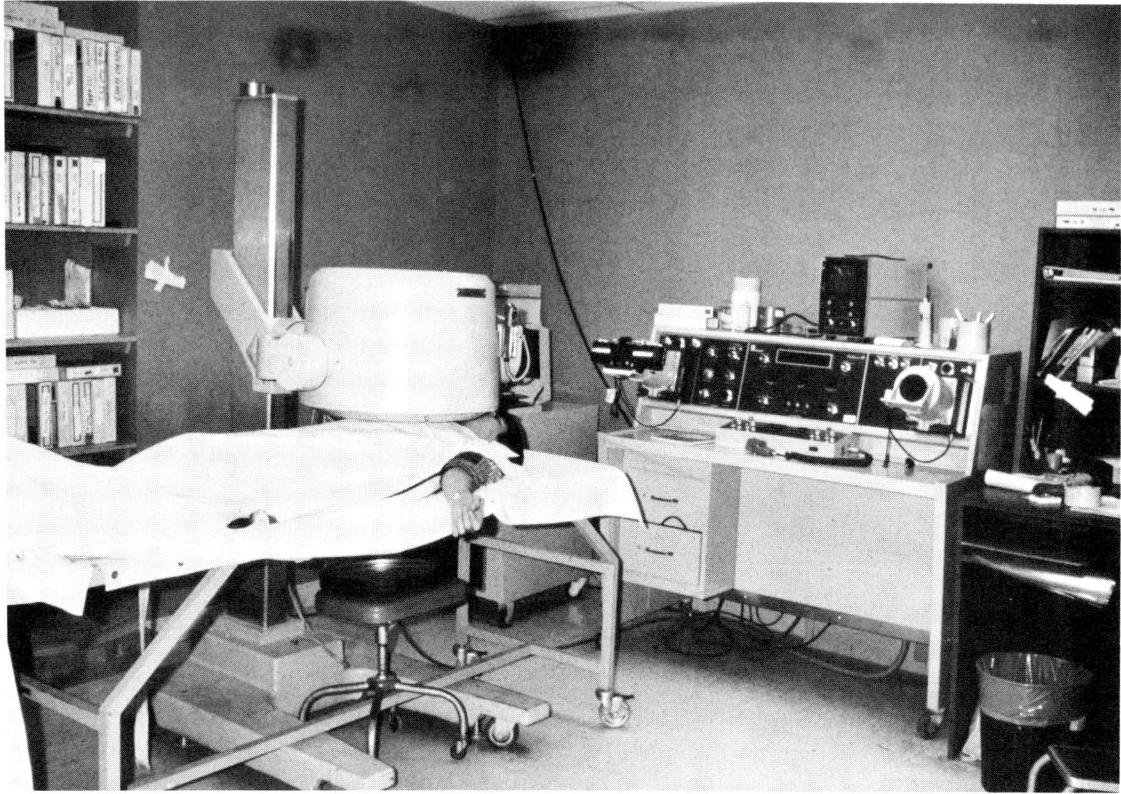

Figure 8-1 *RAC equipment. Anger scintillation camera is in foreground; console to right and tape-recording accessory background at left. Tape storage for previous studies is at far left.*

This chapter presents briefly the practical applications of dynamic radioactive tracer techniques and their interpretation in the evaluation of cardiovascular disorders. Only those areas of practical interest and, for the most part, not requiring data-processing equipment are described. Where appropriate, reference is made to our experience with the combined use of radionuclide angiocardiography (RAC) and echocardiography, since we believe these studies are optimally used in a complementary manner.

Radionuclide Angiocardiography

Indications

At present, RAC is useful for:

- Diagnosis of percardial effusion
- Detection of ventricular aneurysm
- Evaluation of cardiac masses
- Demonstration of acquired and congenital valvular disease
- Dynamic measurement for evaluation of cardiac function
- Detection of intracardiac shunts and differentiation of pulmonary from cardiac cyanosis in neonates
- Detection and differential diagnosis of mediastinal masses
- Demonstration of aortic aneurysm and patency of major vascular channels

Method

The patient is positioned supine beneath the detector of an Anger scintillation camera situated so the cardiopulmonary structures can be viewed from either the anterior or oblique projection (Fig 8-1). Positioning the patient is facilitated by viewing a transmission image of the heart and lungs

Table 8-1. Radiopharmaceuticals Commonly Used in RAC

Radiopharmaceutical	Dose administered (mCi)	Dose to target organ (rad)	Total-body dose (rad)
Sodium pertechnetate Tc 99m	10–20	2.4 (colon)	0.20
HSA Tc 99m	10	0.4 (blood)	0.17
Sulfur colloid Tc 99m	6– 8	1.8–2.4 (liver)	0.048
Transferrin In 113	10	0.6 (blood)	0.17

on a persistence oscilloscope. This transmission image is obtained by placing a plane source of either ^{57}Co or ^{99m}Tc beneath the patient. A static transmission image is also recorded on 35-mm film for later comparison with dynamic and blood pool scans.

A bolus of 10 to 20 mCi of human serum albumin (HSA) Tc 99m or sodium pertechnetate Tc 99m is administered intravenously utilizing a modified Oldendorf technique.[14] The cardiopulmonary transit of the radionuclide is recorded on 35-mm film at one- or two-second intervals (Fig 8-5) for approximately 45 seconds. By planning a suitable frame rate, eg, one frame per second, intracardiac peak-to-peak (mode) transit times can be estimated by visual identification of those frames containing maximal nuclide concentration in the right and left ventricles. This information not only demonstrates abnormal dynamics, but also provides a baseline against which to evaluate future changes. Following the dynamic flow study, without moving the patient, a 400,000-count static image of the cardiac blood pool is recorded (Fig 8-4).

Studies in both the oblique and anterior projections can be made during a single session if 8 mCi of sulfur colloid Tc 99m is used for the first injection with the patient in the oblique position. Within a few minutes most of the colloid is removed by the liver (half-time disappearance of sulfur colloid Tc 99m is four to five minutes) and a second injection of sodium pertechnetate Tc 99m or HSA Tc 99m can be given with the patient in the anterior position. The entire imaging procedure requires about 15 minutes. A 10-mCi dose of sodium pertechnetate Tc 99m results in a total-body dose of 0.12 rad (Table 8-1).

In this laboratory data are also recorded on magnetic videotape for later visual review and are processed by a small on-line computer (Medical Data Systems Nova 1200). Intracardiac transit times, cardiac output, and other quantitative data can be derived through the use of analog records generated by area-of-interest and strip-chart recording accessories to the gamma camera.

Vascular structures distal to the heart are examined utilizing the same injection technique with the area of interest positioned beneath the camera collimator. Two-second frame time is generally used in these studies.

Interpretation

NORMAL HEART

Figures 8-2 through 8-4 illustrate the normal RAC anatomy of the heart. The 35-mm scintiphotos (Fig 8-5) demonstrate prompt transit of a compact radioactive bolus through the superior vena cava and right side of the heart. The right atrium, right ventricle, pulmonary outflow tract, and pulmonary artery are normal in size and the right ventricular outflow tract is not displaced. The right heart and lungs

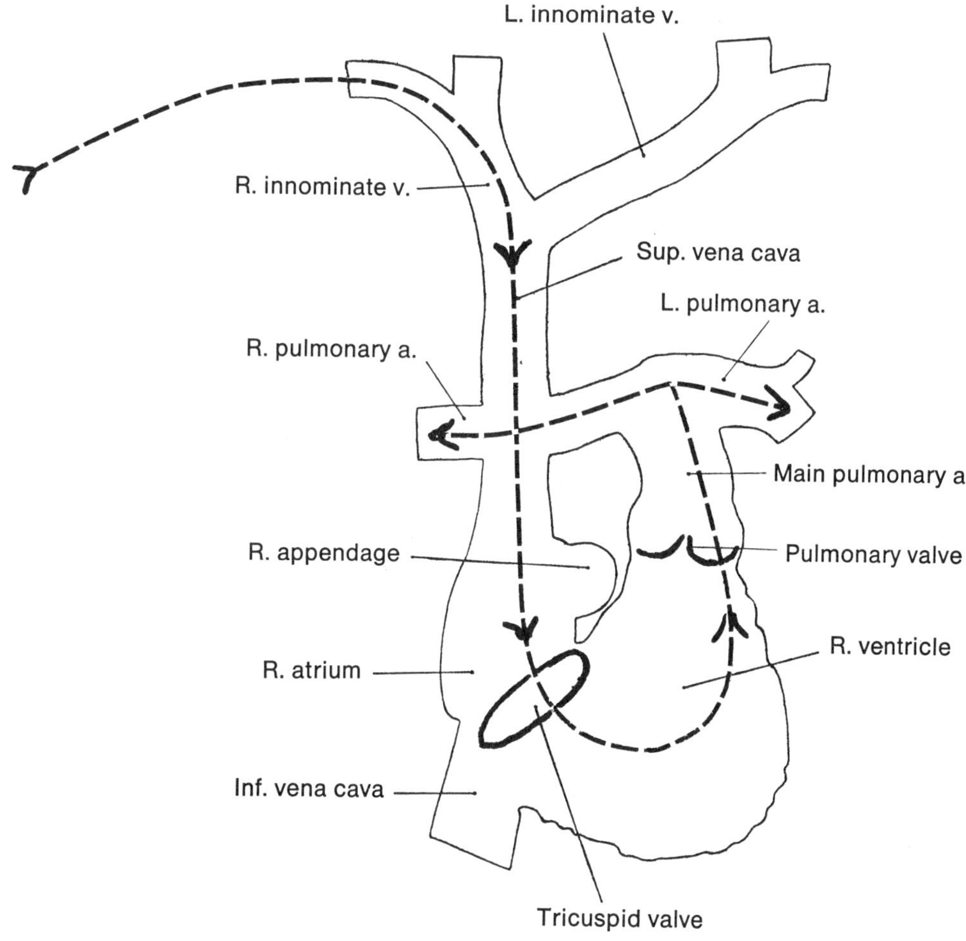

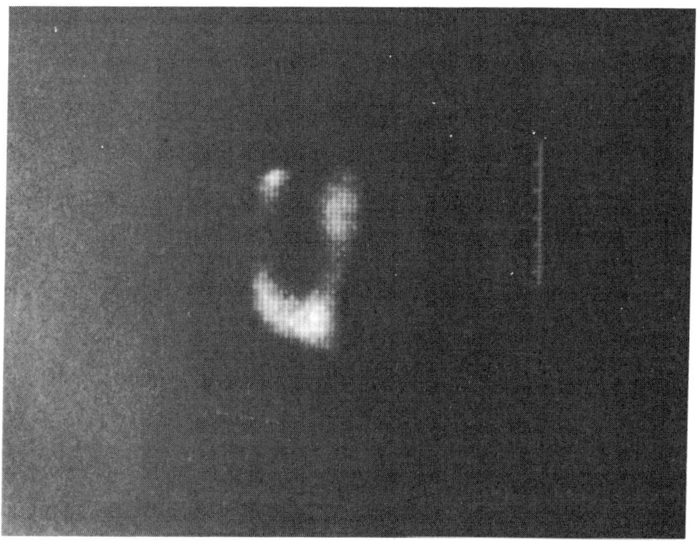

Figure 8-2 *Normal RAC anatomy of right side of heart. (From DeLand FH, Wagner HN:* Atlas of Nuclear Medicine *(II). Philadelphia, Saunders, 1970.)*

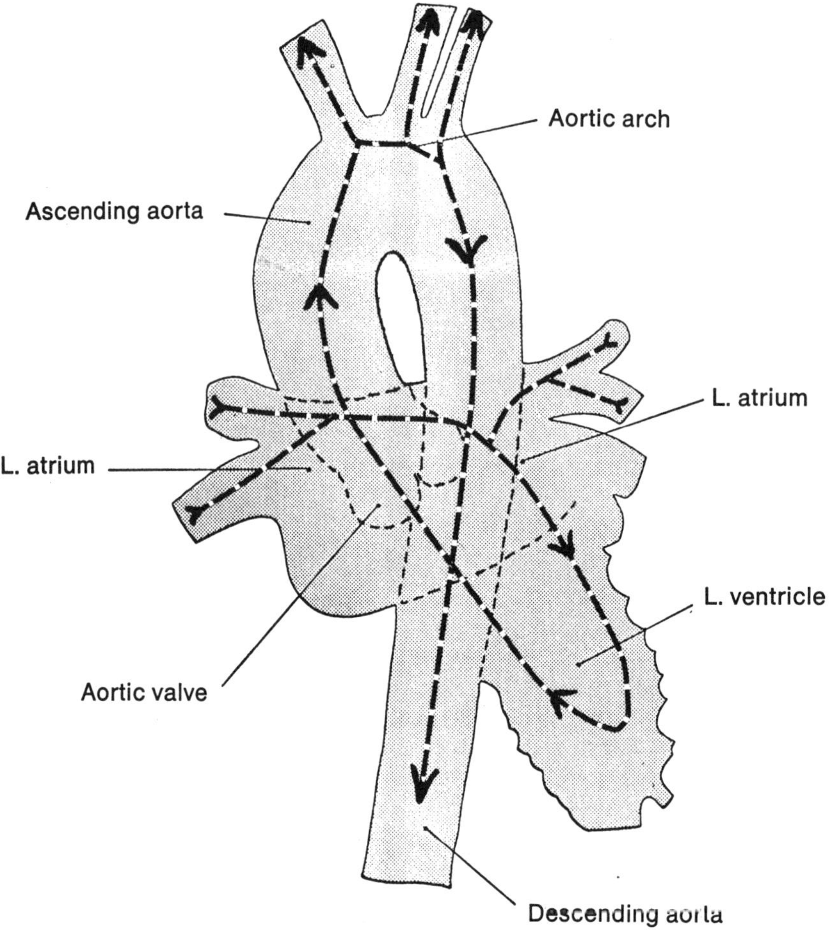

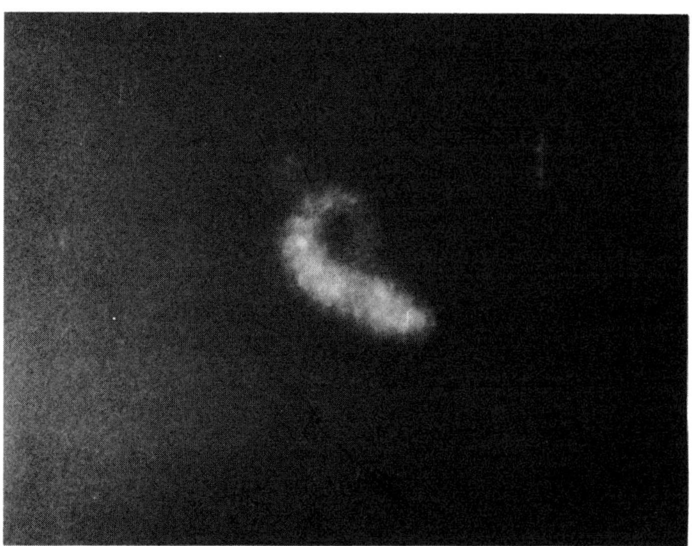

Figure 8-3 *Normal RAC anatomy of left side of heart. (From DeLand FH, Wagner HN:* Atlas of Nuclear Medicine *(II). Philadelphia, Saunders, 1970.)*

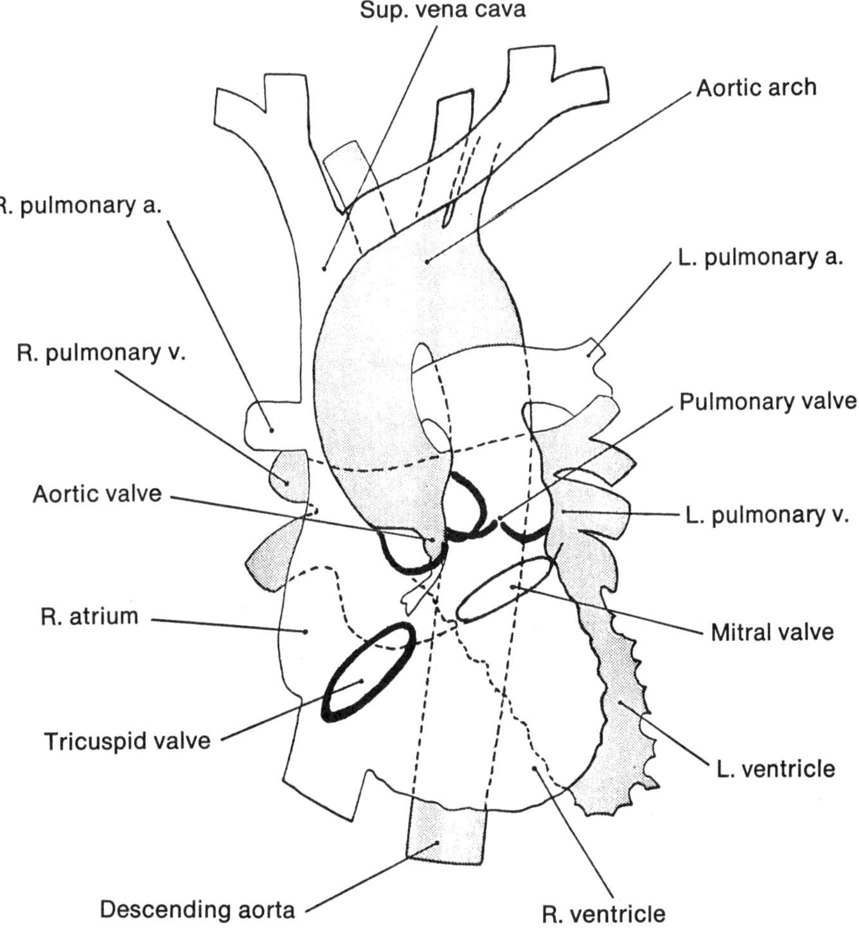

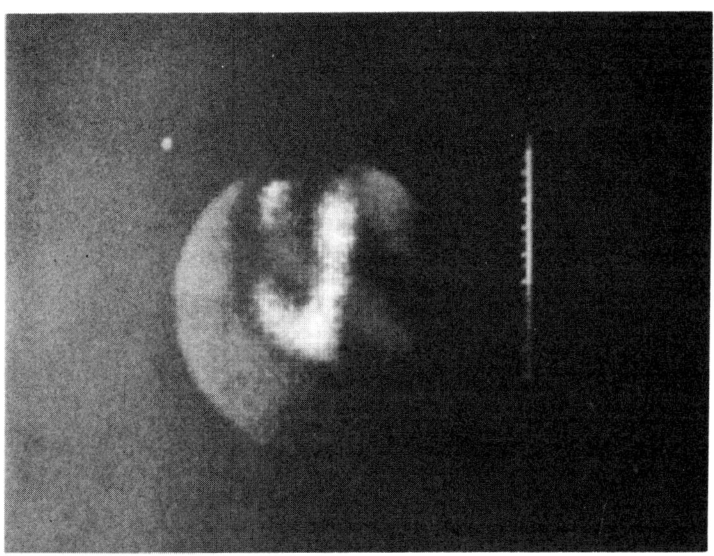

Figure 8-4 *Normal RAC anatomy of left and right sides of heart. (From DeLand FH, Wagner HN:* Atlas of Nuclear Medicine *(II). Philadelphia, Saunders, 1970.)*

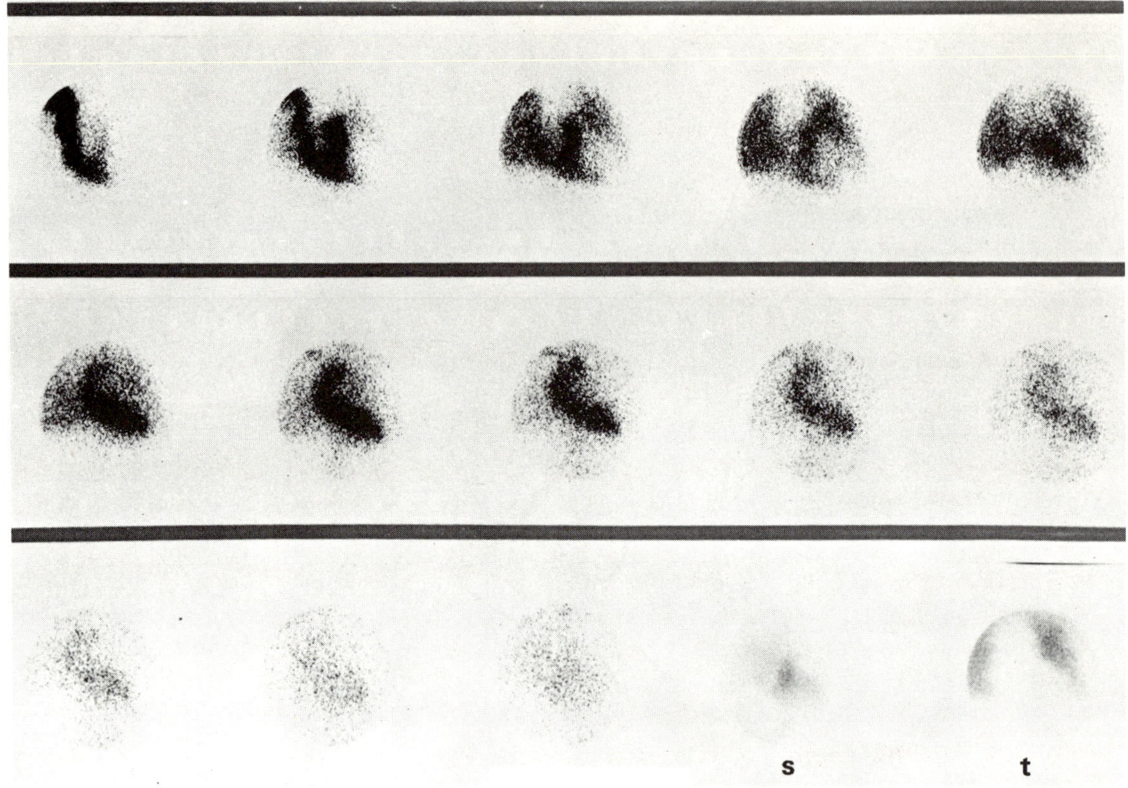

Figure 8-5 *Normal heart. See text for description.*

perfuse and empty in succession, followed by visualization of the left side of the heart and the aorta. The normal peak-to-peak time between the right and left ventricles is four to five seconds. The left ventricle appears ovoid, and radioactivity disappears from it uniformly and without focal areas of prolonged retention. The aortic root occupies the space between the superior vena cava and right ventricular outflow tract and is visualized after the right heart, lungs, and left ventricle. Activity within the cardiac chambers is not separated from activtiy within the lungs or liver.

PERICARDIAL EFFUSION

About 200 ml of pericardial fluid can be detected by RAC or by blood pool scanning. This laboratory prefers the dynamic procedure, which also provides an estimate of intracardiac transit time and demonstrates the pattern of central delivery of the radioactive bolus. Diagnosis of pericardial effusion in both RAC and static studies rests on the demonstration of an abnormal separation of activity within the heart from activity within the pulmonary and hepatic blood pools (Fig 8-6). Figure 8-7 shows the RAC obtained in a patient with cardiomegaly and congestive heart failure. Reflux into the innominate vein and inferior vena cava suggests elevation in right heart pressures. There is no evidence of pericardial effusion. When a rectilinear device is used, the size of the cardiac blood pool must be compared with the cardiac silhouette outlined on a chest roentgenogram made at a distance of six feet with the patient supine (Fig 8-8). If the ratio of the maximum transverse diameters is less than 0.8, pericardial effusion is present. When a small amount of pericardial fluid potentially of diagnostic sig-

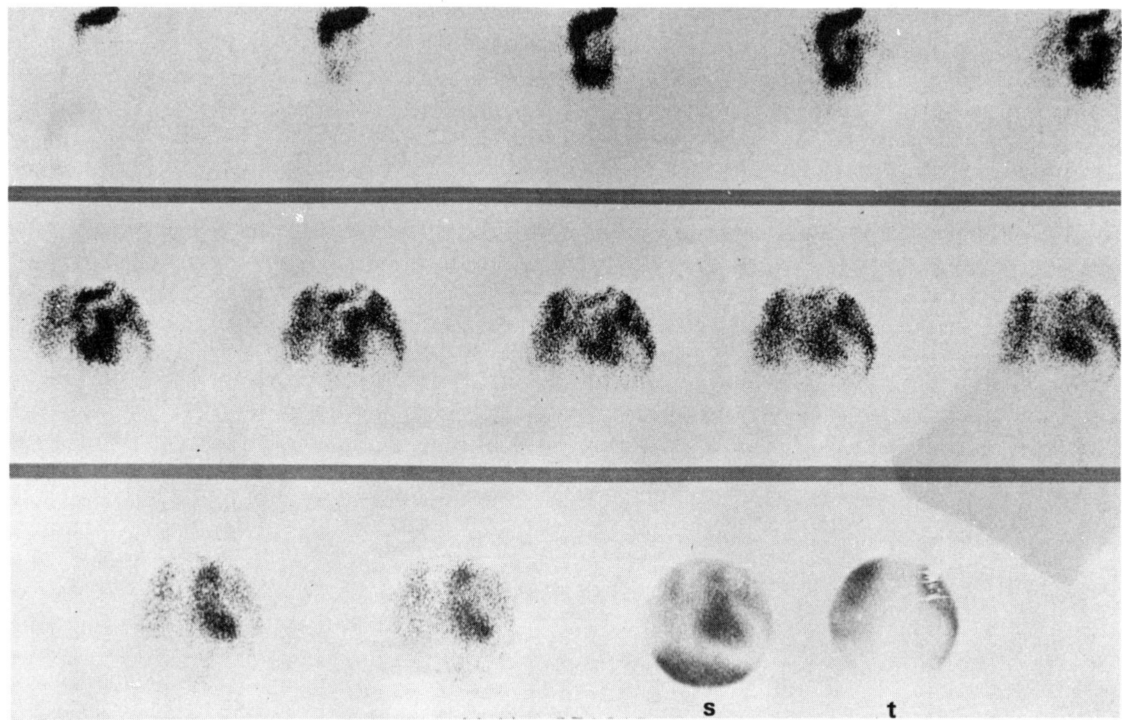

Figure 8-6 *Pericardial effusion. Each frame represents two seconds of elapsed time. Delivery of bolus is prolonged. In dynamic images activity within heart is separated from activity wthin pulmonary and later hepatic blood pools (s). Heart chambers are normal in size.* s, *400,000-count static image;* t, *transmission image.*

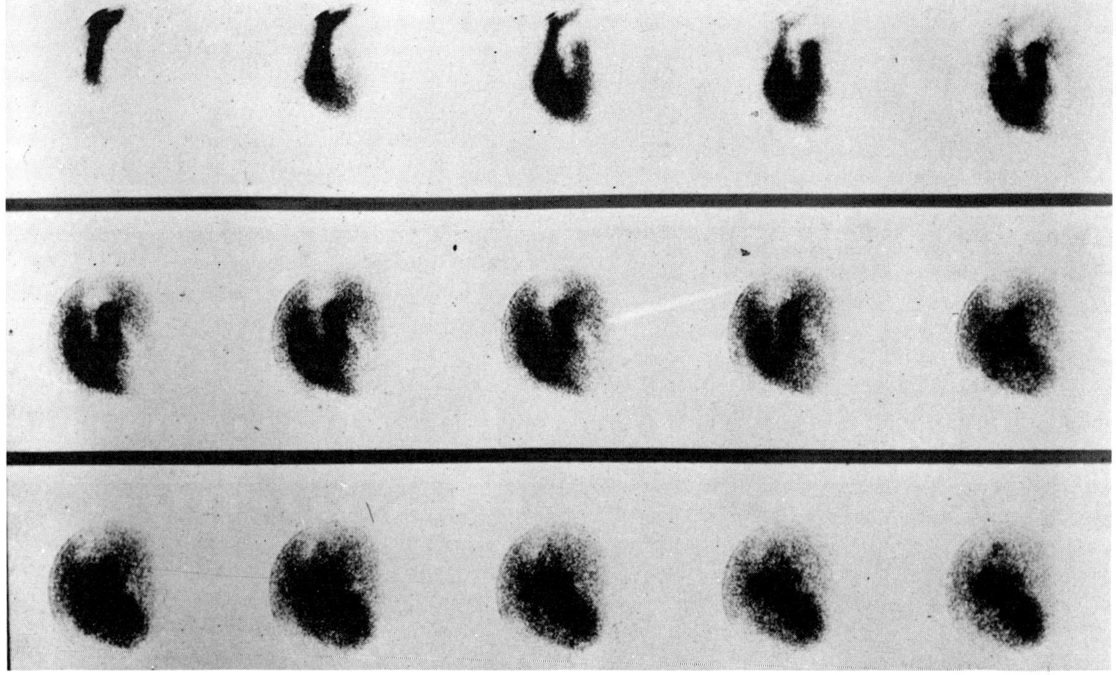

Figure 8-7 *Cardiomegaly with congestive heart failure. Each frame represents two seconds of elapsed time. Intracardiac transit of radioactive bolus is prolonged. Reflux of activity into innominate vein suggests increased right heart pressures. Cardiac chambers are dilated.*

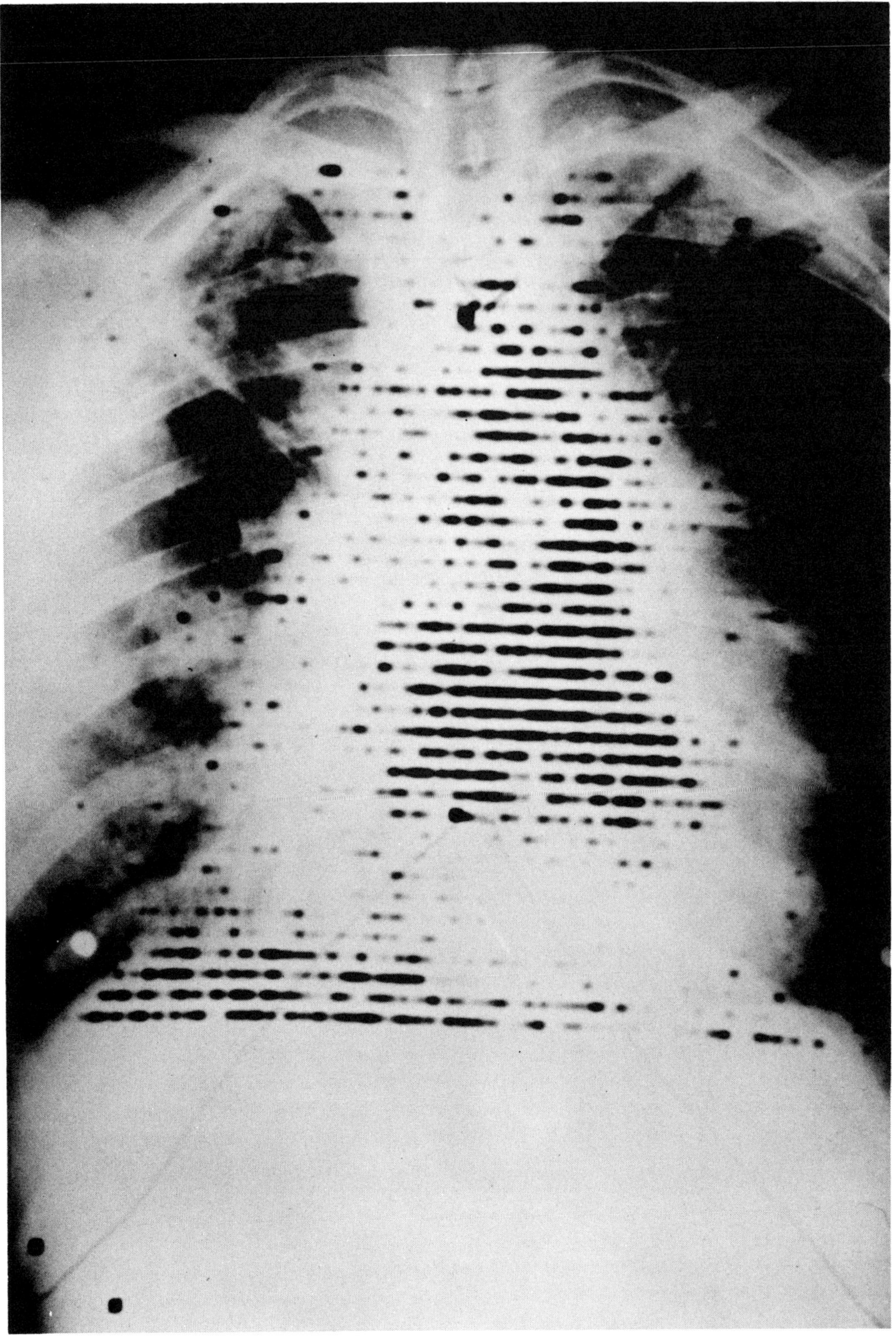

Figure 8-8 *Pericardial effusion demonstrated by superimposed rectilinear blood pool scan and chest roentgenogram. Halo of nonactivity separates margins of cardiac blood pool from outer margin of cardiac silhouette on the roentgenogram.*

Conditions Evaluated by RAC and RA

- Pericardial effusion
- Ventricular aneurysm
- Aortic aneurysm
- Intracardiac mass
- Valvular disease
- Intracardiac shunting
- Cardiac function

nificance is suspected, this laboratory uses echocardiography, since this technique is the more sensitive.

Diagnostic information about the cause of cardiomegaly, effusion, or hemodynamic difficulties is frequently available from the dynamic scintiphotos (Fig 8-9). Patients in whom malignant effusion is considered, patients with chronic right heart failure (Fig 8-10), and patients with pericardial effusion in whom dynamic information is important are selected for radionuclide examination. Loculated effusions are frequently best studied by a combination of these procedures.

VENTRICULAR ANEURYSM

About 15% of patients develop a ventricular aneurysm after infarction. Usually the aneurysm involves the anterolateral, apical, or inferior left heart wall. On the RAC a ventricular aneurysm appears as a focal bulge of the left ventricle (Fig 8-11) compared with the normally ovoid contour (Fig 8-5). While static blood pool scanning is sometimes useful in demonstrating the lesion, we have found RAC more valuable. Localized abnormalities of ventricular contractility frequently produce well-defined areas of prolonged nuclide retention during washout (Fig 8-12). The Johns Hopkins group[17] has reliably demonstrated the presence of regional akinesis and dyskinesis with gated blood pool scans depicting the left ventricle in systole and diastole. By comparing measurements of predetermined axes, they were able not only to detect areas of abnormal myocardial contraction, but to estimate left ventricular volume, cardiac output, and ejection fraction. A

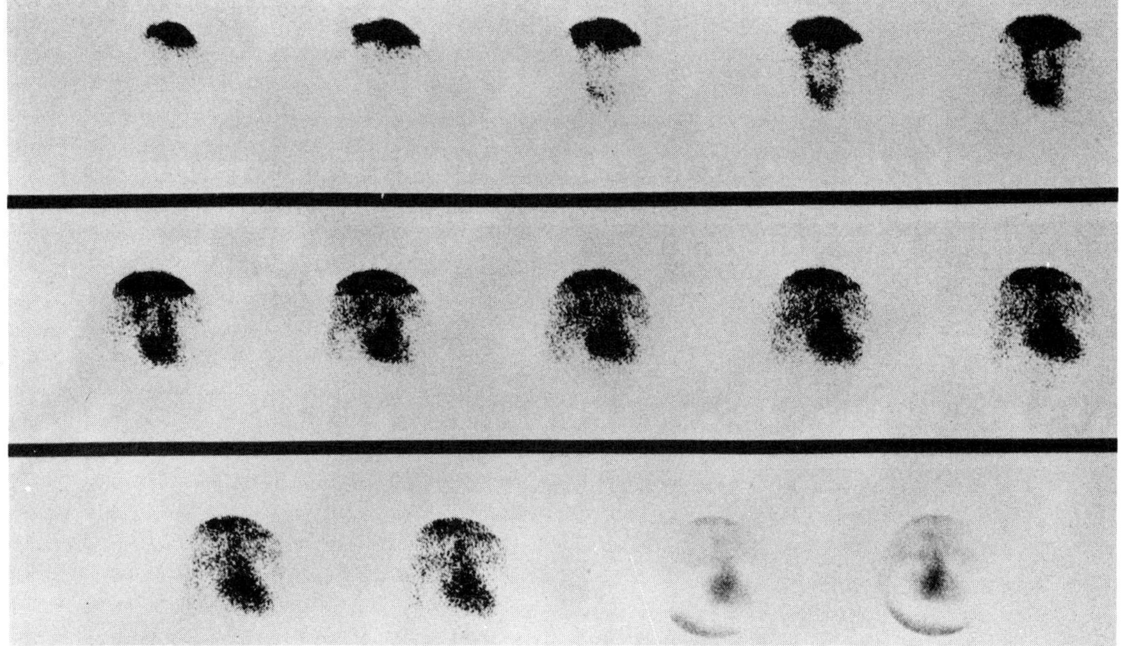

Figure 8-9 *Partial obstruction of superior vena cava suggesting presence of mediastinal mass. Pericardial effusion is also present.*

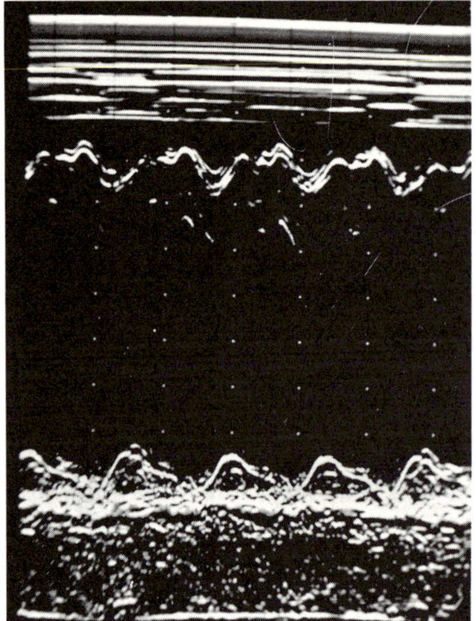

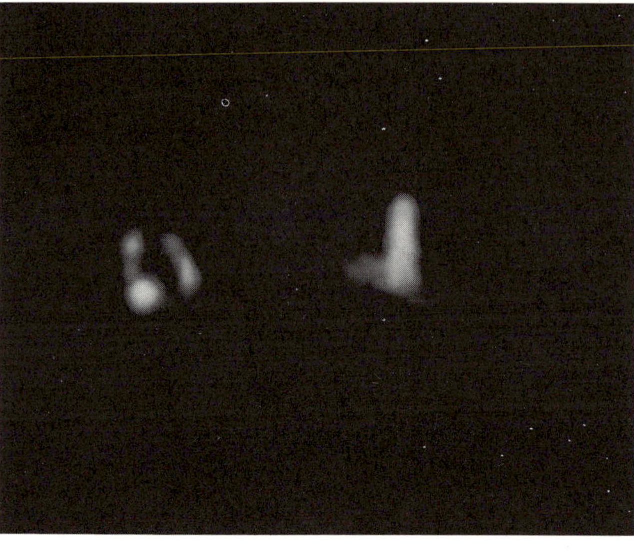

Figure 8-10 *Right heart failure.* A. *Echocardiogram demonstrates anteriorly located pericardial fluid indicated by separation of anterior myocardium from anterior pericardium. No definable fluid is seen posteriorly. At surgery 250 ml of fluid was removed.* B. *RAC demonstrates partial obstruction of right ventricular inflow tract suggesting a constricting band or intracardiac mass. A fibrous pericardial band secondary to previous tuberculous pericarditis was removed at surgery.*

clot within an aneurysmal segment is visualized as an avascular mass. Nuclide disappearance from the left ventricle may still be abnormal, however, suggesting abnormal myocardial contraction.

CARDIAC MASSES

The cause of masses associated with the cardiac silhouette can be studied in relation both to the continuity of the mass with

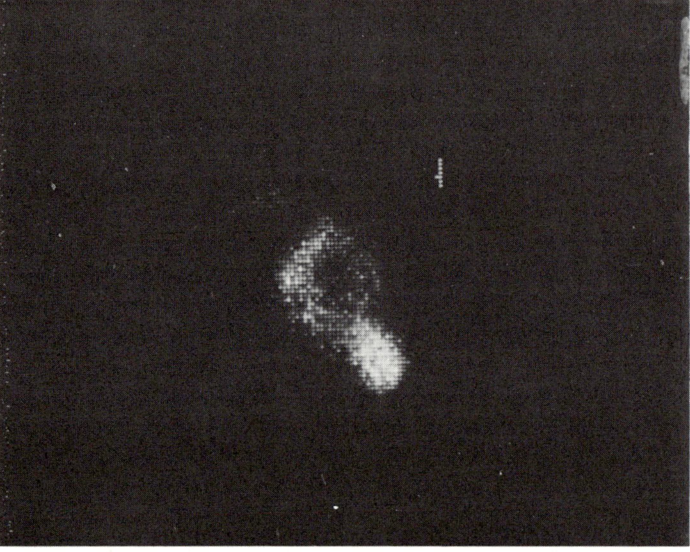

Figure 8-11 *Ventricular aneurysm indicated by large and apical bulge in left ventricular contour.*

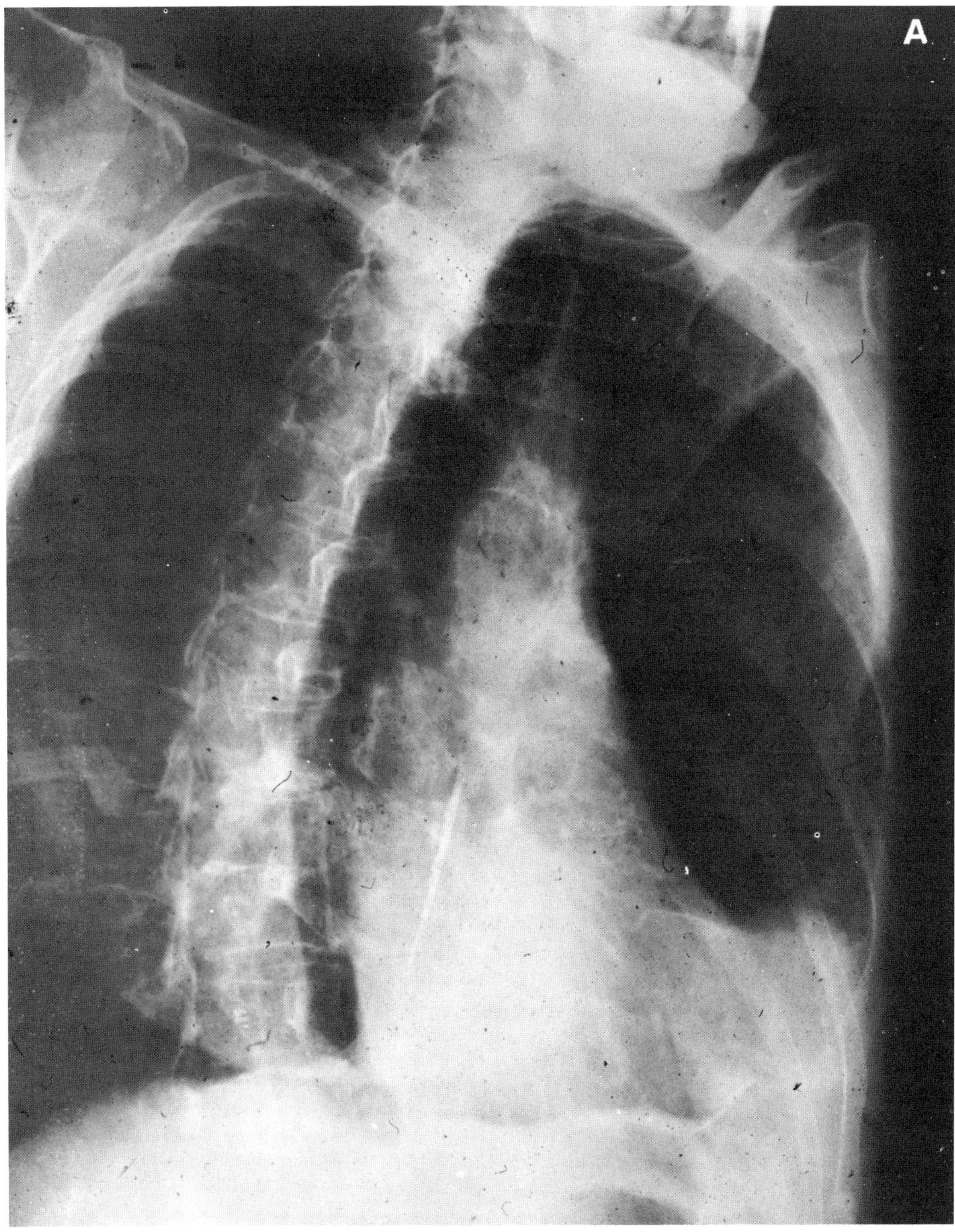

Figure 8-12 *Ventricular aneurysm. A. Chest roentgenogram, right anterior oblique projection, shows mass continuous with anterior apical portion of left ventricle. Rim-like calcifications are also evident. B. Echocardiogram demonstrates the mass in question to be solid and also suggests calcification. C. RAC demonstrates noncontinuity of cardiac blood pool with mass. Focal nuclide retention in left ventricle suggests abnormality of contraction. The three studies point to a thrombosed ventricular aneurysm as most likely lesion.*

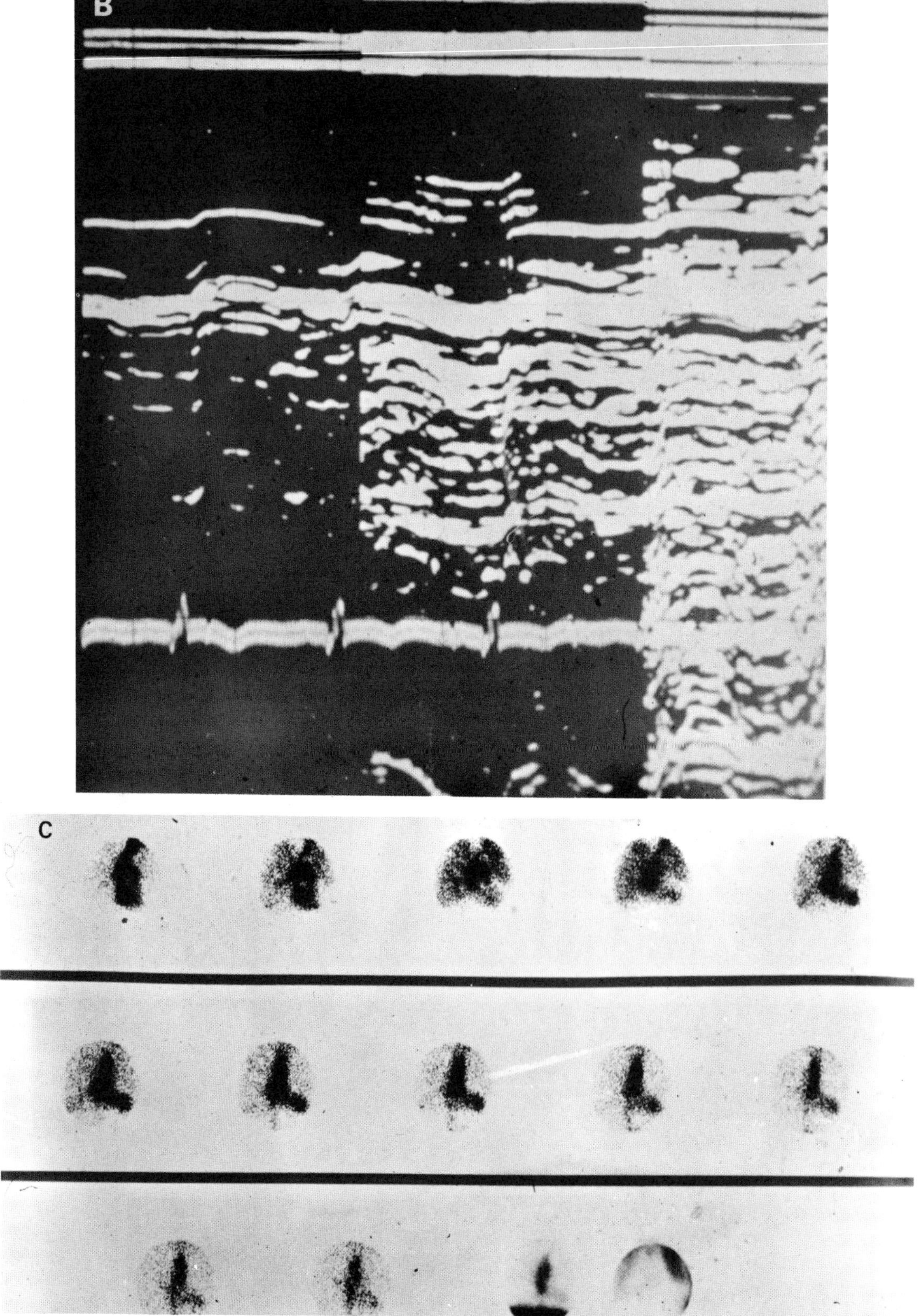

Figure 8-12 *Continued.*

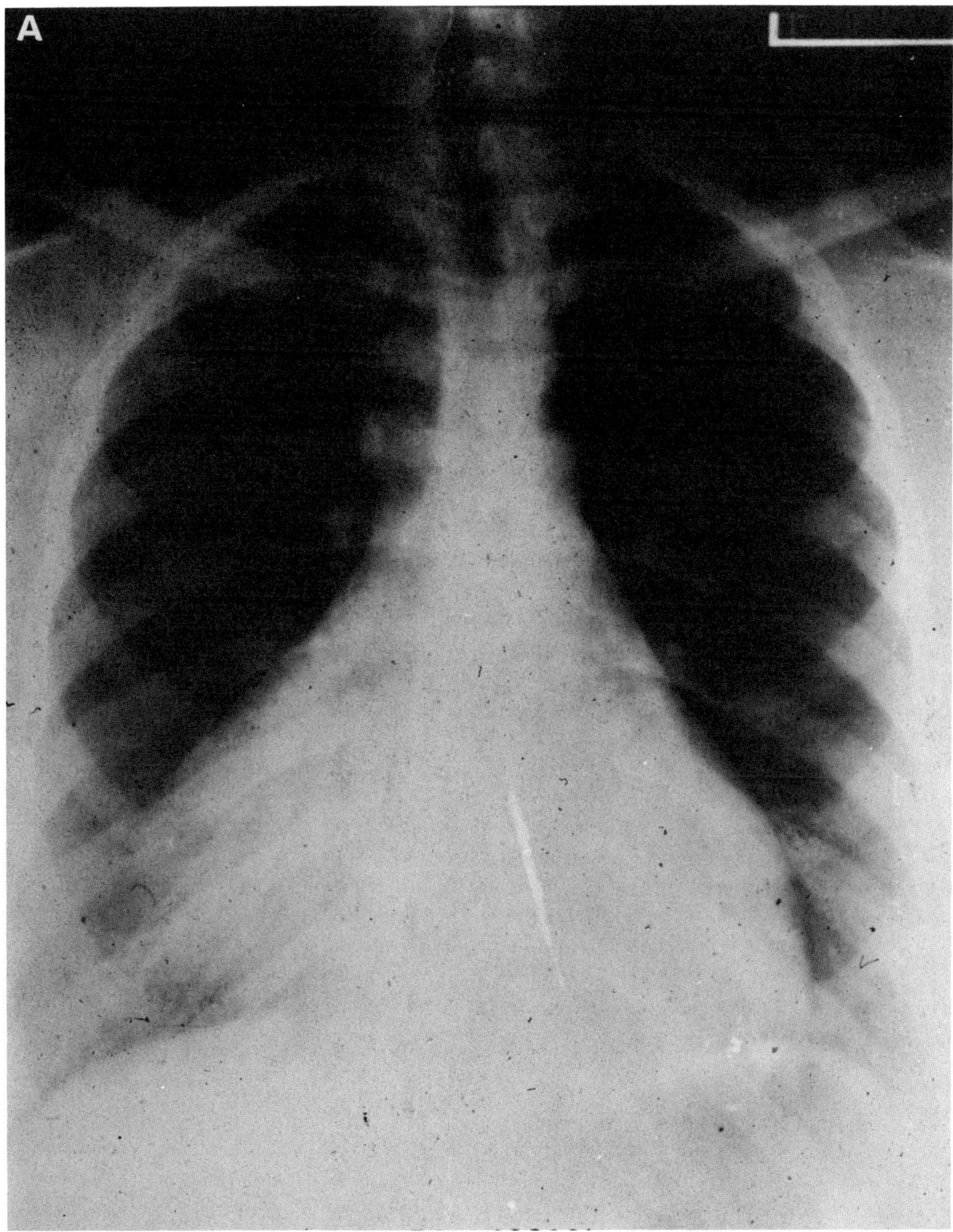

Figure 8-13 *Pericardial cyst. A. Chest roentgenogram demonstrates mass adjacent to right cardiophrenic border. B. RAC shows mass is avascular and not continuous with cardiac blood pool. C. Echocardiogram defines cystic nature of lesion.*

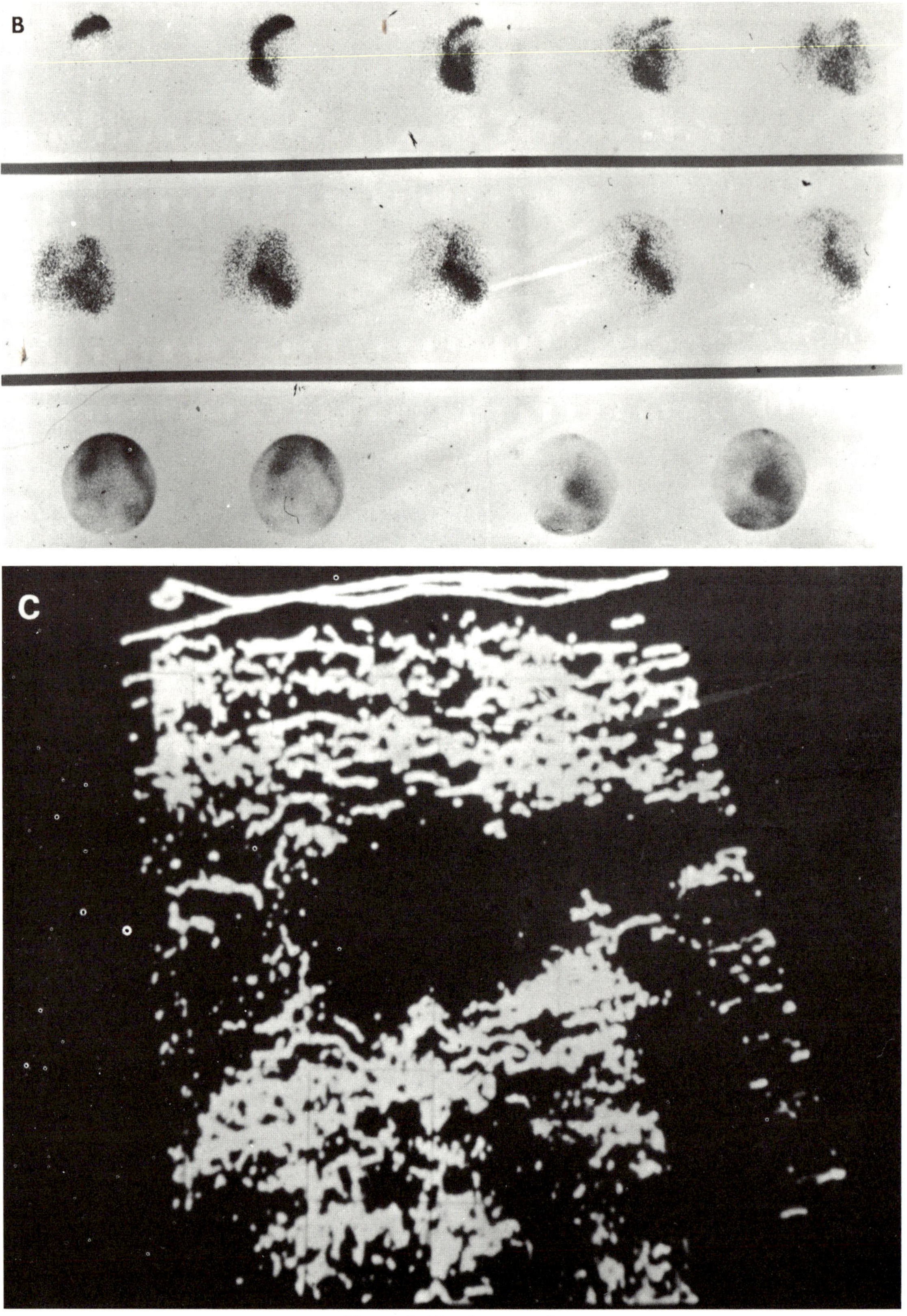

Figure 8-13 *Continued.*

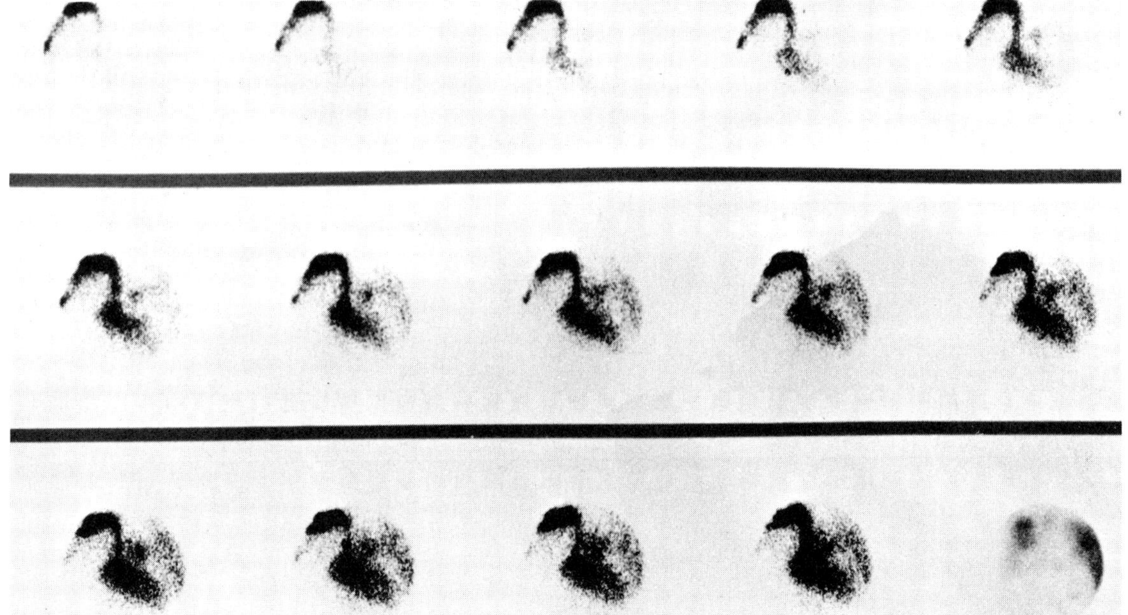

Figure 8-14 *Mass in right ventricular outflow tract. Note narrowing and displacement of right ventricular outflow tract and obstruction of right pulmonary artery. Autopsy disclosed carcinoma of lung obstructing right pulmonary artery and invading right venticular outflow tract.*

the cardiac blood pool and to the blood supply of the mass itself. Diagnostic ultrasound is frequently of complementary value in establishing the cystic or solid nature of a mass demonstrated by RAC to be avascular (Fig 8-13).

Intracardiac masses, particularly those involving the right heart, can be demonstrated by RAC and should be suspected in patients with chronic right heart failure. Detection is facilitated by the high count density in the right heart and the absence of radioactivity within superimposed vascular structures in the early phases of the study (Figs 8-14 through 8-17). Detection of left heart masses has been more difficult in our experience and frequently requires generation of computer-processed images. Zaret et al[16] have demonstrated a left atrial myxoma with the use of gated systolic and diastolic cardiac images. We have found echocardiography perferable in the demonstration of left atrial masses.

VALVULAR DISEASE

Kriss et al[6] have described what they feel are characteristic findings in acquired valvular disease. The examples presented here are those of tricuspid and mitral stenosis (Figs 8-18 and 8-19). Each lesion is associated with prolonged retention of nuclide in an enlarged chamber proximal to the valvular narrowing. Echocardiography is well suited to assessment of valve function, but evaluation of right heart structures is frequently difficult by this technique. Here RAC may be of considerable value. The tricuspid stenosis shown in Figure 8-18 was first demonstrated by RAC. Only by reexamining the patient in light of the information contained in the RAC was the tricuspid stenosis demonstrated echographically, and with some technical difficulty.

CARDIAC FUNCTION

Intracardiac mean and peak-to-peak (mode)

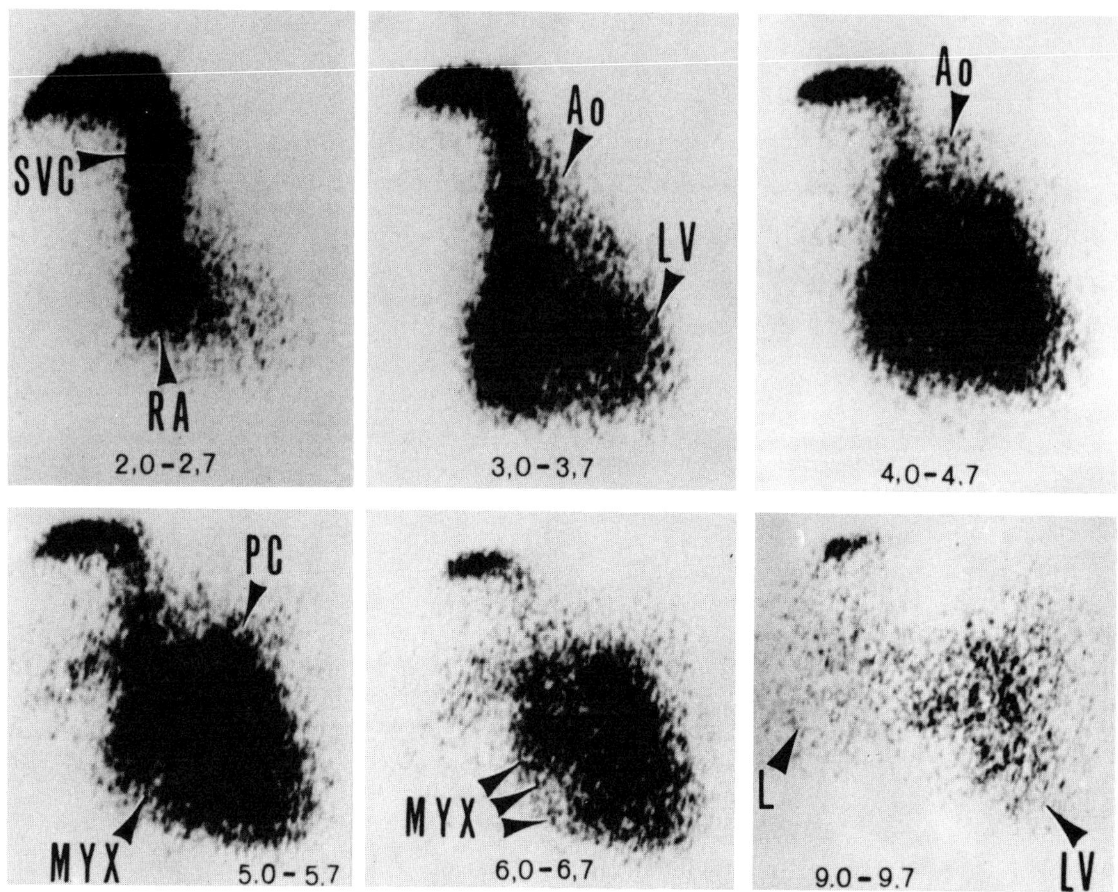

Figure 8-15 *Right atrial myxoma. Selected frames from RAC show partial obstruction to passage of radionuclide through right heart, suggesting mass (MYX). Activity is seen in aorta* (Ao) *and left ventricle (LV) prior to pulmonary perfusion, indicating right-to-left shunting.*

transit times can be determined by analysis of time-activity curves obtained over the various heart chambers (Fig 8-20). When a tracer confined to the intravascular compartment is used, cardiac output can also be calculated (Fig 8-21). By dilution principles, cardiac output (CO) is determined as:

$$CO = \frac{Cf}{A} \cdot BV$$

where Cf is the height of the curve when the tracer has achieved equilibrium; A is the area beneath the curve describing the first transit of the tracer, obtained by extrapolating the descending limb to the baseline as a single exponential function; and BV is the patient's blood volume. These curves may be generated by on-line computer facilities or region-of-interest and ratemeter printout accessories to the gamma camera. Such systems allow optimal placement of electronic cursors, thereby reducing the contribution by scattering from regions outside the area of immediate concern. A single precordial probe coupled to a strip-chart recorder can also be used; however, limitations related to probe placement, collimation, and inability to image are evident.

The mean transit time $\bar{t}$ (time when about half the injected bolus passes the site of

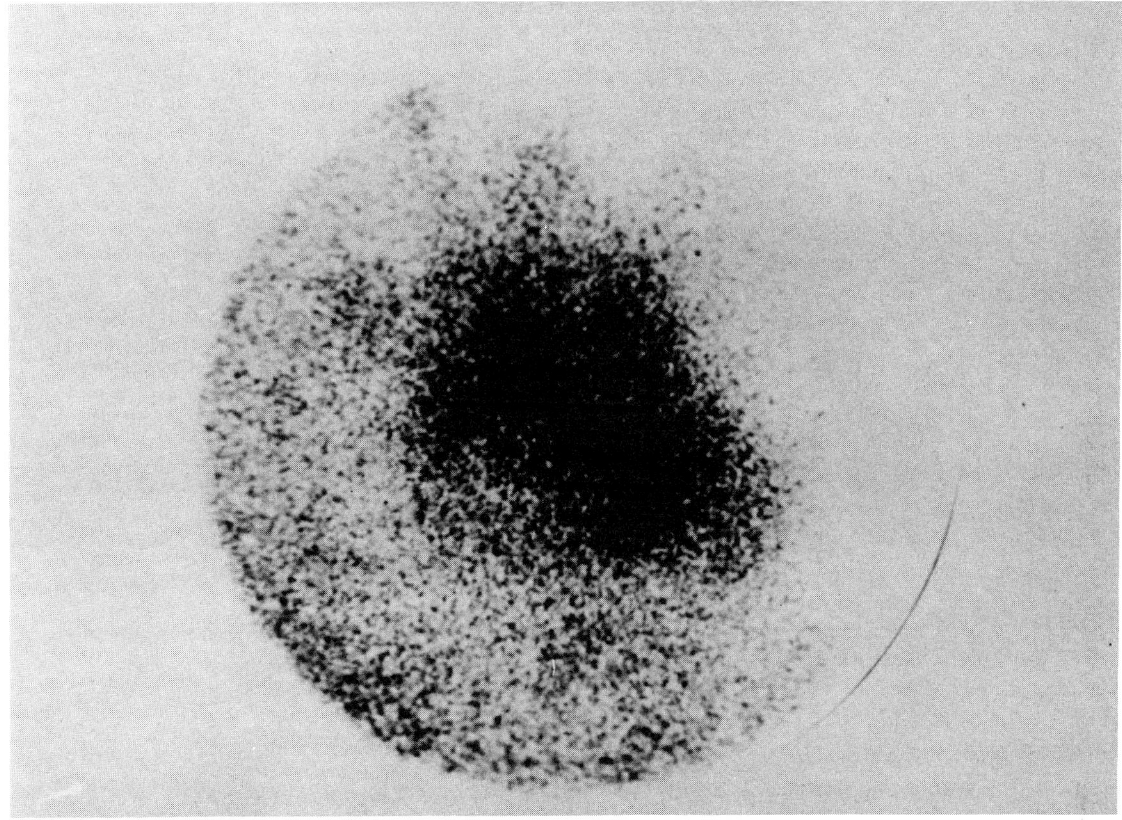

Figure 8-16 *Right atrial myxoma. Static image shows large mass in the right atrium. At surgery myxoma was removed from right atrium and secundum atrial septal defect was repaired.*

sampling) is particularly important since it alone relates volume (V) to flow (F) and is therefore physiologically and mathematically definable, as:

$$\bar{t} = V/F$$

Thus, if flow (cardiac output) and mean transit time are known, the volume between two points of sampling can be calculated. For example, pulmonary blood volume can be estimated as the product of the mean pulmonary transit time and the cardiac output.

Many laboratories also calculate by different methods left ventricular end-systolic and end-diastolic volumes, stroke volume, and ejection fraction. Most of the techniques involve assessment, either in digital or analog form, of left ventricular systolic and diastolic count rate differences or scintigraphic changes in left ventricular size.[1,5,13,15]

Of particular interest, Strauss and coworkers[11] have utilized the gating method for acquiring images of the left ventricle during systole and diastole. By assuming an ellipse of rotation, these two-dimensional images can be used to estimate left ventricular end-diastolic volume (*EDV*) and end-systolic volume (*ESV*). Stroke volume (*SV*) reduces to $EDV - ESV$, ejection fraction (*EF*) *to* SV/EDV, and cardiac output to heart rate (HR) $\times$ SV.

The time and equipment needed plus the requirement that the patient be physically within the nuclear medicine facility will probably limit application of this tech-

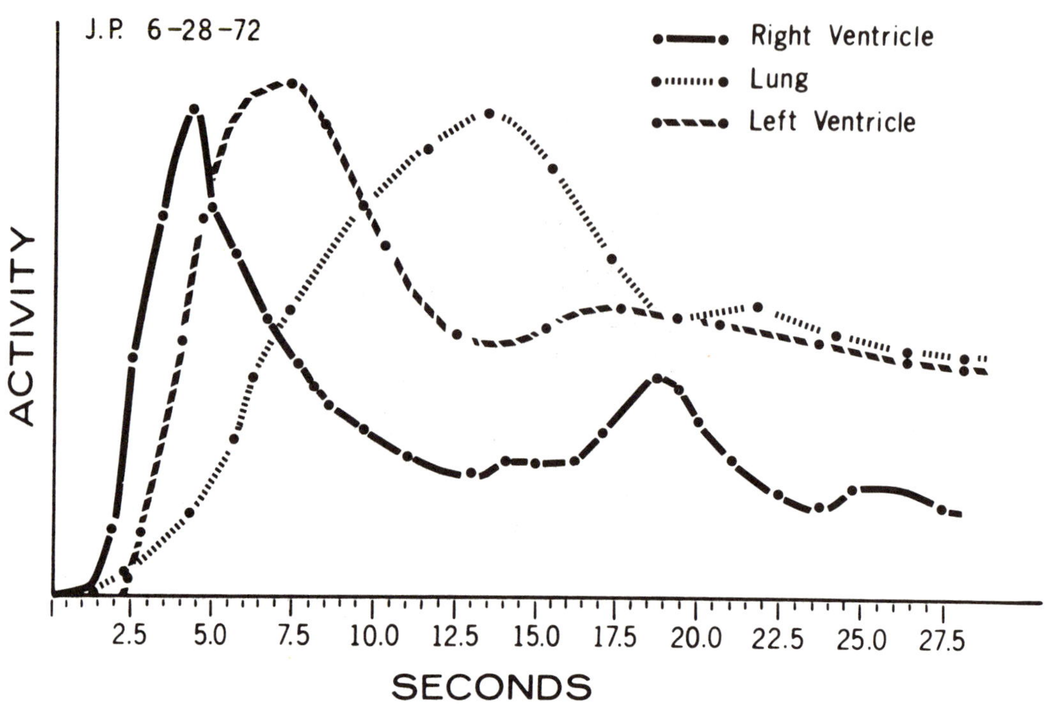

Figure 8-17 *Right atrial myxoma. Time-activity histograms demonstrate appearance of left heart activity prior to pulmonary perfusion, documenting right-to-left shunting.*

Figure 8-18 *Tricuspid stenosis. RAC shows partial obstruction to bolus transit between dilated right atrium and right ventricle.*

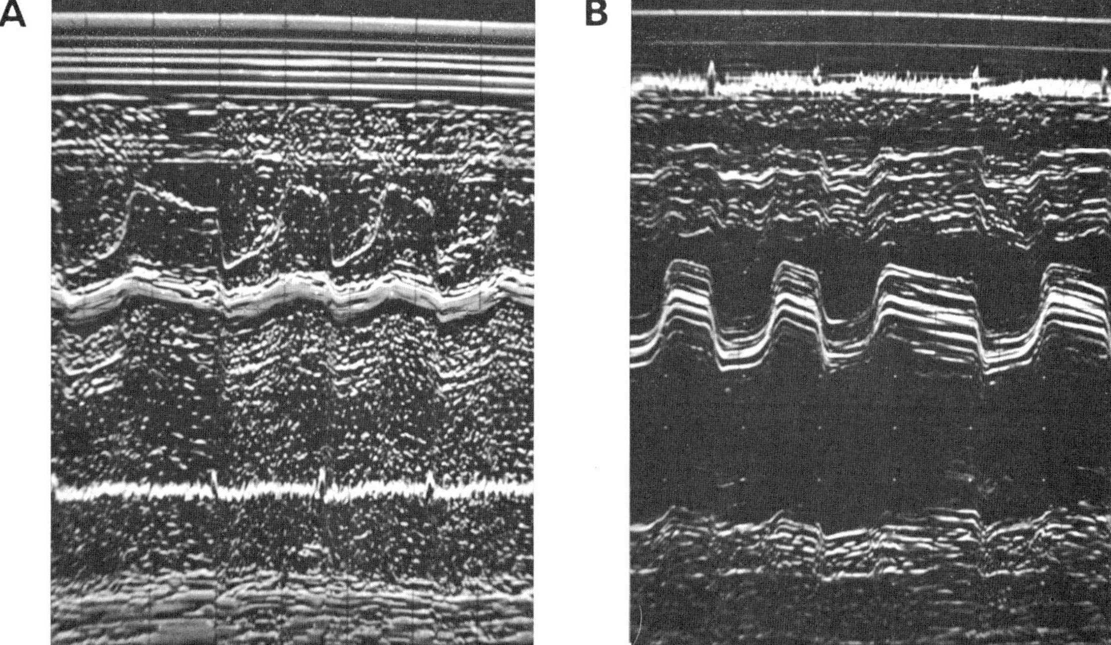

Figure 8-19 *Mitral stenosis and tricuspid stenosis in same patient as Fig 8-18. A. Demonstrates pattern of tricuspid stenosis. B. Demonstrates pattern of mitral stenosis.*

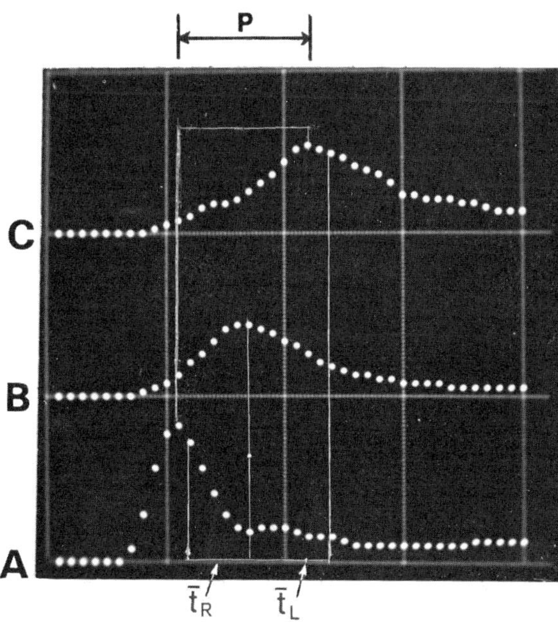

Figure 8-20 *Time-activity histograms obtained from right heart (A), lung (B), and left ventricle (C). Areas of interest indicated have been normalized to uniform area. P, peak-to-peak right-to-left ventricle 5.5 seconds. $\bar{t}_R$, 2.5-second and mean transit time between right heart and lung. $\bar{t}_L$, 3.5-second mean transit time between lung and left ventricle. Each data point represents 0.5 second and full scale on ordinate is 250 counts.*

nique. Results obtained by this method compare favorably with similar measurements made by dye-dilution and contrast angiography. Van Dyke,[12] recognizing the limitations and attempting to make these techniques available to critically ill patients, has recorded left ventricular curves

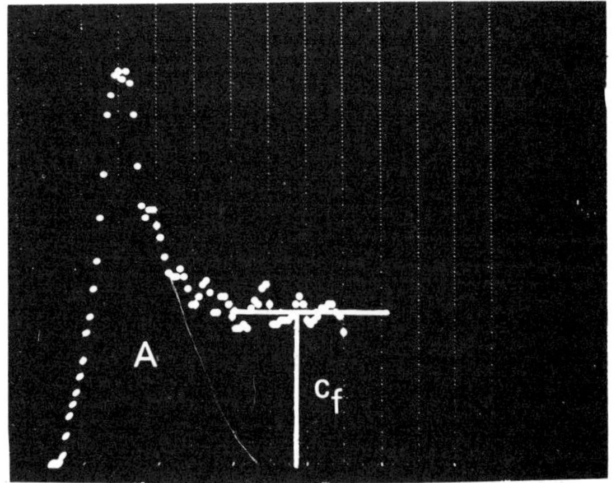

Figure 8-21 *Time-activity histogram obtained from left ventricle. Cardiac output is calculated as c_f on final blood concentration at equilibrium divided by area beneath primary bolus peak. This quantity is multiplied by separately determined blood volume.*

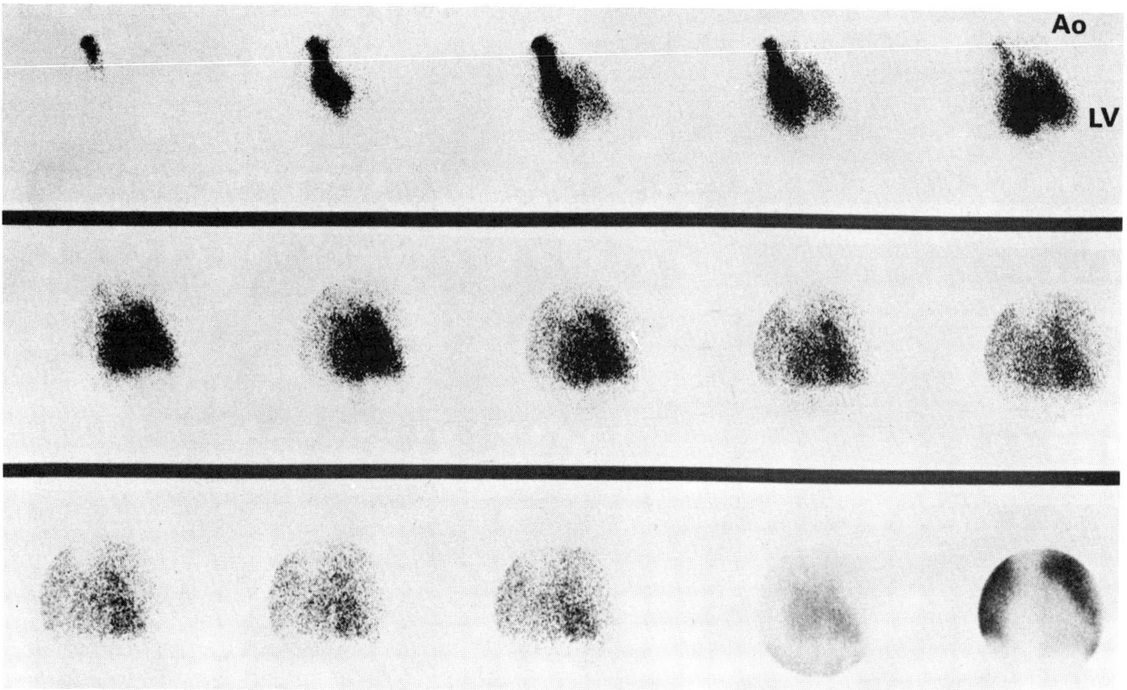

Figure 8-22 *Ebstein's anomaly. Right atrium is enlarged and passage of radioactive bolus is partially obstructed at tricuspid level. Activity within left ventricle and aorta prior to pulmonary perfusion indicates right-to-left shunting.*

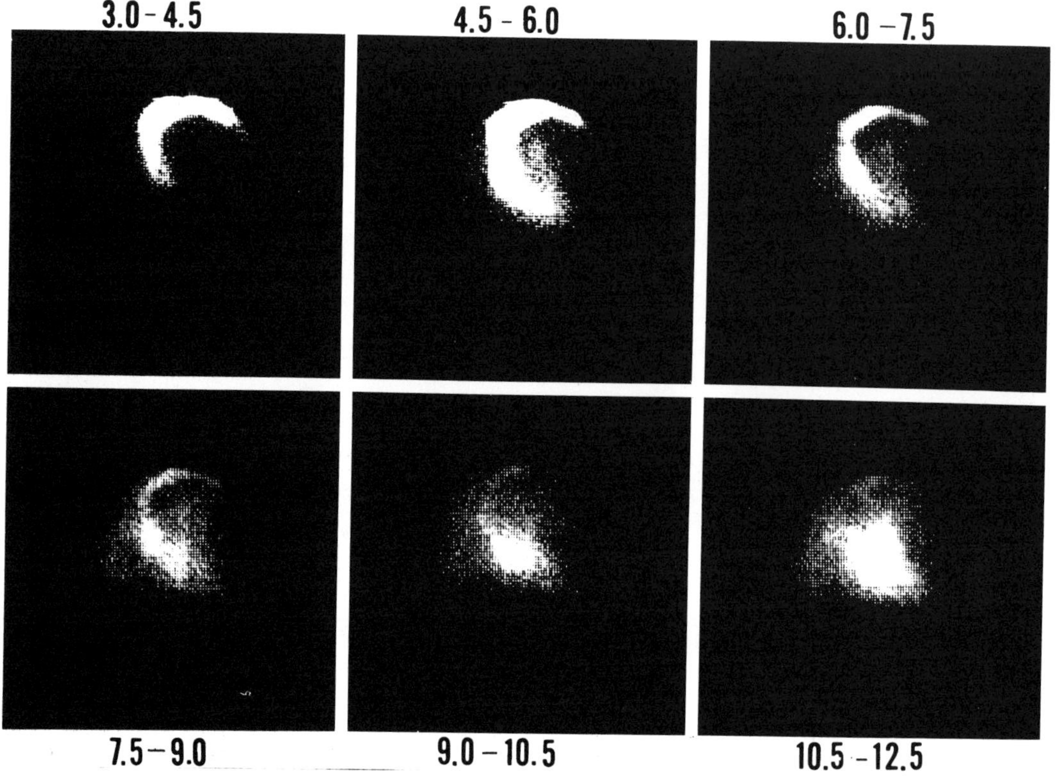

Figure 8-23 *Atrial septal defect. RAC shows poorly defined left heart. Recirculation of activity in all four cardiac chambers and lungs creates a smudge pattern.*

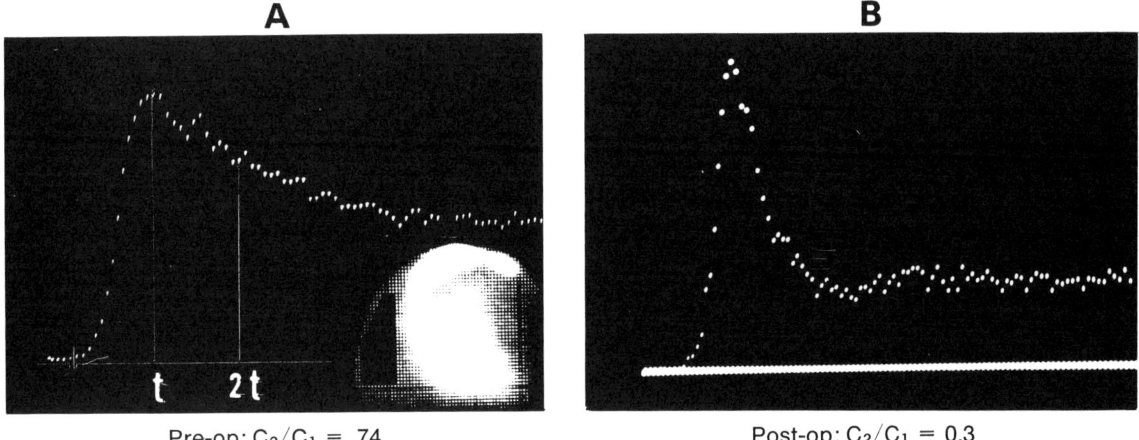

Figure 8-24 *Atrial septal defect. A. Preoperative time-activity histogram obtained from lung. C_2/C_1 ratio is 0.74 and indicates left-to-right shunt. B. Postoperative pulmonary time-activity histogram indicates closure of defect with no residual shunting.*

with careful placement of a single collimated precordial probe. His somewhat empirical analysis of high-frequency data results in the same measurements obtained within clinically acceptable periods of time while the patient remains within the intensive care facility.

INTRACARDIAC SHUNTING

RAC offers several advantages over cardiac catheterization as a first approach toward evaluating a patient with suspected shunting:

- Arterial puncture not required

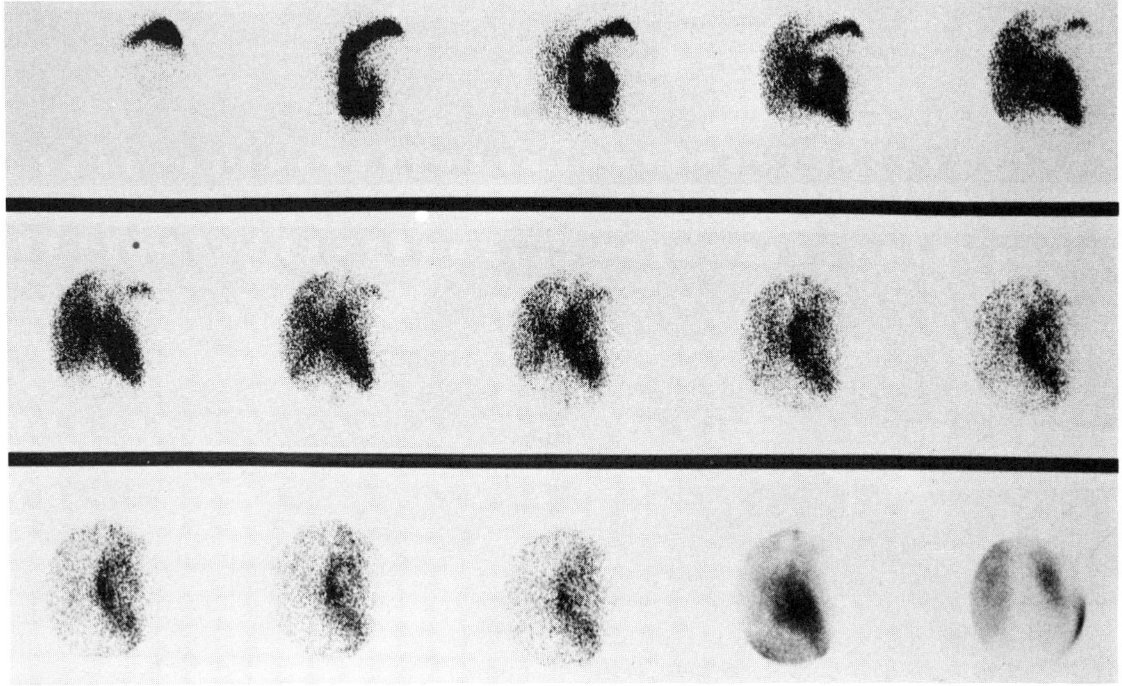

Figure 8-25 *Tetralogy of Fallot with patent Blalock anastomosis. A large pulmonary conus is visible, but no evidence of right-to-left shunting. Right lung perfuses normally but left lung is seen to perfuse through surgically created shunt coincident with and following visualization of left ventricle.*

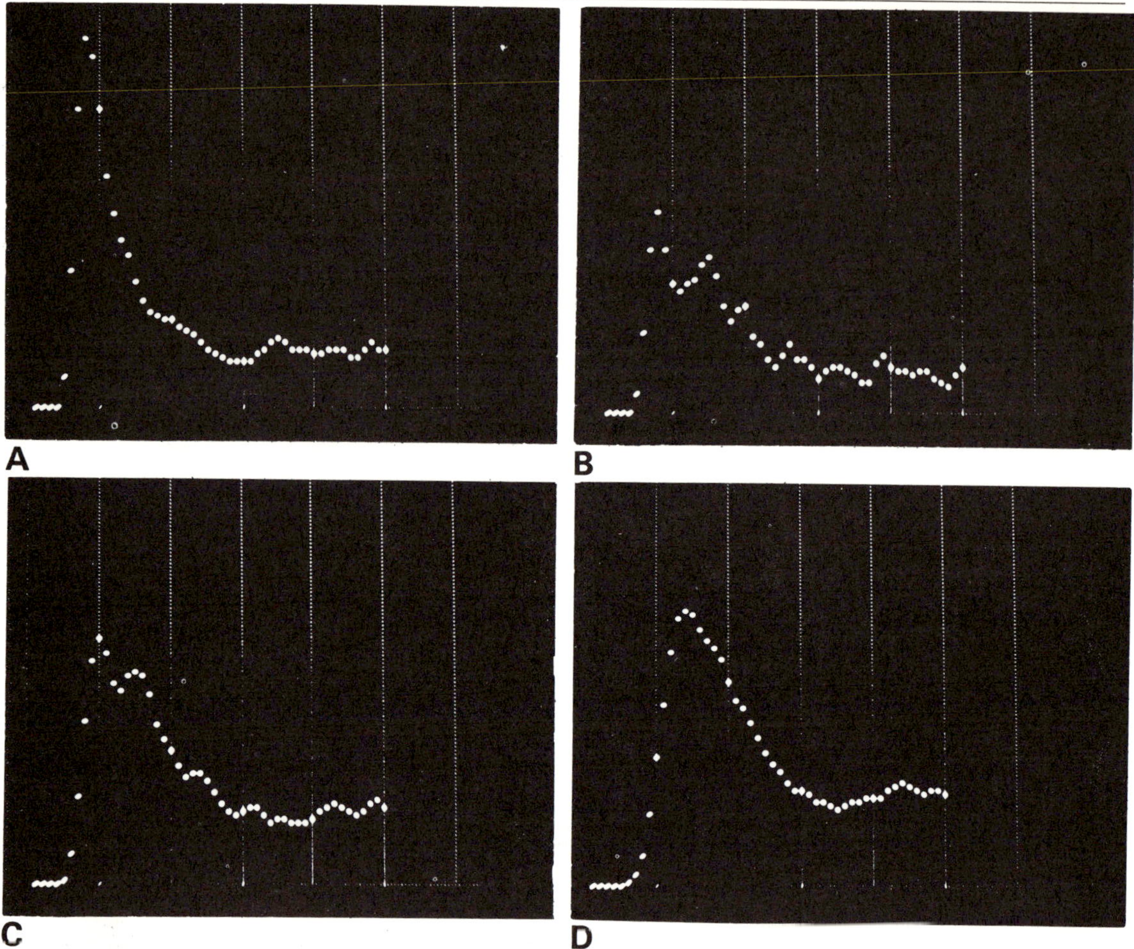

Figure 8-26 *Partial anomalous pulmonary venous return. Passage of administered radioactive bolus through upper portion of superior vena cava. No recirculation peak is seen (A). Abnormal, rapid-appearing recirculation peak is seen in lower superior vena cava (B) and right atrium (C), which corresponds in time to primary lung peak (D). There are 2.5 seconds between primary right atrial and pulmonary peaks and 2.5 seconds between primary and recirculation peaks in lower superior vena cava and right atrium.*

- Performable on outpatient basis
- Repeatable if necessary
- Reliable
- Performable in patients sensitive to contrast material
- Safe
- Useful to select patients for further invasive study or to obviate need for further study

A right-to-left shunt can be detected and quantitated by a variety of techniques. The appearance of radioactivity within the left heart or aorta prior to pulmonary perfusion indicates such a shunt (Figs 8-15, 8-16, 8-17, and 8-22). Quantitation may be accomplished by administration of high-specific-activity albumin microspheres (Tc99m) (Figs 8-18 and 8-19) or macroaggregated albumin Tc 99m.[3] Percentage of shunting is estimated by relating the total amount of activity present to that contained within the lungs. Visualization of renal activity following injection of such particles generally indicates right-to-left shunting in excess of 15%. Differentiation between cardiac and pulmonary cause for cyanosis in the acutely ill neonate is of considerable importance to rational selection of patients for catheterization. Interestingly, some apparently normal neonates demonstrate right-to-left shunting through a patent foramen ovale. This is secondary to elevated right atrial pressures related to increased pulmonary vascular resistance.[4]

Left-to-right shunting can be detected by imaging and analysis of isotope-dilution curves. Shunts as small as 1.2:1 pulmonary/systemic flow ratio have been detected.[9] Imaging techniques involve demonstration of abnormal recirculation of radioactivity within the cardiac chambers[6] and lungs (Fig 8-23). The level of the defect determines the chambers in which activity persists. Supracristal ventricular septal defects and patent ductus arteriosus produce no visible evidence of right ventricular recirculation, but abnormal pulmonary perfusion is present. The adequacy of shunt repair and the patency of surgically introduced shunts can also be assessed (Fig 8-25).

Isotope-dilution curves obtained over the lungs and cardiac chambers provide another means of establishing the presence of left-to-right shunting. One popular method involves calculation of C_2/C_1 ratios obtained from lung histograms.

C_1 is defined as the maximum height of the pulmonary curve occurring at time t after the first appearance of activity within the region of interest; C_2 is the height of the same curve at twice the time (t). Different C_2/C_1 values have been reported by several investigators. Greenfield and Bennett[4] state that the maximum normal C_2/C_1 ratio is 0.35, while Rosenthall[8] suggests that C_2/C_1 ratios less than 0.6 do not indicate significant shunting. Cardiac failure and insufficiency of the tricuspid or

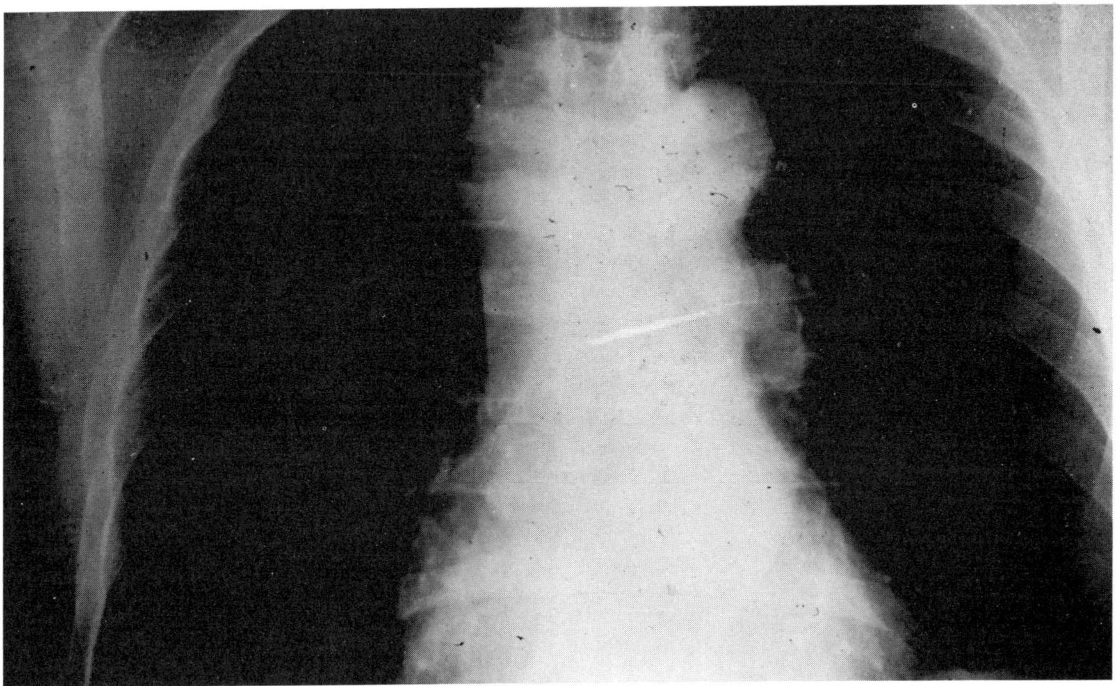

Figure 8-27 *Mass adjacent to proximal aorta. Roentgenographic appearance.*

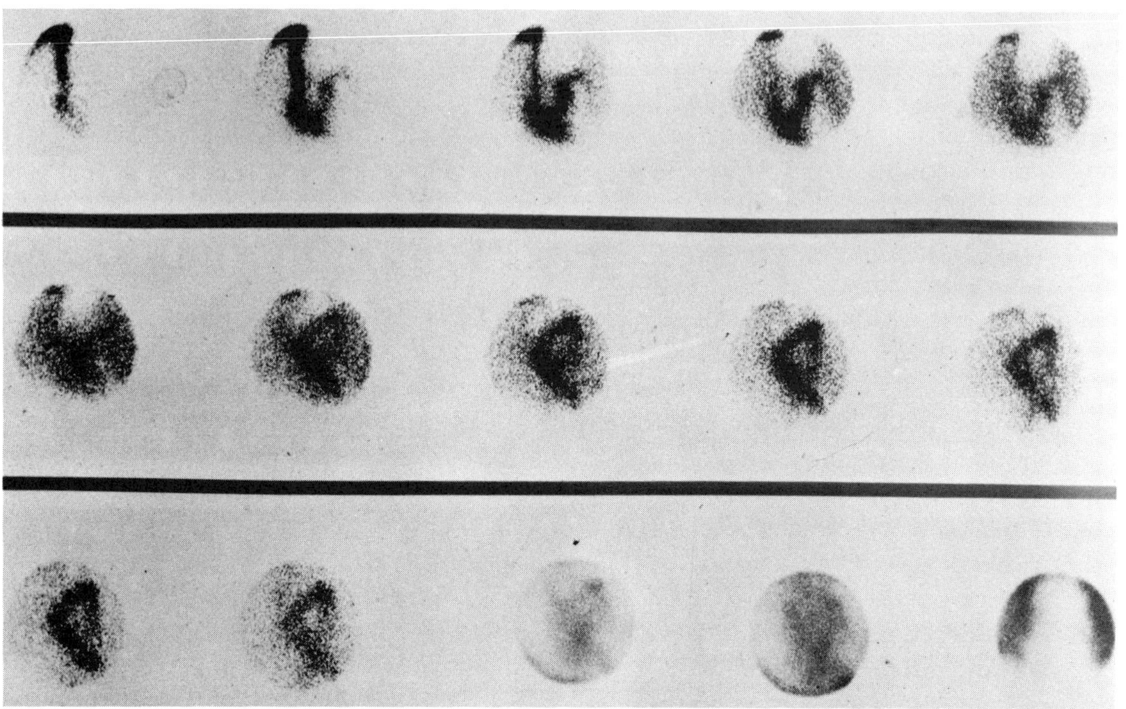

Figure 8-28 *Mass adjacent to proximal aorta. RAC shows displacement of otherwise normal appearing ascending aorta by relatively hypovascular mass (second row of scintiphotos).*

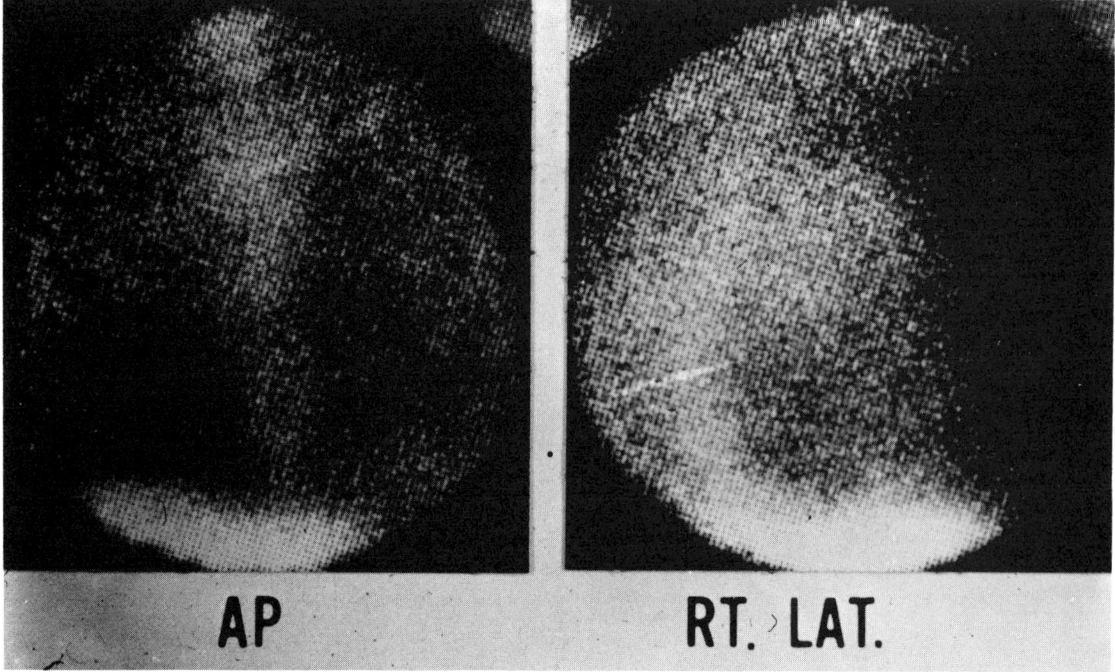

Figure 8-29 *Mass adjacent to proximal aorta. Indium 111 scan shows abnormal accumulation of tracer within well-defined area of mediastinum, best seen in lateral projection (arrow). A neoplastic mass is suggested.*

pulmonary valve may also produce elevated C_2/C_1 values. This ratio cannot be used to quantitate the degree of shunting. The presence of abnormal recirculation peaks in the time-activity curves over various heart chambers and lung also indicate left-to-right shunting. We have found this method quite tedious and time consuming; however, it is occasionally the method of choice (Fig 8-26). Comparison of the area under the recirculation peak with the area under the primary peak results in a reasonable approximation of percentage of shunting.

Radionuclide Angiography of Mediastinum and Great Vessels

The radionuclide angiogram (RA) is helpful in detecting mediastinal masses, establishing their relative vascularity, and demonstrating their relation to adjacent vascular structures. Figure 8-27 demonstrates roentgenographically a mass associated with the proximal aorta. For technical reasons it was desirable to exclude the possibility of aortic aneurysm prior to bronchoscopy. This was accomplished by combined isotope studies, which demonstrated displacement of an otherwise normal-appearing aorta (Fig 8-28) by a mass which concentrated chloride In 111, a tumor-seeking nuclide (Fig 8-29). Subsequent biopsy revealed undifferentiated carcinoma of the lung. Superior vena cava obstruction is easily and atraumatically documented (Fig 8-9).

Aneurysms of either the thoracic or the abdominal aorta appear as localized areas of luminal widening frequently associated

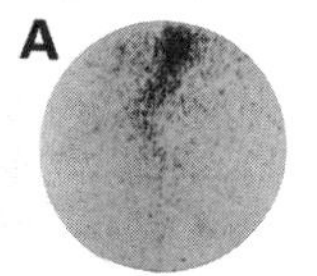

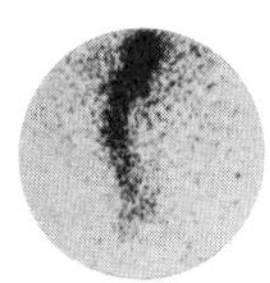
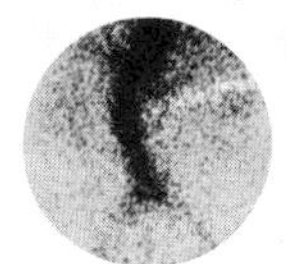
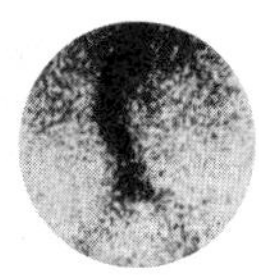
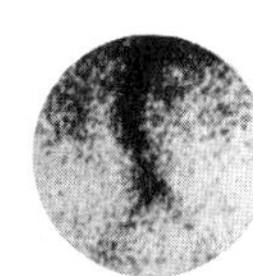
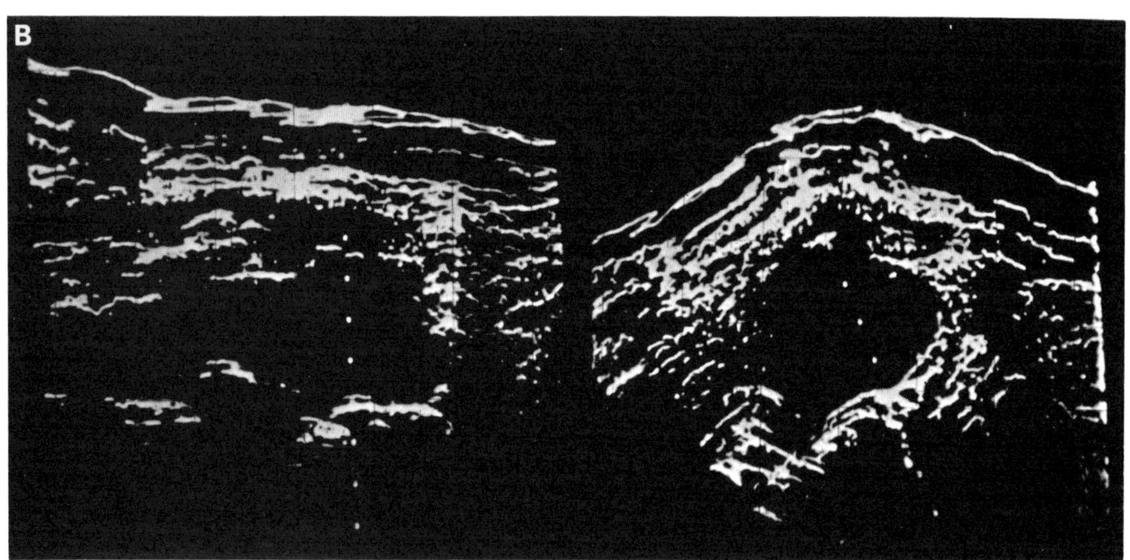

Figure 8-30 *Aneurysm of abdominal aorta. A. RA shows a mildly dilated lumen in abdominal aorta and poor distal runoff into common iliac arteries. B. Sagittal and transverse echoaortograms indicate aneurysmal widening in distal aorta. Presence of circumferential thrombus can be inferred from the two studies.*

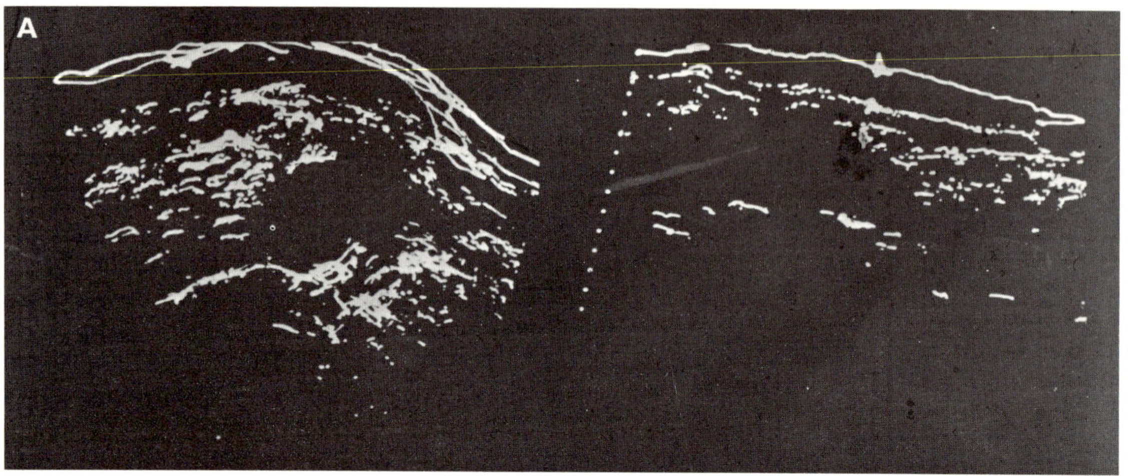

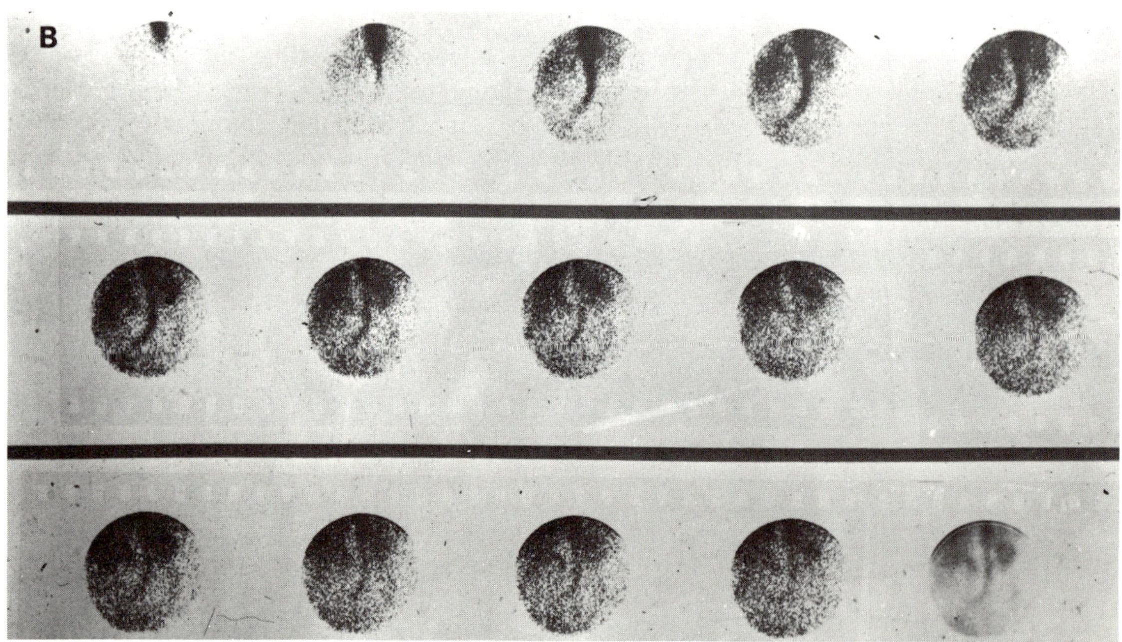

Figure 8-31 *Aneurysm of abdominal aorta.* A. *Echoaortogram demonstrates aneurysm involving proximal abdominal aorta.* B. *RA shows area of widening in proximal aorta and occlusion of left common iliac artery.*

with an abnormal flow pattern in comparison with adjacent vascular segments. The same principles which apply to contrast angiography are true for the radionuclide studies. Specifically, a normal-appearing lumen does not exclude the presence of aneurysm and may simply reflect recanalization or circumferential thrombus (Fig 8-30). The complementary information provided by ultrasonography frequently clarifies these complexities. The morphologic anatomy of an aneurysm can be demonstrated by ultrasonography (Fig 8-31*A*), while effective lumen and branch vessel occlusions are evident on dynamic isotope examination (Fig 8-31*B*).

References

1. Ashburn WL, Kostuk WJ, Karliner JS, et al: Left ventricular volume and ejection fraction determination by radionuclide angiography. *Semin Nucl Med* 3:165–176, 1973.
2. Blumgart HL, Yens C: Studies on the velocity of blood flow. 1. The method utilized. *J Clin Invest* 4:1, 1927.
3. Gates GF, Orme HW, Dore EK: Measurement of cardiac shunting with technetium labeled albumin aggregates. *J Nucl Med* **12**:746, 1971.
4. Greenfield LD, Bennett LR: Detection of intracardiac shunts with radionuclide imaging. *Semin Nucl Med* 3:139–151, 1973.
5. Jones RH, Sabisto DC, Bates BB: Quantitative radionuclide angiocardiography for determination of chamber to chamber cardiac transit times. *Am J Cardiol* **30**:855–864, 1972.
6. Kriss JP, Enright LP, Hayden WG, et al: Radioisotope angiocardiography: Wide scope of clinical applicability in diagnosis and evaluation of therapy in diseases of the heart and great vessels. *Circulation* **43**:792, 1971.
7. Prinzmetal M, Corday E, Sprintzler J, et al: Radiocardiography and its clinical applications. *JAMA* **139**:617, 1949.
8. Rosenthall L: Nucleographic screening of patients for left-to-right cardiac shunts. *Radiology* **99**:601, 1971.
9. Stocker FP, Kinser J, Weber JW: Pediatric radioangiography: Shunt diagnosis. *Circulation* **47**:819, 1973.
10. Strauss HW, Hurley PJ, Rhodes BA, et al: Quantification of right to left transpulmonary shunts in man. *J Lab Clin Med* **74**:597, 1969.
11. Strauss HW, Zaret BE, Hurley PJ: A scintiphotographic method for measuring left ventricular ejection fraction in man without cardiac catheterization. *Am J Cardiol* **28**:575, 1971.
12. Van Dyke D: Scintiphotographic analysis of left ventricular function. Presented at nuclear cardiology symposium, Johns Hopkins University, April 12–14, 1973.
13. Van Dyke D, Anger HO, Sullivan RW, et al: Cardiac evaluation from radioisotope dynamics. *J Nucl Med* **13**:585, 1972.
14. Watson DD, Nelson J, Gottlieb S: Rapid bolus injections of radioisotopes. *Radiology* **106**:347, 1973.
15. Weber PM, Dos Remedios LV, and Josko IA: Quantitative radioisotope angiocardiography. *J Nucl Med* **13**:815–822, 1972.
16. Zaret BL, Hurley PJ, Pitt B: Non-invasive scintiphotographic diagnosis of left atrial myxoma. *J Nucl Med* **13**:81–84, 1973.
17. Zaret BL, Strauss HW, Hurley PJ, et al: A noninvasive scintiphotographic method for the testing of ventricular dysfunction in man. *N Engl J Med* **284**:1165, 1971.

Radionuclide scanning detects areas of increased bone metabolism suggestive of such abnormalities as neoplastic disease, trauma, aseptic necrosis, inflammatory disease, and metabolic disturbance.

9
The Skeletal System

Aldo N. Serafini

Principles

Accretion and resorption of bone is a continuous metabolic process. Proliferating osteoblasts deposit hydroxyapatite crystals onto a matrix of osteoid tissue. Bone responds to a wide variety of noxious stimuli by new bone formation. In disease this metabolic turnover may be increased either at the site of a lesion (as in metastases or fractures) or throughout the skeletal system (as in hyperparathyroidism).

Bone scanning exploits the fact that bone lesions are areas of disturbed metabolism that accumulate radionuclides more than does normal bone.

The radionuclides used in bone scanning localize in metabolically active regions, and thus an area of increased metabolism attracts greater amounts of the tracers. The degree of radionuclide uptake at the site of the lesion depends on two main factors: blood flow to the area and reactivity of the newly forming bone. Figure 9-1, a photomicrograph from a patient with Paget's disease, illustrates these factors. Bone-scanning techniques detect these regions of increased metabolic turnover.

Logically the radionuclides used in bone scanning should be made from those elements in the hydroxyapatite crystals which are deposited onto the osteoid tissue in the turnover process. These crystals include calcium, phosphorus, oxygen, carbon, and hydrogen. However, the radioactive isotopes of most of these elements are not satisfactory for bone scanning because they do not possess the physical properties necessary for external detection. Consequently, other radionuclides with more appropriate photon energies and half-lives have been developed for bone scanning. These include strontium 85, strontium 87m, fluorine 18, and technetium 99m labeled compounds. Less commonly used are calcium 47, gallium 68, barium 131, barium 135, and dysprosium 157.[1,2]

Radionuclides Used in Bone Scanning

- Strontium 85
- Strontium 87m
- Fluorine 18
- Technetium 99m Labeled Phosphate Compounds

Some of these bone-seeking agents have characteristics similar to the elements of

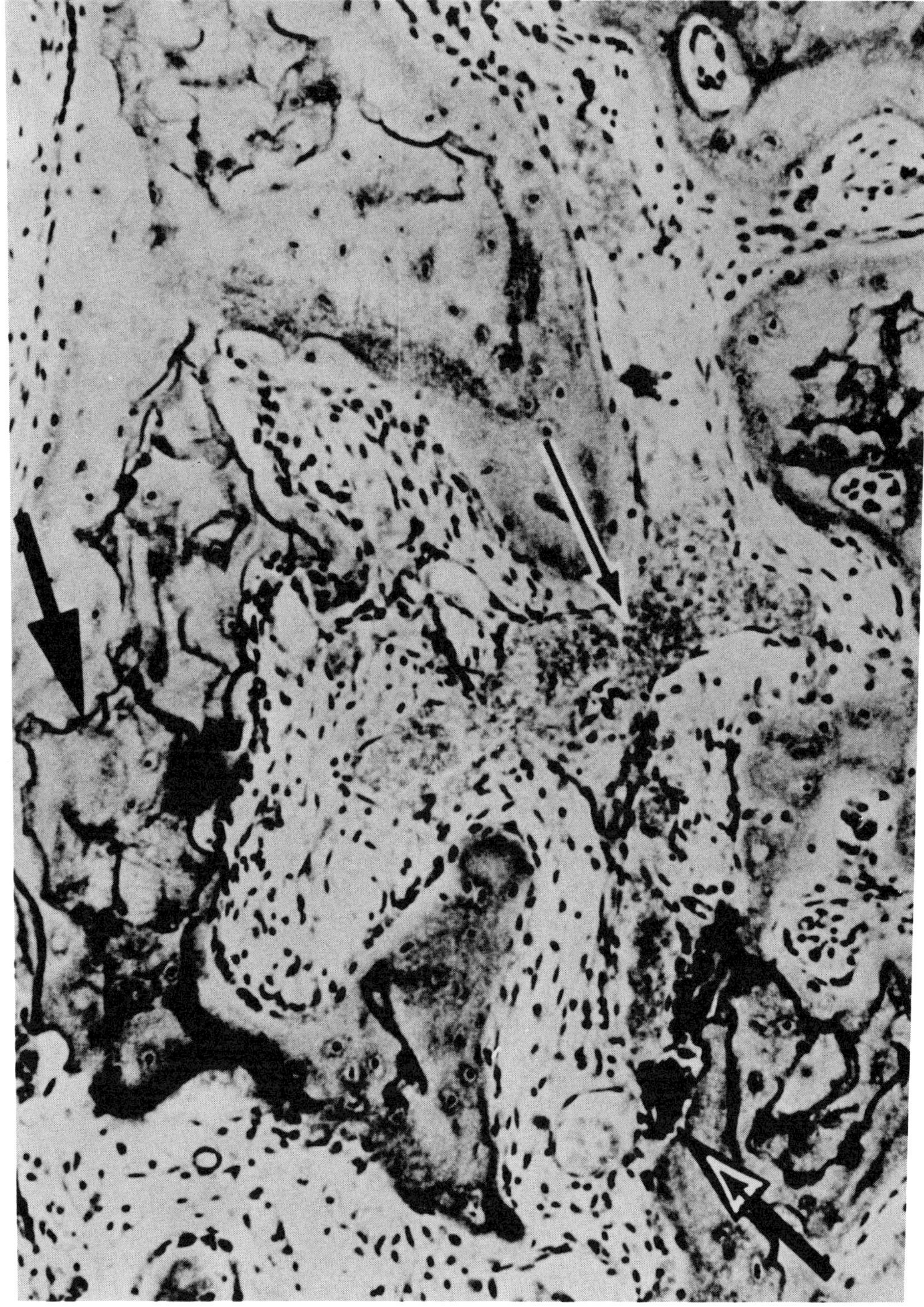

Figure 9-1 *Photomicrograph of bone in a patient with Paget's disease shows blood supply and reactive osteoblasts on which local accumulation of bone-seeking radionuclides is dependent. Black arrow points to mosaic pattern characteristic of Paget's disease, black arrow with white insert indicates reactive osteoblast, white arrow with black insert points to a vascular channel. (Courtesy of Arkadi M. Rywlin.)*

the hydroxyapatite crystals. For example, the distribution and kinetics of strontium are similar to those of calcium, and strontium is taken up in new bone in place of calcium. Fluorine is believed to substitute for the hydroxyl ions in the hydroxyapatite crystal and has been shown to be dependent on the blood flow to the area. Tc 99m polyphosphate and Tc 99m diphosphonate are thought to localize by chemisorption, but in addition may depend upon the regional bone blood flow. [3,49,50]

Radiopharmaceuticals

STRONTIUM 85

Strontium 85 is a pure gamma emitter with a photon energy of 514 kev and a physical half-life of 64 days. The usual dose is 100 μCi injected intravenously in the form of citrate or nitrate. Bone scanning is best performed with a rectilinear instrument, and studies are usually made 48 to 72 hours after injection. Because of the long half-life of ^{85}Sr, scanning can be done or delayed up to two weeks after injection to detect bone tumors with a slow metabolic rate.

Because the fecal excretion is fairly significant, a laxative the night before scanning and a high colonic enema the morning of the study are recommended.[4,5,6]

The main advantage of ^{85}Sr is its long shelf life—of real importance to a small laboratory doing few scans and in regions where shorter-lived radionuclides are not available. In addition, it is comparatively inexpensive.

Disadvantages relate mainly to the low photon flux from the small dose administered. Because of the long biologic half-life, the radiation dose to the patient is 1 to 4 rads. Use of ^{85}Sr is therefore restricted to patients with known malignancy.

STRONTIUM 87m

Strontium 87m is a pure gamma emitter with a photon energy of 388 kev and a physical half-life of 2.8 hours. It is eluted from a commercially available sterile yttrium 87 generator with a physical half-life of 80 hours. The usual dose is 1 to 4 mCi injected intravenously. Scanning is done with either a rectilinear scanner or an Anger scintillation camera with a high-energy collimator, usually one to three hours postinjection.

Because of the shorter physical half-life, the radiation dose to the bone is lower than that of ^{85}Sr and therefore ^{87m}Sr is approved for use in benign as well as malignant conditions in children and adults. In addition, a higher administered dose is permissible, allowing rapid scanning times. Disadvantages relate to its slow urinary excretion. This, associated with the shorter half-life, requires scanning while blood and body background activity is still high. A high incidence of false-positive and false-negative scans may result, especially if scans are begun earlier than recommended.

FLUORIDE F18

Fluorine 18, a positron emitter, produces annihilation photons of 510 kev. The physical half-life is 110 minutes. From 1 to 4 mCi is injected intravenously or given orally. Scanning is best carried out one to four hours later. A rectilinear scanner (Fig 9-2) or an Anger scintillation camera with a high-energy diverging-hole collimator or tungsten pinhole collimator can be used. Uptake by bone is prompt, and by 60 to 100 minutes a plateau is reached, with little further rise. The unfixed Fuorine 18 is excreted rapidly in the urine, and the bladder should be emptied prior to scanning; the patient is encouraged to drink water so as to reduce the radiation dose to the bladder.

Fluorine localizes rapidly in bony sites and accumulates significantly more in diseased than in normal bone. Clearance from the soft tissues and blood is rapid, giving a higher bone-to-background ratio. Be-

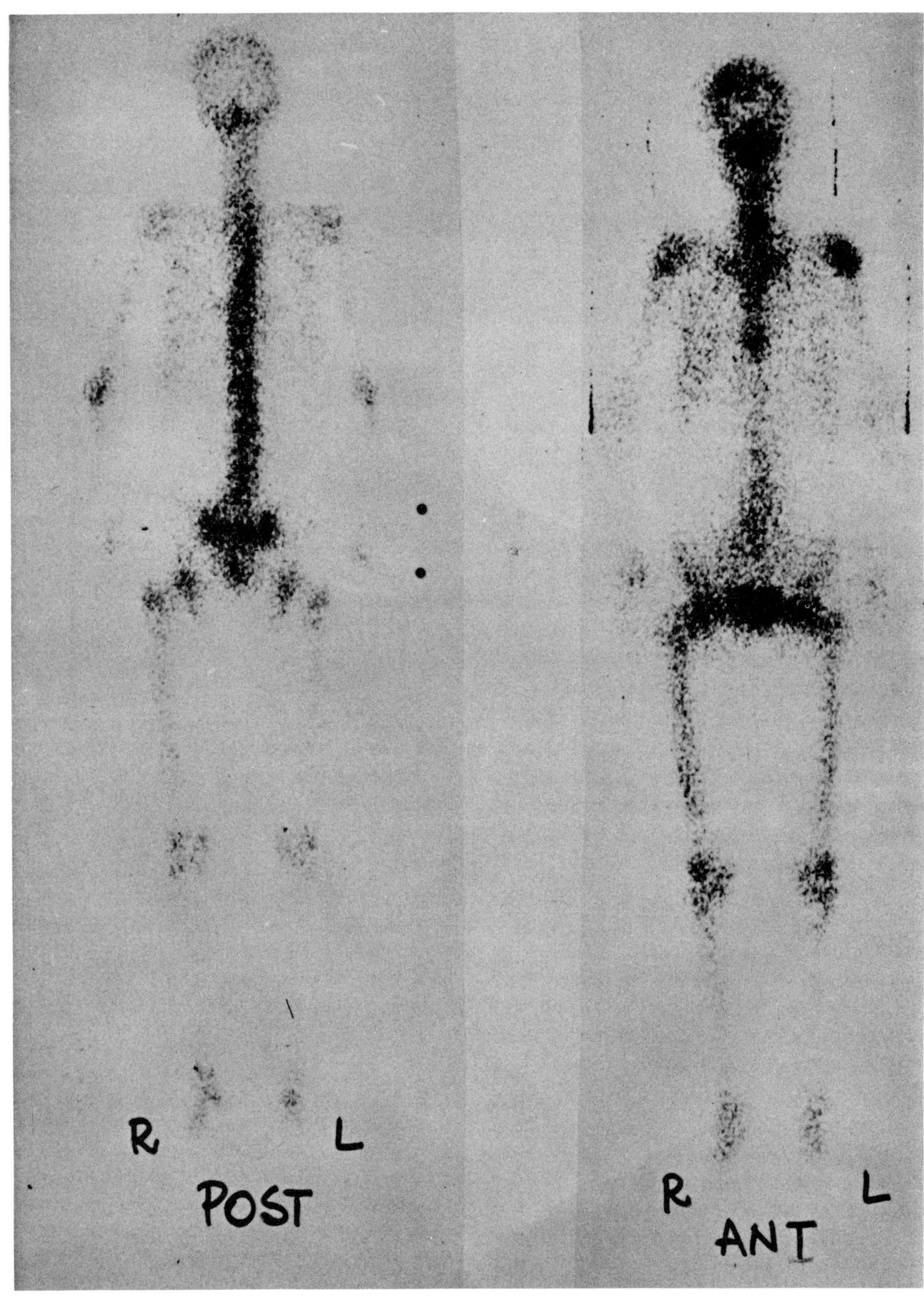

Figure 9-2 *Metastatic lesion to scalp. Study done with fluoride F18 and dual probe rectilinear scanner.*

cause of the short half-life, the radiation dose is less and larger amounts can be administered.[7,8]

Disadvantages relate at present to its relative expense and difficult availability.

Tc 99m POLYPHOSPHATE

This monoenergetic gamma emitter has a photon energy of 140 kev and a 6.4 hour physical half-life. From 10 to 15 mCi is injected intravenously, and scanning is done three to six hours postinjection using either the Anger scintillation camera or a rectilinear scanner.

The chief advantage of Tc 99m polyphosphate is a bone background ratio reported to be as favorable as that of fluorine. In addition, the physical properties of ^{99m}Tc are ideally suited to present-day scanning equipment. Owing to the short physical half-life, the administered dose may be as high as 10 to 15 mCi with little radiation to the patient compared with the longer-lived radionuclides.

Unfortunately, not all patients consistently give high bone/background ratios because incomplete tagging of the polyphosphate with the technetium moiety allows free technetium to be distributed within the tissues. These problems arise mainly from the presence of oxidizing agents or unsuitable chain lengths of polyphosphate.

Tc 99m DIPHOSPHONATE

Tc 99m diphosphonate has many of the properties associated with Tc 99m polyphosphate. Ethane-1-hydroxy-1, 1-diphosphonate (EHDP) has been shown to chemisorb specifically to bone, particularly to newly formed bone surfaces.

A number of advantages attributed to Tc 99m diphosphonate relate to its stability. The diphosphonate does not appear to be degraded by the body. Also, although the percentage of activity accumulating in bone is comparable with the two agents, urinary clearance of the unfixed free portion is greater for Tc 99m diphosphonate than

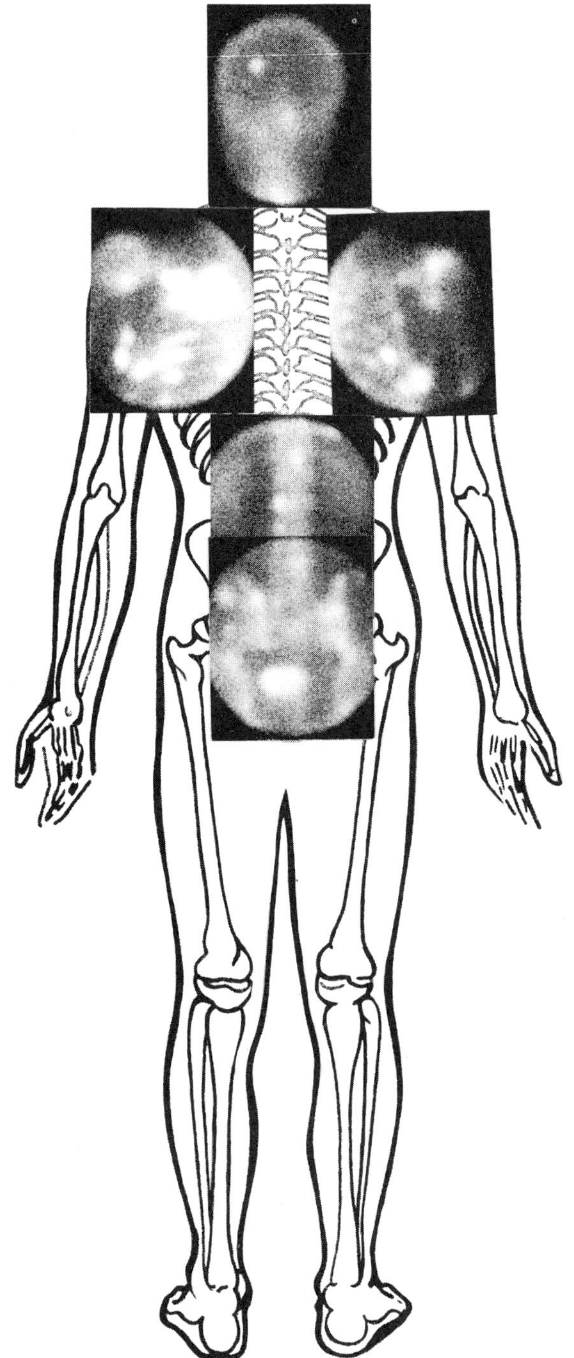

Figure 9-3 *Multiple metastases to bone from primary carcinoma of prostate. Study done with Tc 99m diphosphonate on Anger scintillation camera.*

Indications for Bone Scanning

- Neoplastic disease
- Trauma
- Aseptic Necrosis
- Inflammatory disease
- Metabolic disorder

for polyphosphate, so that soft tissue activity is significantly lower (Fig 9-3).

Indications and Application

Bone scanning has an important role in the diagnosis and evaluation of neoplastic disease, trauma, aseptic necrosis, inflammatory disease, and various metabolic disorders. Specific applications are outlined in Table 9-1.

DIAGNOSIS OF NEOPLASTIC DISEASE

Bone scanning can be used in children to detect primary bone tumors and to differentiate between malignant and benign tumors. Diagnosis is based on the relative intensity of radionuclide uptake in the sus-

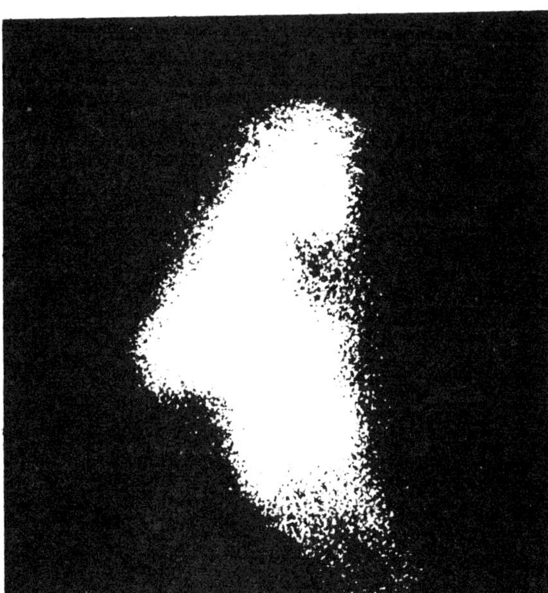

Figure 9-4 *Osteogenic sarcoma. Polyphosphate scan shows uptake in lower femur and upper tibia in 11-year-old patient.*

Table 9-1. Indications for and Application of Bone Scanning

Neoplastic disease
- Diagnosis
  - Detection of primary bone tumor
  - Differentiation of benign from malignant bone tumors
  - Demonstration of spread of bony tumor
  - Localization of lesion following complaint of bone pain
  - Detection of bone invasion by adjacent tumor
  - Differentiation of bone from intracerebral metastases
  - Detection of early metastatic lesions
- Selection of therapy
  - Planning radiotherapy portals
  - Selection of additional forms of therapy
  - Selection of bone biopsy site for confirmation of clinical diagnosis of malignancy with metastases when primary tumor is occult
  - Definition of level for amputation of extremity or for radiotherapy of primary tumor
- Evaluation of response of skeletal metastases to therapy
- Trauma
  - Estimation of age of fracture of axial skeleton
  - Differentiation of pathologic from traumatic fracture
  - Detection of basal skull fracture
  - Detection of impending fracture in multiple myeloma
- Aseptic necrosis
  - Inflammatory bone disease
- Bone islands
- Metabolic disorders

pected lesion compared with the epiphyses of the long bones (Fig 9-4). An accuracy of 92% has been reported.[31]

The procedure can also demonstrate the spread of a bony tumor, either to the skeletal system (eg, Ewing's sarcoma) or to the viscera or soft tissue (eg, osteogenic sarcoma).[33-35]

When a patient known to harbor a malignant tumor complains of bone pain, scanning can demonstrate metastases which may be responsible. If scanning does not reveal bone metastases, another cause for the pain should be sought. Scanning can also evidence metastatic bone lesions that are not painful and that would otherwise not be detected,[29] and it can demonstrate occult invasion of bone by an adjacent tumor, usually carcinoma of the oral cavity, head, or neck.[26,27] The procedure can show whether a tumor metastatic to the cranium involves the bone or the brain.[28]

Bone scanning is more sensitive than roentgenography for detecting early metastatic bone lesions.

Bone scanning is a more sensitive method than roentgenography for detecting early metastatic bone lesions.[4-8] For roentgenographic visualization, such a lesion must be larger than 1.5 cm in diameter and must be demineralized more than 50%.[9,10] Three stages of metastatic bone lesions can be identified:

- Stage 1: Scan shows increased radionuclide concentration indicative of new bone formation; roentgenogram does not show the new bone.
- Stage 2: Both scan and roentgenogram are showing positive evidence of mixed bone destruction and reactive bone formation.
- Stage 3: Scan shows no evidence of reactive bone formation; roentgenogram shows a dense sclerotic lesion which is inactive.

Stage 1 is characteristic of an early lesion; new bone deposition is too small to be visualized as increased density on the x-ray film, but increased uptake of radioactivity by the new bone is detectable by scanning. Stage 2 is characteristic of older lesions, and Stage 3 is one pattern displayed by metastases so old that the new bone has matured and new bone formation has decreased, so that scanning shows no abnormality while the x-ray film records a dense lesion.

Rate of accuracy Since most destructive bone metastases have an associated reactive component,[12] about 95% are detected by scanning. In only about 5% of such patients does the x-ray film show radiolucencies while bone scan results are normal. In 10% to 52% of patients with neoplasms of the lung, prostate, breast, head, or neck, bone scanning shows evidence of metastases while the roentgenographic appearance of the bones is normal.[4-6,16-20] In 10% to 70% of patients with lymphomatous disease, the same discrepancy occurs.[6,21-23] In addition, while 45% to 60% of patients show evidence of metastases on both roentgenograms and scans, a third of these have further abnormalities revealed by the scan but not the roentgenogram.[6,18]

False-negative bone scans are occasionally associated with multiple myeloma, breast carcinoma, anaplastic tumor, and indolent tumor such as thyroid carcinoma.[7,13]

SELECTION AND EVALUATION OF TREATMENT FOR NEOPLASTIC DISEASE

Bone scanning can delineate the region affected by malignant disease and enhance the accuracy of radiotherapy application.[24]

The procedure is also useful in determining whether phosphorus 32 therapy will benefit a particular patient with bone metastases from prostatic cancer. ^{32}P therapy is more likely to be successful if scanning indicates reactive bone to which the radioactive isotope will be attracted.[25]

When bone biopsy is contemplated to confirm a clinical diagnosis of metastatic malignancy from an occult primary tumor, bone scanning is a valuable aid in selecting the site for biopsy. Similarly, scanning can define the proper level for extremity amputation or for the application of radiotherapy in a patient with a primary bone tumor.[24,32]

In advanced bone cancer, scanning provides a quick, reliable means of evaluating tumor response to therapy.

In advanced bone cancer, scanning provides a guide and reliable means of evaluating the tumor's response to therapy. If response is lacking, alternate treatment can be promptly tried and in turn evaluated.[16,29,30]

EVALUATION OF TRAUMA

Bone scanning allows estimation of the age of fractures of the axial skeleton—information sometimes needed for medicolegal purposes. Compression fractures of the vertebrae display increased radionuclide uptake as early as five days and as late as 19 months following insult.[36,37]

Basal skull fracture, notoriously difficult to detect by roentgenography, can sometimes be confirmed or denied by the additional evidence of bone scanning.[38]

The procedure is useful in differentiating pathologic from traumatic bone fractures. If scanning indicates additional areas of increased radionuclide uptake, pathologic fracture due to metastatic carcinoma should be suspected. Similarly, scanning can warn of impending fracture in a patient with multiple myeloma[39] or osteoporosis.

DIAGNOSIS OF ASEPTIC NECROSIS

Bone scanning offers a means for early diagnosis of aseptic necrosis—before gross structural changes detectable by roentgenography have occurred. Early treatment may prevent serious damage.[40,41]

DETECTION OF INFLAMMATORY BONE DISEASE

Bone scanning can detect evidence of tuberculosis, osteomyelitis, ankylosing spondylitis, and mastoiditis[42-45] at an earlier stage than can be identified by roentgeno-

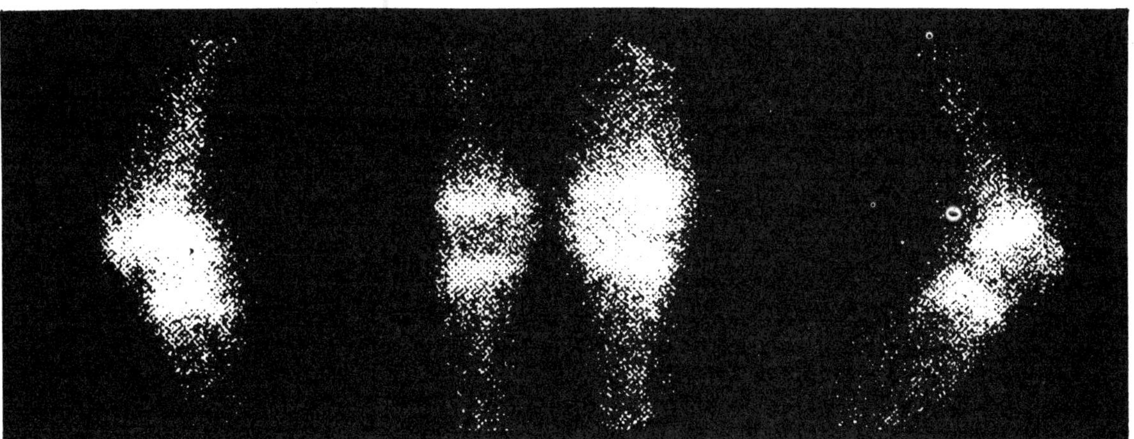

Figure 9-5 *Spread of septic arthritis of left knee to involve lower end of femur and upper end of tibia. Study done with strontium 87m.*

graphy (Fig 9-5). The procedure is also useful to evaluate response to therapy and to detect recurrence of the inflammatory process.

IDENTIFICATION OF BONE ISLANDS

Differentiation of a bone island from a metastatic lesion is difficult by roentgenography. Since a bone island does not concentrate the radionuclide, bone scanning can facilitate diagnosis.

EVALUATION OF METABOLIC DISORDERS

Bone scanning is a useful adjunct in the evaluation of the therapeutic response of such disorders as Paget's disease,[46] transient osteoporosis,[47,48] and renal osteodystrophy. Scanning can detect such conditions as osteoarthritis, fibrous dysplasis, hyperostosis frontalis interna, and eosinophilic granuloma.

Summary

Abnormal uptake of a bone-scanning agent is based on a disturbance of bone mineral metabolism. A bone scan that indicates such a disturbance is not pathognomonic of any specific disease; it merely records the dynamic state of the bone. Correlation of data obtained from roentgenography, clinical and laboratory examination, and bone scanning can suggest the nature of the bone lesion.

Bone scanning alone is rarely diagnostic. With data from roentgenography and clinical and laboratory evaluations, it can suggest the nature of the lesion.

References

1. O'Mara RE, Subramian G: Experimental agents for skeletal imaging. *Semin Nucl Med* 2:38, 1972.
2. Spencer RP, Lange RC, Treves S: Use of ^{135m}Ba and ^{131}Ba as bone scanning agents. *J Nucl Med* **12**:216, 1971.
3. Subramanian G, McAfee JG, Bell EG, et al: $^{99}{}_{m}$Tc labeled polyphosphate as a skeletal imaging agent. *Radiology* **102**:701, 1972.
4. Sklaroff DM, Charkes ND: Bone metastases from breast cancer at the time of radical mastectomy. *Surg Gynecol Obstet* **127**:763, 1968.
5. Sklaroff DM, Charkes ND: Early detection of bone lesions by photoscanning with radioactive strontium. *Cancer* **20**:734, 1967.
6. DeNardo GL, Jacobson SJ, Raventos A: ^{85}Sr bone scans in neoplastic disease. *Semin Nucl Med* **2**:18, 1972.
7. French RJ, McCready VR: The use of ^{18}F for bone scanning. *Br J Radiol* **40**:655, 1967.
8. Blaufox M, Ganatra R, Bender MA: ^{18}F—fluoride for bone imaging. *Semin Nucl Med* **2**:31, 1972.
9. Bachman AL, Sproul EE: Correlation of radiographic and autopsy findings in suspected metastases in the spine. *Bull NY Acad Med* **31**:146, 1955.
10. Edelstyn GA, Gillespie PJ, Grebell FS: The radiological demonstration of osseous metastasis: Experimental observations. *Clin Radiol* **18**:158, 1967.
11. Charkes ND, Young I, Sklaroff DM: The pathologic basis of the strontium bone scan. *JAMA* **206**:2482, 1968.
12. Milch RA, Changus GW: Response of bone to tumor invasion. *Cancer* **9**:340, 1956.
13. Charkes ND, Sklaroff DM, Young I: A critical analysis of strontium bone scanning for detection of metastatic cancer. *J Roentgenol* **96**:647, 1966.
14. Krishnamurthy GT, Walsh C, Winston MA, et al: Comparison of fluorine-18 bone studies obtained with rectilinear scanner and scintillation camera equipped with high-energy diverging collimator. *Radiology* May, 365, 1972.
15. Weber DA, Greenberg EJ, et al: Kinetics of radionuclides used for bone studies. *J Nucl Med* **10**:8, 1969.
16. Galasko CS: Skeletal metastases and mammary cancer. *Ann R Coll Surg Engl* **50**:3, 1972.
17. Rubin P, Ciccio S: Status of bone scanning for bone metastases in breast cancer. *Cancer* **24**:1338, 1969.
18. Milner TH, Maynard CD, Cowan RJ: Evaluation of strontium-85 bone scans and roentgenograms in 100 patients. *Arch Surg* **103**:371, 1971.
19. Rubin P: Cancer of the urogenital tract–prostatic cancer. Comment: The detection of occult metastatic cancer by radioactive bone scans. *JAMA* **210**:1079, 1969.
20. Roy RR, Nathan BE, et al: ^{18}Fluorine total body scans in patients with carcinoma of the prostate. *Br J Urol* **43**:58, 1971.

21. Harbert JC, Ashburn WL: Radiostrontium bone scanning in Hodgkin's disease. *Cancer* **22**:58, 1968.
22. Weber WG, DeNardo GL, Bergin JJ: Scintiscanning in malignant lymphomatous involvement of bone. *Arch Intern Med* **121**:433, 1968.
23. Dworkin HJ, Filmanowicz EV: Radiofluoride scanning of bone for reticulum cell sarcoma: Early detection of bone involvement. *JAMA* **198**:985, 1966.
24. Schmidt J: Use of scintigraphy for diagnosis and case control during radiotherapy of bone tumors. *Strahlentherapie* **141**:69, 1971.
25. Maxfield WS, Watson JD Jr: Strontium-85 bone scans as an aid in the selection of patients for phosphorus-32 therapy of skeletal metastasis. *J Nucl Med* **8**:390, 1967.
26. Vera R, Mineiro L, et al: Determination of occult invasion of bone by adjacent tumors. *Radiology* **101**:125, 1971.
27. Mashberg A, Strauss H, et al: Use of scintillation scanning for the early detection of bone involvement by squamous cell carcinoma of the oral mucosa: Preliminary report. *J Am Dent Assoc* **79**:1151, 1969.
28. Tow DE: Differentiation of brain and bone tumors with combined radionuclide technique. *Semin Nucl Med* **1**:85, 1971.
29. Galasko CS, Doyle FH: The role of scintigraphy in the assessment of response to therapy of skeletal metastases from mammary cancer. *Br J Surg* **57**:859, 1970.
30. Kampffmeyer HG, Dworkin H, Carr EA Jr: The effect of drug therapy on the uptake of radioactive fluorine by osseous metastases. *Clin Pharmacol Ther* **8**:647, 1967.
31. Samuels LD: Diagnosis of malignant bone disease with strontium-87m scans. *Can Med Assoc J* **104**:411, 1971.
32. Komitowski D, Potryn A, Wojciechowski J: Histolophathologieczne badania przydatnosci Strontu-85 dla okreslenia rozleglosci nacieku nowotoworowego miesakow kosci. *Chir Narzadow Ruchu Ortop Pol* **33**:537, 1968.
33. Schall GL, Zeigler L, et al: Uptake of ^{85}Sr by osteosarcoma metastatic to lung. *J Nucl Med* **12**:131, 1971.
34. Schall GL, Larson SM, De Lellis R: Pathogenesis of the positive bone scan and its implications for the detection of metastatic osteosarcomas. *J Surg Oncol* 3:673, 1971.
35. Samuel LD: Lung scanning with Sr-87m in metastatic osteosarcoma. *Am J Roentgenol Radium Ther Nucl Med* **104**:766, 1968.
36. Affram PA, Lindberg L: External counting of ^{85}Sr in vertebral fractures. *J Bone Joint Surg* **50**-A:563, 1968.
37. Flipse RC, Gilson AJ, Hall MF: Sequential studies of vertebral trauma employing strontium-85. *J Nucl Med* **7**:351, 1966.
38. Rosenthal L: The use of strontium-85 for the detection of bone lesions. *J Can Assoc Radiol* **15**:53, 1964.
39. Charkes ND, Durant J, Barry W: Sequential strontium-87m bone scans in multiple myeloma. *J Nucl Med* **9**:308, 1968.
40. Crutchlow WP: Sr-85 scintimetry of the hip in osteoarthritis and osteonecrosis. *Am J Roentgenol Radium Ther Nucl Med* **109**:803, 1970.
41. Cameron RB: Strontium-85 scintimetry in nontraumatic necrosis of the femoral head. *Clin Orthop* **65**:243, 1969.
42. Dymling JF, Wendenberg B: External counting of ^{85}Sr and ^{47}Ca in localized bone infections. *Acta Orthop Scand* 36:8, 1965.
43. Fellander M, Lindberg L: Clinical use of radiostrontium in evaluation of spondylitis. *J Bone Joint Surg (Am)* **48**:1585, 1966.
44. Harma R, Rekonen A, Suurkari SO: Uptake of radioactive strontium (Sr-85) in inflamed mastoid process. *Acta Otolaryngol (Stockh)* **71**:34, 1971.
45. Webb J, Collins LT, Southwell PB, et al: Fluorine-18 isotope scans in the early diagnosis of sacroilitis. *Med J Aust* **2**:1270, 1971.
46. Klein EW, Lung RR: Strontium-85 photoscanning in Paget's disease: With comments on several other skeletal problems. *Am J Roentgenol Radium Ther Nucl Med* **92**:195, 1964.
47. Hunder GG, Kelly PJ: Bone scans in transient osteoporosis. *Ann Intern Med* **75**:134, 1971.
48. O'Mara RE, Pinals RS: Bone scanning in regional migrating osteoporosis: Case report. *Radiology* **97**:579, 1970.
49. Francis MD: Inhibition of calcium hydroxyapatite crystal growth by polyphosphonates and polyphosphates. *Calcif Tissue Res* 3:151–162, 1969.
50. Yano Y, McRae Y, Anger HO: Technetium-99m labeled stannous ethane-1-hydroxy-11-diphosphonate: A new bone scanning agent. *J Nucl Med* **14**:73, 1973.

Radionuclide scanning is a safe, reliable procedure for plancental localization. Radioimmunoassays can detect abnormal hormone levels that warn of fetal distress and can monitor hormone levels that indicate ovarian function.

10
The Reproductive System

Alex A. Bezjian

Nuclear Medicine in Obstetrics and Gynecology

Dangers

Radioactive isotopic scanning in obstetrics has not paralleled the rapid progress of nuclear procedures in other medical fields. In the pregnant woman radioactive isotopes, either for diagnostic or therapeutic purposes, have been employed cautiously and reluctantly because of the danger of radiation damage to the fetus caused by passage of the radionuclide from the maternal to the fetal circulation through the placenta. It is generally believed[1] that as the mechanism of placental transfer does not attain full development before the 50th day of life, true radioactive contamination cannot occur before that time. Fortunately by the 50th day the embryo has already passed the two most sensitive developmental phases—the primordial organ and organogenesis phases.

Sternberg[1] reviewed the effect on the human fetus of contamination with different radionuclides. Iodine 131 administered in therapeutic doses after the 12th week of gestation can produce a severe and irreversible glandular destruction, exophthalmos, and anencephaly. Before the third month of gestation (ie, prior to the onset of thyroid function in the fetus) the ^{131}I is distributed mainly in the fetal liver, gut, brain, and muscle, and the distribution pattern dilutes the isotope and reduces the risk of radiation damage to the thyroid. Liver scanning with colloidal gold Au 198 or colloidal sulfide Tc 99m may be safely performed during pregnancy as these substances do not cross the placental barrier. Labeled rose bengal used for dynamic studies and ^{197m}Hg used for kidney and brain scanning also remain confined to the maternal compartment and thus are safe to use.

Pancreas scanning with selenomethionine Se 75 is hazardous during pregnancy as about 1.5% of the radioactive material injected intravenously crosses the placenta and accumulates in the fetus. The same applies to the in vivo uptake tests using labeled iron (ie, determination of red cell volume, red cell survival time, and iron-binding capacity in serum), as iron is freely transferred to the fetus and has a long biologic half-life. Bone scanning with carbon 47 and strontium 85 is forbidden during pregnancy as these elements cross the placenta freely and are readily taken up by the fetal skeletal system.

Uses

The most common use of radionuclide scanning in obstetrics today is for placental

The radiation dose to the fetus from any nuclear placentography procedure is 1/50 to 1/100 of that produced by x-ray pelvimetry.

localization. Regardless of technique and radionuclide used, the dose of radiation to the fetus from any nuclear placentography procedure is about 1/50 to 1/100 of that produced by a single roentgenographic examination.

In vitro radioimmunoassay techniques are increasingly being applied to the measurement of most of the reproductive hormones. Some procedures are still confined to experimental laboratories, but others are presently available to hospital laboratories in the form of kits produced by pharmaceutical companies.

Placental Localization with Radioactive Isotopes

Indications

Recent advances in obstetrics have increased the need for accurate localization of the placenta. Localization is important, for example, when amniocentesis is to be performed and when vaginal bleeding occurs in the third trimester.

AMNIOCENTESIS

Amniocentesis is frequently done to obtain a sample of the amniotic fluid for estimation of fetal maturity and detection of Rh incompatibility. Previous knowledge of the placental implantation site prevents transplacental insertion of the needle and minimizes the danger of partial placental separation, fetomaternal transfusion, or both.

THIRD TRIMESTER BLEEDING

Although third trimester bleeding occurs in about 3% of pregnancies, the incidence of placenta previa is only 0.4%. Vaginal bleeding is easily managed in a patient with a mature baby, as gentle vaginal examination provides the final diagnosis and a double setup in the operating room allows prompt delivery if necessary. It is in the patient with a small baby that knowledge of the placental site is useful. The patient with placenta previa is kept on strict bed rest, while the woman without placenta previa need not follow such a strict course.

Methods

Current methods for placental localization are (1) plain film roentgenography, (2) amniography, (3) pelvic angiography, (4) thermography, (5) ultrasonic placentography, and (6) isotopic placentography. The two most commonly used are ultrasonic and isotopic placentography.

X-ray placentography gives reliable results in 95% to 97% of patients.[2] Soft tissue roentgenography gives poor results in polyhydramnios, multiple gestation, and transverse lie of the fetus, and its reliability decreases with decreasing gestational age. Arteriography, on the other hand, has a diagnostic reliability of 97% regardless of the length of gestation.[3] However, arteriography is a tedious procedure and, like soft tissue placentography, exposes the fetus to x-radiation.

In comparing isotopic placentography with amniography, Drukhen et al[4] concluded that the former is preferable and that amniography should be used only when isotopic placentography is not available.

Therography, most authors agree, is not a sufficiently reliable method for placental localization.[5]

Ultrasonography is harmless to the fetus[10] and its accuracy in placental localization compares favorably with that of isotopic scanning. Aiers et al,[11] in comparing ultrasonic and isotopic scanning for placental localization, concluded that the ultrasonic technique has the advantages of (1) defining accurately the margins of the placenta and the extent to which it covers the uterine cervix, and (2) avoiding radiation exposure to the fetus and mother. However, localization of a posterior placenta previa is sometimes difficult because of the overlying fetal presenting part, and isotopic scanning is helpful in these cases.

Radiopharmaceuticals

In 1950 Browne and Veall[12] described a radioactive isotopic method using sodium 24 for the diagnosis of placenta previa. Their technique was based on the principle that since the placenta is a vascular, space-occupying organ that represents a pool of maternal blood, any radioactive tracer injected intravenously produces an area of increased radioactivity over the placental site. Weinberg et al[13] in 1957 used human serum albumin (HSA) I 131. Since then, HSA I 132, and HSA 1 125, chromium 51, technetium 99m, and indium 113m have been investigated.

> Since the placenta is a vascular, space-occupying organ that represents a pool of maternal blood, an intravenously injected tracer produces an area of increased radioactivity over the placental site.

Radionuclides for Placental Localization

- Iodine 131
- Iodine 125
- Chromium 51
- Technetium 99m
- Indium 113m

IODINATED SERUM ALBUMIN

Both HSA I 131 and HSA I 125 dissociate into the free form. Thus every patient receiving either isotope should be given iodine; either Lugol's solution (orally) or 100 mg of sodium iodide (intravenously) to block the maternal and fetal thyroid. Lugol's solution should be administered for five days after the examination. HSA I 131 is considered superior to HSA I 125 because it is a pure gamma emitter. However, both isotopes must be given in small doses (5μCi) as their half-lives are 8.2 and 60 days respectively.

HSA I 132 can be given in a dose of 50 μCi to 100 μCi without thyroid blocking because its half-life is short (2.5 hours). It emits beta radiation, however. Only multiple-point counting can be done with the iodine preparations.

CHROMIUM 51

^{51}Cr has a half-life of 27.8 days and can be given in a 20 μCi dose. It can be tagged to either albumin or red blood cells. When tagged to erythrocytes, red blood cell volume can be determined simultaneously.

TECHNETIUM 99m

^{99m}Tc is a pure gamma emitter, has a six-hour half-life, and can be given in a dose of 500 μCi to 1000 μCi. A scanning rather than a point-count technique is possible, the quality of the image is better than with iodine preparations, and the radiation to the patient is less. Since technetium concentrates in the thyroid glands of mother and fetus, preliminary preparation with potassium perchloride is required. Since

Table 10-1. Radiation Dose from Placentography

	Relative radiation dose (mrad)		
Procedure	**Maternal ovaries**	**Fetal thyroid gland**	**Fetal gonads**
Soft tissue roentgenography	1000	1000	1000
HSA I 131, 5 μCi (with Lugol's preparation)	15	4900	7
Technetium 99m, 1 mCi (with $KClO_4$ preparation)	13	5	14
Indium 113m	10	8	8
Background radiation in one year	100	100	100

technetium is excreted in the urine it can accumulate in the bladder and interfere with interpretation of the scan.

INDIUM 113m

This too is a pure gamma emitter, has a 1.7-hour half-life, and can be given in a dose of 500 μCi to 1000 μCi. A scanning technique is utilized, and the quality of the scan is comparable to that obtained with technetium. Urinary excretion of indium is insignificant and does not interfere with scan interpretation.

Radiation Dosage

The radiation dose to both mother and fetus from isotopic placentography is small and, as mentioned earlier, is about 1/50 to 1/100 of the dose delivered to the fetus by x-ray pelvimetry (Table 10-1).

Procedures

MULTIPLE-POINT COUNTING

The abdomen of the gravid patient is marked off into 9 or 12 anatomic areas and the thyroid gland is blocked with ten drops of Lugol's solution given orally. After intravenous injection of 5 μCi of albumin I 131 about two minutes is allowed for the tracer to mix in the circulating blood. A scintillation probe is then placed over the center of each of the 9 or 12 areas and the radioactivity is measured in each. Radioactivity is also measured over the xiphoid before and after the uterus is scanned; this is used as a reference point as count rates over the uterus vary widely among patients. The recorded radioactivity over the xiphoid is arbitrarily designated to represent 100% and the counts per minute in each abdominal area are then expresed as a percentage of the counts recorded over the xiphoid. The entire procedure requires about 15 minutes.

SCANNING

The patient is placed on a scanning table in the supine position and 500 μCi to 1000 μCi of either albumin Tc 99m or gelatin In 113m is injected intravenously. These agents remain in the maternal vascular space. Immediately after the injection, scanning is started using a rectilinear scanner with a 5-inch sodium iodide crystal and a high-resolution focused collimator. The positions of the symphysis pubis, umbilicus, and the fundus of the uterus are marked. The abdomen is scanned from the level above the uterine fundus to about 3 or 4 cm below the level of the symphysis

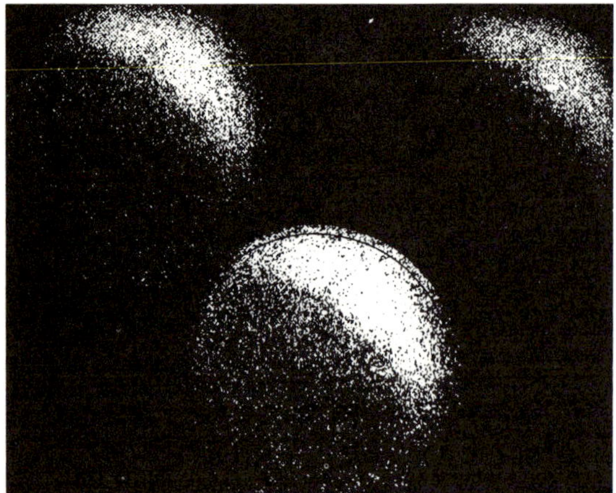

A

B

Figure 10-1 *Left fundal implantation of placenta visualized by scanning.* A. *In anterior view increased uptake of radioactivity is noted in area of uterine fundus, toward left.* B. *In left lateral view area of increased uptake of radioactivity at left of scan represents spleen and liver. Placenta is seen inferior and posterior to that area in fundus of uterus.*

pubis. Following the anterior view, a lateral is obtained with the detector placed on that side of the uterus where the anterior view shows the placenta to be lying. On both projections the placenta is visualized as an area of increased radioactivity (Fig 10-1). Total time for the procedure is 20 minutes with a scintillation camera, 50 minutes with a rectilinear scanner.

With this scanning technique, determination of the relation between the placenta and the internal cervical os is sometimes difficult, as the only point of reference used is the symphysis pubis, the relation of which to the uterine cervix varies from one patient to another. A marker consisting of 50 μCi of ^{99m}Tc (for patients studied with indium) or ^{113m}In (for patients studied with technetium) placed at the tip of a sealed polyethylene tube can be inserted into the posterior fornix of the vagina by the obstetrician to localize the cervical os. Care must be taken to avoid entering the cervical os. Estimated dose to the fetus from such a marker is 17 mrad at 2 cm and 0.03 mrad at 40 cm.

DYNAMIC IMAGING

Use of a diffusible agent such as sodium pertechnetate allows dynamic visualization of the placenta with the scintillation camera.

With the patient either standing or lying supine on the stretcher, the detector head of the Anger scintillation camera is placed over the pregnant uterus. Sodium pertechnetate Tc 99m (1 mCi) is rapidly injected intravenously as a bolus. Sequential scintophotographs are taken at two- to three-second intervals. The bolus is visualized within the abdominal aorta and subsequently noted to bifurcate at the femoral level. The placental bed is then seen to be perfused and its relation is noted to certain standard anatomic structures (symphysis pubis, umbilicus, and xiphoid) which have been premarked with a small quantity of radionuclide. Although the usual technique is to obtain a series of 30-second exposures after injection of the radionuclide bolus, our results have been more satisfactory with two- to three-second exposures. The scintophotographs obtained within the first 30 seconds of the study are much more informative than the ones obtained after that period. The placental bed is first seen within 10 to 15 seconds after injection of

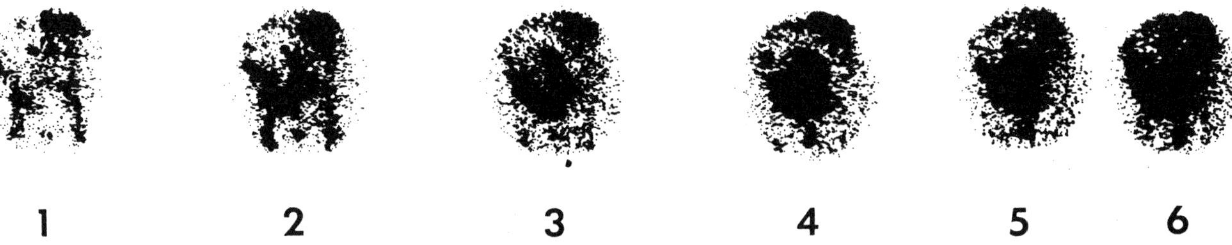

Figure 10-2 *Low-lying placenta on right side of uterus visualized by dynamic imaging. Serial scintiphotographs at three-second intervals starting at 12 seconds after bolus injection. Note femoral vessels seen at 12 seconds and gradual visualization of placenta in right lower part of uterus in subsequent scintiphotographs.*

the radionuclide and is well outlined within the following 10 to 15 seconds, making a total of 30 seconds (Fig 10-2). After that the pertechnetate usually diffuses through the uterine vasculature, making definite identification of the placenta more difficult.

Once the dynamic imaging is completed, a static view is obtained by accumulating 300,000 to 400,000 counts and taking anterior and left or right lateral scintophotographs of the uterus to determine whether the placenta lies anteriorly or posteriorly within the uterine cavity.

Radioimmunoassay

Clinical Use

Since its introduction by Yalow and Berson 13 years ago, radioimmunoassay has probably had a greater impact than almost any other single development in the history of gynecologic endocrinology. Today this technique is utilized to measure pituitary and chorionic gonadotropins, the ovarian steroids, human placental lactogen, oxytocin, and prostaglandins.

Hormones Identified by Radioimmunoassay

- Human placental lactogen (HPL)
- Human chorionic gonadotropin (HCG)
- Estrogens
- Progesterone
- Follicle-stimulating hormone (FSH)
- Luteotropic hormone (LH)

However, the transition of radioimmunoassay from the research laboratory to routine clinical application has been slow, owing as much to financial as to operational obstacles. Some assays are required on a regular and large-scale basis, while others are only infrequently requested for clinical use. For each assay, antigens must be labeled isotopically every two to eight weeks, and specific reagents must be produced. Since results are usually wanted quickly, accumulating requests and running the procedure once a week is not feasible. Small hospitals have therefore been forced to use the services of a centralized laboratory. Recently developed kits containing both the specific antibodies and the reagents allow these hospitals to provide daily radioimmunoassay services of their own.

Radiommunoassays are used in obstetrics and gynecology to determine:

- Human placental lactogen (HPL)
- Human chorionic gonadotropin (HCG)
- Estrogen
- Progesterone
- Follicle-stimulating hormone (FSH)
- Luteotropic hormone (LH)

Procedures have also been developed for prostaglandin F[16] and for oxytocin[17] determinations, but at present these two assays are not used clinically.

HPL DETERMINATION

HPL, also known as purified placental protein (PPP) and human chorionic somatomammotropin (HCS), is structurally similar to human growth hormone (HGH) and is synthesized and stored in the syncytiotrophoblasts of the placenta. It is secreted into the intervillous space of the maternal blood pool, and very little reaches the fetal compartment.[18]

Determination of serum HPL allows detection of threatened abortion, hypertensive toxemia, intrauterine growth retardation, and signs of fetal distress—all conditions that affect fetal survival.

In normal pregnancy the serum HPL level is detectable after only four or five weeks of gestation and gradually rises until about 35 weeks. After that, values of 7.7 ± 0.2 μg/ml persist until delivery (Fig 10-3). After 30 weeks of gestation, an HPL value less than 4 μg/ml constitutes evidence of fetal danger.[19] A falling or stationary HPL level together with bleeding or cramping usually indicates threatened abortion.[20] A low HPL level is often associated with toxemia and may herald fetal death on this basis.[18,19] Intrauterine growth retardation is often manifested by a low HPL level.[21] While no correlation exists between HPL level and fetal heart rate patterns or five-minute Apgar scores, there is a significant relation between low HPL

A low HPL level is often associated with toxemia and may herald fetal death.

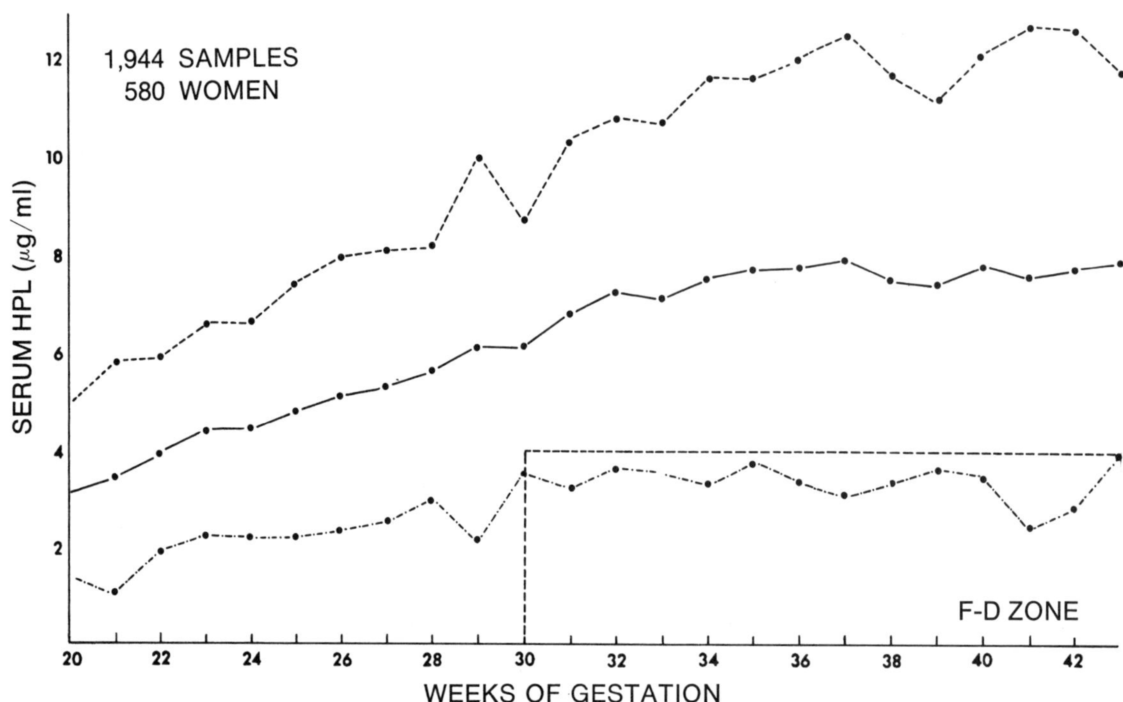

Figure 10-3 *Mean (± 2 SD) curve for serum HPL in normal late pregnancy. (From Spellacy WN:* Clin Obstet Gynecol ***16****:301, 1973.)*

value and meconium passage in vertex presentations and between low HPL level and the one-minute Apgar score.[22,23] Neither diabetes mellitus nor Rh sensitization is associated with a consistently abnormal serum HPL value.

HPL levels in amniotic fluid have been studied in all the above mentioned conditions, but the value of amniotic fluid HPL as a clinical tool remains to be established.

HCG DETERMINATION

Determination of plasma HCG is the most important test for the diagnosis, treatment, and follow-up of patients with trophoblastic disease. Radioimmunossay is a more rapid

> **Determination of plasma HCG is the most important test for trophoblastic disease.**

and sensitive method than bioassay or agglutination-inhibition tests. Levels as low as 4 to 5 mIu/ml of plasma can be detected. Several techniques are available, but differences in methodology and lack of an international reference standard for radioimmunoassay make comparative results difficult to interpret.[25]

Until recently, cross reactivity prevented differentiation between HCG and human luteinizing hormone HLH by radioimmunoassay techniques. Now Vaitukaitis et al[26] have developed a procedure that selectively measures HCG in samples containing both HLH and HCG. Furthermore, the specific HCG assay is sufficiently sensitive to measure plasma HCG levels even when these fall within the range of serum HLH levels observed in regularly cycling women. In plasma samples obtained from a patient undergoing chemotherapy for choriocarcinoma, HCG remained detectable at a time when urinary gonadotropin excretion determined by bioassay was within the range for normally menstruating women—a point at which chemotherapy would usually have been stopped (Fig 10-4).

In our institution the recommended protocol for follow-up of a patient with trophoblastic disease is:

- Plasma HCG is determined weekly
- When HCG level is undetectable, assay is repeated for two more consecutive weeks
- Plasma HCG is determined monthly for 6 to 12 months
- If patient remains disease-free, she is allowed to become pregnant after 6 to 12 months
- If HCG level increases or plateaus for two consecutive weeks, patient is reevaluated

ESTROGEN DETERMINATION IN PREGNANCY

Both plasma and urinary estrogen levels are known to increase with advancing pregnancy.[27] Though more than 20 estrogens have been identified in the human, the most frequently described during pregnancy are estrone, estradiol, and estriol. Since over 90% of the estrogen present in pregnancy is estriol or its conjugates, most clinical laboratory tests measure the total estrogen present rather than specific estrogens. These tests are relatively simple, inexpensive, and rapid, but are not specific.

Recently several radioimmunoassay procedures have been described for the measurement of urinary and plasma estrogens in general and estriol in particular.[29,30] These procedures are simple and rapid and their sensitivity is in the picogram range. The correlation between values obtained by radioimmunoassay and by gas-liquid chromatography is excellent,[31] However, the radioimmunoassay is so specific that it can be performed only on samples that

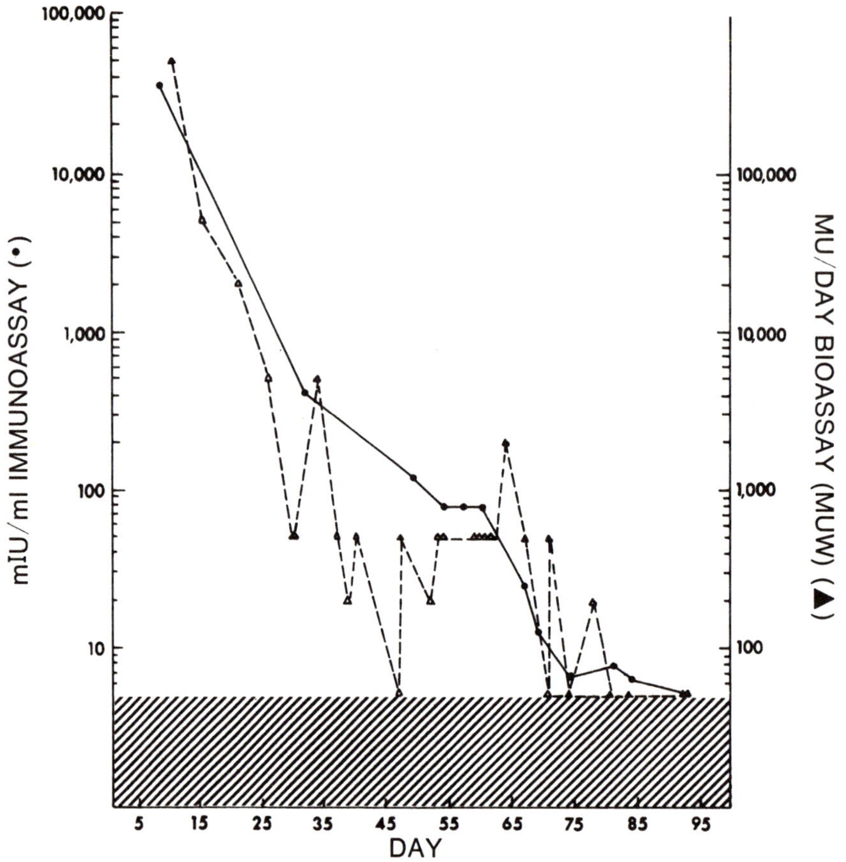

Figure 10-4 *Plasma HCG levels and daily gonadotropin excretion in patient undergoing therapy for gestational choriocarcinoma. Shaded area represents level below lower limit of HCG radioimmunoassay. (From Vaitukaitis J, Braunstein G, Ross G:* Am J Obstet Gynecol *113:756, 1972.)*

have been purified and the individual estrogens separated.

In normal pregnancy urinary estriol increases 1 mg every two weeks (4 mg at the 24th, 6 mg at the 28th, 8 mg at the 32nd, 10 mg at the 36th, and 12 mg at the 40th week). Any value below these can be considered abnormal if technical and iatrogenic influences have been eliminated.[32] Green et al[33] have shown that at term a 24-hour urinary estriol value less than 2 mg suggests that fetal death has occurred; a value greater than 4 mg but less than 12 mg is inconclusive; and a value greater than 12 mg suggests normality. A 50% reduction in the urinary estriol value is considered significant and suggests fetal distress.

Estriol determination in pregnancy is most helpful in detecting chronic distress states that cause placental insufficiency (ie, poor maternal nutrition, maternal vascular and renal disease, subacute and chronic toxemia). In toxemia, both low normal and significantly reduced levels of urinary estriol have been reported.[32]

In intrauterine fetal growth retardation, the urinary estrogen level is usually low, and as pregnancy advances does not rise as sharply as in normal pregnancy.[34] Prospective monitoring of urinary estrogen levels can assist in the determination of the optimum time for delivery of such an infant.

When diabetes mellitus is associated with pregnancy, urinary estrogen level is not always a reliable monitor of fetal well-being. Sudden fetal death can occur despite recent normal urinary estrogen levels.[35] Lundy et al[32] therefore recommend that women with overt diabetes be delivered at or before the 37th week of pregnancy and that prospective monitoring of urinary estrogen values be performed in the woman with gestational diabetes.

ESTROGEN DETERMINATION IN THE NONPREGNANT STATE

In the nonpregnant state, estradiol and estrone are the dominant circulating estrogens in the body, and radioimmunoassay procedures are presently available to measure each separately or together as total estrogens. These procedures allow rapid and accurate measurement of estrogens in the range of nanograms per 100 ml of plasma. Using this procedure, several investigators[36,37] have serially measured plasma estrogen, progesterone, and LH levels during the normal menstrual cycle. These studies have shed further light on the mechanism of ovarian function and ovulation. They have also shown no diurnal

Abnormally low urinary estriol levels identify chronic distress states that cause placental insufficiency.

variation in plasma estrogen level during a normal menstrual cycle,[38] and hence a blood sample for plasma estrogen determination can be obtained at any time during the day.

Serial determination of plasma estrogen levels is clinically useful to detect ovarian hypofunction, either primary or secondary to pituitary-hypothalamic failure. It is also useful to monitor estrogen levels following induction of ovulation and subsequent

Serial determination of plasma estrogen levels is clinically useful to detect ovarian hypofunction.

pregnancy in amenorrheic and anovulatory women. Fertility achieved by the sequential administration of human menopausal gonadotropin (HMG) and HCG is sometimes asociated with multiple fetuses, ovarian cyst formation, and ascites—all directly related to high estrogen levels.[39] Close monitoring of estrogen levels prior to HCG administration minimizes or prevents these effects of severe ovarian overstimulation.[40]

PROGESTERONE DETERMINATION

Plasma progesterone determination has today replaced urine pregnanediol measurement as a test for corpus luteum function. Several rapid and precise radioimmunoassay procedures are available for plasma progesterone measurement and have been widely used to study the physiology of ovulation and the function of the corpus luteum both in the nonpregnant and pregnant states. Serial plasma progesterone determinations can identify ovulation. The level rises substantially following ovulation, plateaus at 10 to 20 ng/ml, and falls to less than 1 ng/ml at the onset of menstruation (Fig 10-5).

GONADOTROPIN DETERMINATION

Radioimmunoassays for FSH and LH are replacing bioassays; they are more rapid and more sensitive, and can be performed on a larger scale. Their use has enhanced understanding of the normal menstrual cycle as well as menstrual abnormalities.

Gonadotropin assays are clinically useful in monitoring ovulation in a patient with irregular menses who desires pregnancy and in evaluating pituitary-hypothalamic function in an anovulatory patient.

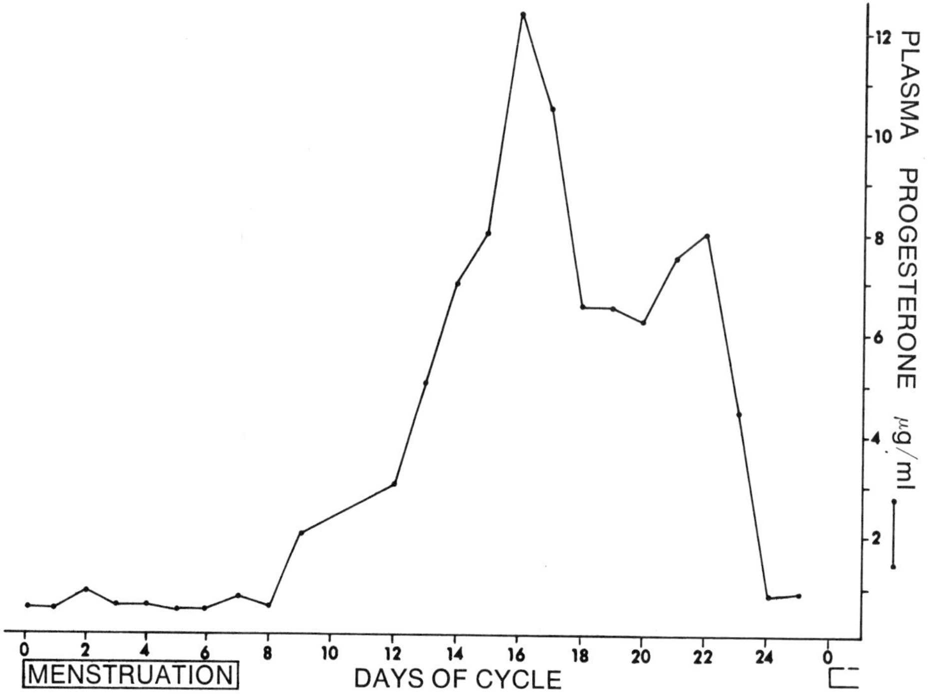

Figure 10-5 *Plasma progesterone levels in normal menstrual cycle measured by competitive protein-binding radioassay. (From Somerville BW:* Am J Obstet Gynecol ***111**:* *422, 1971.)*

At the midpoint of a normal menstrual cycle a sudden surge of both LH and FSH secretion occurs.[41] The serum LH level peaks 12 to 24 hours prior to ovulation.[42] This knowledge allows timing insemination in a patient with irregular menses who wishes to become pregnant.

Since the mechanism of ovulation depends on a delicate balance between the functions of the pituitary-hypothalamic unit and the ovary, any disruption in this balance can result in anovulation and menstrual disorders. It has been shown[42] that anovulation and secondary oligomenorrhea or amenorrhea can occur with low, normal, or high serum gonadotropin levels. Thus, in evaluating a patient with infertility or menstrual distrurbance, a knowledge of endocrine function is desirable.

For most anovulatory patients with no other signs of pituitary failure, clomiphene administration induces ovulation—as evidenced by basal body temperature, menstruation, plasma progesterone level, and plasma LH level between days 9 and 15 after clomiphene. In patients with sustained low gonadotropin and estrogen levels and no evidence of hypopituitarism who do not respond to clomiphene, further differentiation between pituitary and hypothalamic failure is indicated. The administration of LH-releasing factor will no doubt be the diagnostic test for such a differentiation in the future.

References

1. Sternberg J: Radiation risk in pregnancy. *Clin Obstet Gynecol* **16**:235, 1973.
2. Sanders B: Placentography by ultrasound. *Acta Obstet Gynecol Scand* **49**:179, 1970.
3. Borell U, Ferstrom I, Ohlson L: Diagnostic value of arteriography in cases of plascenta previa. *Am J Obstet Gynecol* **86**:535, 1963.
4. Drukhen B, Reynolds W, Orteg E, Hosey J: Pla-

cental localization. *Am J Obstet Gynec* **110**:9, 1971.
5. Reynolds WA, Ayers MA, Parker GM: Thermoplacentography. *Radiology* **19**:825, 1967.
6. Donald I: On launching a new diagnostic science. *Am J Obstet Gynecol* **103**:609, 1969.
7. Thompson J, Makowski E: Estimation of birth weight and gestational age. *Obstet Gynecol* **37**:44, 1971.
8. Gottesfeld K, Thompson HE, Holmes JH, et al: Ultrasonic placentography: A new method for placental localization. *Am J Obstet Gynecol* **96**:538, 1966.
9. Thompson H, Holmes J, Gottesfeld K, et al: Ultrasound as a diagnostic aid in diseases of the pelvis. *Am J Obstet Gynecol* **98**:472, 1967.
10. Bobrow M, Blackwell N, Nnrau A, et al: Absence of any observed effect of ultrasonic irradiation on human chromosomes. *J Obstet Gynaecol Br Commonw* **78**:730, 1971.
11. Aiers M, Evered DC, Smith AH: Placental localization by the use of ^{132}I-human serum albumin and by ultrasonic scanning. *J Obstet Gynaecol Br Commonw* **76**:220, 1969.
12. Browne JCM, Veall N: Method of locating the placenta in the intact uterus by means of radioactive sodium. *J Obstet Gynaecol Bri Emp* **57**:566, 1950.
13. Weinberg A, Rizzi J, McManus R, et al: Localization of the placental site by radioactive isotopes. *Obstet Gynecol* **9**:695, 1957.
14. Johnson P, Chao S, Reilly J: Placental imaging with ^{113m}In. *Radiology* **103**:359, 1972.
15. James AE, Strauss HW, Fischer K, et al: Placental imaging with ^{113m}In transferrin and ^{99m}Tc serum albumin. *Obstet Gynecol* **37**:602, 1971.
16. Caldwell B, Burstein S, Brock WA, et al: Radioimmunoassays of the F prostaglardin. *J Clin Endocrinol Metab* **33**:171, 1971.
17. Boyd NRH, Chard T: Human urine oxytocin levels during pregnancy and labor. *Am J Obstet Gynecol* **115**:827, 1973.
18. Spellacy WN: Human placental lactogen (HPL): The review of a protein hormone important to obstetrics and gynecology. *South Med J* **62**:1054, 1969.
19. Spellacy WN, Teoh ES, Buhi WC, et al: Value of human chorionic somatomammotropin in managing high risk pregnancies. *Am J Obstet Gynecol* **109**:588, 1971.
20. Spellacy WN: Human placental lactogen in high-risk pregnancy. *Clin Obstet Gynecol* **16**:298, 1973.
21. Vauna K, Driscoll SG, Emerson KJ, et al: Clinical and pathologic evaluation of serum immunoreactive human placental lactogen (IR-HPL) in abnormal pregnancy. *Obstet Gynecol* **38**:487, 1971.
22. Spellacy WN: *Clinical Significance of Human Placental Lactogen Measurements.* Fourth International Congress on Endocrinology. Amsterdam, Excerpta Medica, 1972.
23. Spellacy WN, Buhi WC, Birk SA, et al: Human placental lactogen levels and intrapartum fetal distress: Meconium stained amniotic fluid, fetal heart rate patterns with Apgar scores. *Am J Obstet Gynecol* **114**:803, 1972.
24. Taynor ML: Bioassay and immunoassay of human chorionic gonadotropin (HCG). *Clin Obstet Gynecol* **10**:303. 1967.
25. Varma K, Larraga L, Selenkow H: Radioimmunoassay of serum human chorionic gonadotropin during normal pregnancy. *Obstet Gynecol* **37**:10, 1971.
26. Vaitukaitis J, Braunstein G, Ross G: A radioimmunoassay which specifically measures human chorionic gonadotropin in the presence of human luteinizing hormone. *Am J Obstet Gynecol* **113**: 751, 1972.
27. Beischer NA, Brown JB: Studies in prolonged pregnancy. *Am J Obstet Gynecol* **103**:485, 1969.
28. Timonen S, Hirvonen E, Sokhanen R: Urinary volume and excretion of estrogens in late pregnancy. *Acta Endocrinol* **49**:393, 1965.
29. Goebelsmann U, Thornegeroft I, Nakimura R, et al: Estriol in pregnancy. *Am Obstet Gynecol* **112**: 802, 1972.
30. Tulchinsky D, Abraham G: Radioimmunoassay of plasmal estriol. *J Clin Endocrinol Metab* **33**:775, 1971.
31. Gurpide E, Giebenhaim N, Tseng L, et al: Radioimmunoassay for estrogens in human pregnancy urine, plasma and amniotic fluid. *Am J Obstet Gynecol* **109**:897, 1971.
32. Lundy L, Wu C, Lee S: Estrogen assessments in high risk pregnancy. *Clin Obstet Gynecol* **16**:279, 1973.
33. Greene JW, Smith K, Kyle CG: Use of urinary estriol in the management of pregnancies complicated by diabetes mellitus. *Am J Obstet Gynecol* **91**:684, 1965.
34. Klopper H: The assessment of feto-placental function by estriol assay. *Surgery* **27**:813, 1972.
35. Buscher NA, Brown JB: Current status of estrogen assays in obstetrics and gynecology. *Obstet Gynecol Surv* **27**:303, 1972.
36. Sommerville BW: Daily variation in plasma levels of progesterone and estradiol throughout the menstrual cycle. *Am J Obstet Gynecol* **111**:419, 1971.
37. Wu CH, Lundy LE, Lee SG: A rapid radioimmunoassay for plasma estrogen. *Am J Obstet Gynecol* **115**:169, 1973.
38. Baird DT, Guevara A: Concentration of unconjugated estrone and estriol in peripheral plasma in nonpregnant women throughout the menstrual cycle, castrate and postmenopausal women and in men. *J Clin Endocrinol Metab* **29**:149, 1969.
39. Taynor ML: Gonadotropin therapy. *JAMA* **203**: 362, 1968.
40. Karam KS, Taynor ML, Gerger MJ: Estrogen monitoring and the prevention of ovarian overstimulation during gonadotropin therapy. *Am J Obstet Gynecol* **115**:972, 1973.
41. Boon RC, Schalch DS, Lee LA, et al: Plasma gonadotropin secretory patterns in patients with functional menstrual disorders and Stein-Levanthal syndrome: Response to clomiphene treatment. *Am J Obstet Gynec* **112**:736, 1972.
42. Migata J, Taynor ML, Levesque L, et al: Timing of ovulation by a rapid luteinizing hormone assay. *Fertil Steril* **21**:748, 1970.

Triple scanning with Hg 197 chlormerodrin, I 131 orthohippuric acid, and Tc 99m pertechnetate allows localization and visualization of the kidneys and evaluation of renal function and blood flow.

11 The Renal System

Aldo N. Serafini

Renal Scintigraphy

This discussion is restricted to studies employing the triple renal scintigraphic technique performed with Hg 197 chlormerodrin, I 131 orthohippuric acid, and Tc 99m pertechnetate. These agents are characterized in Table 11-1.

Table 11-1. Characteristics of Radioactive Isotopes Used in Renal Scanning

Characteristic	^{197}Hg	^{99m}Tc	^{131}I
Dose	100–150μCi	15 mCi	400μCi
Half-life	2.7 days	6 hours	8 days
Energy	77 kev	140 kev	364 kev
% Abundance	118	90	82

A number of newer radiopharmaceuticals have low particulate radiations and shorter half-lives—characteristics that allow larger doses to be administered, increasing the available photon flux. Increased photon flux improves counting statistics, decreases duration of studies, and considerably reduces radiation exposure to the patients. These new materials include iron Tc 99m iron complex, Tc 99m DTPA, Yb 169 DTPA, In 113m DTPA.[5] Their increased commercial availability will make them agents of choice for renal scanning in the future.

Triple Scanning

Triple scanning combines the use of three different radionuclides to evaluate the functional and anatomical statue of the urinary system. Each radionuclide serves a specific purpose as outlined below. Together with the clinical and radiological data, it plays an important role in the evaluation of patients suffering from diseases of the urinary system.

The Triple Scanning Procedure

- Hg 197 Chlormerodrin
  - Kidney localization, visualization
  - Indirect assessment of renal function and blood flow
- I 131 Orthohippuric acid
  - Direct assessment of renal function
  - Indirect evaluation of renal vascular hypertension
- Tc 99m Pertechnetate
  - Kidney visualization
  - Evaluation of blood flow to specific lesion identified by other radionuclides
  - Evaluation of renovascular hypertension

Hg 197 chlormerodrin

This radionuclide is used to localize and image the kidneys (Fig 11-1). It concen-

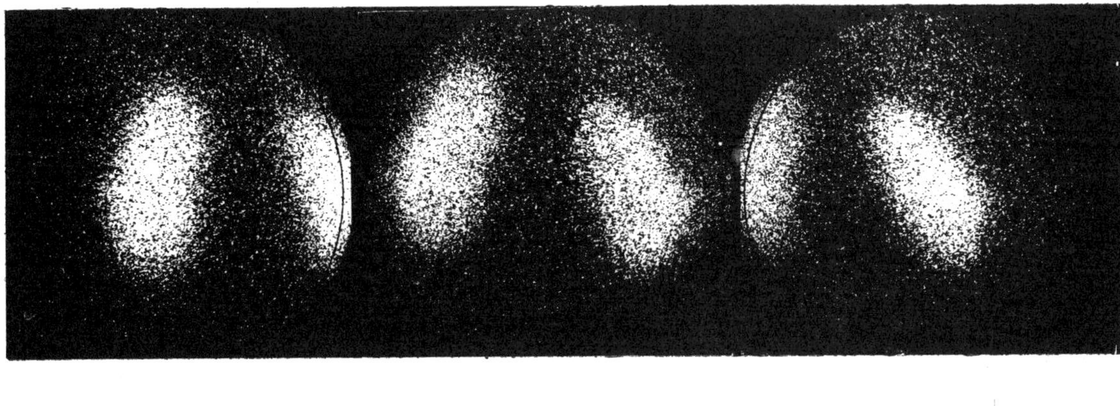

Figure 11-1 *Normal renal uptake and distribution of Hg 197 chlormerodrin. Left posterior oblique, posterior, and right posterior oblique views.*

trates in the proximal tubules by sulfhydryl binding and is temporarily stored and subsequently excreted. This behavior allows differentiation of areas of normal functioning tissue from areas of nonfunctioning tissue. In addition, the degree of accumulation of mercury within the kidneys provides an index of renal blood flow and renal function.[10] From 100 μCi to 150 μCi is injected intravenously, and imaging is started with either a rectilinear or a stationary imaging device approximately one hour later. In uremic patients the delay before scanning should be increased to enhance kidney visualization.

I 131 ORTHOHIPPURIC ACID

This agent is used to evaluate renal function. Since function depends on blood flow, one can also evaluate renal vascular hypertension.[6] It behaves similarly to paraaminohippuric acid (PAH), 85% to 90% being secreted by the proximal renal tubules and the remainder by glomerular filtration.

In normal patients I 131 orthohippuric acid passes rapidly through the kidneys, which can be satisfactorily visualized by Anger camera scintiphotography at two-minute intervals. Radioactivity first appears within the cortico-medullary regions. With increased trapping by the renal tubules, the peak of concentration shifts to the medullary region. As the tubular cells excrete the tracer into the tubular lumen, the material is cleared by the urine flow in these tubules which is dependent on the prevailing glomerular filtration rate. The tracer is then carried on toward the collecting tubules and renal pelvis.

The patient should be adequately hydrated before the procedure, and the studies should be done before or at least 24 hours after intravenous pyelography, retrograde pyelography, or arteriography since contrast material temporarily impair trapping of the orthohippuric acid (Fig 11-2).

The patient is placed prone or supine under the camera. Abdominal compression is avoided. The 400 μCi dose of the tracer is rapidly injected intravenously as bolus, with care to avoid extravasation. With the gamma crystal in the divided modes, scintillation photographs at two- to four-minute intervals are obtained, recording the intrarenal passage of the tracer for 20 minutes or longer. If the data are recorded directly on to a videotape system or a small on-line computer, a histogram can be obtained of the radioactivity recorded over each kidney during this period. When the

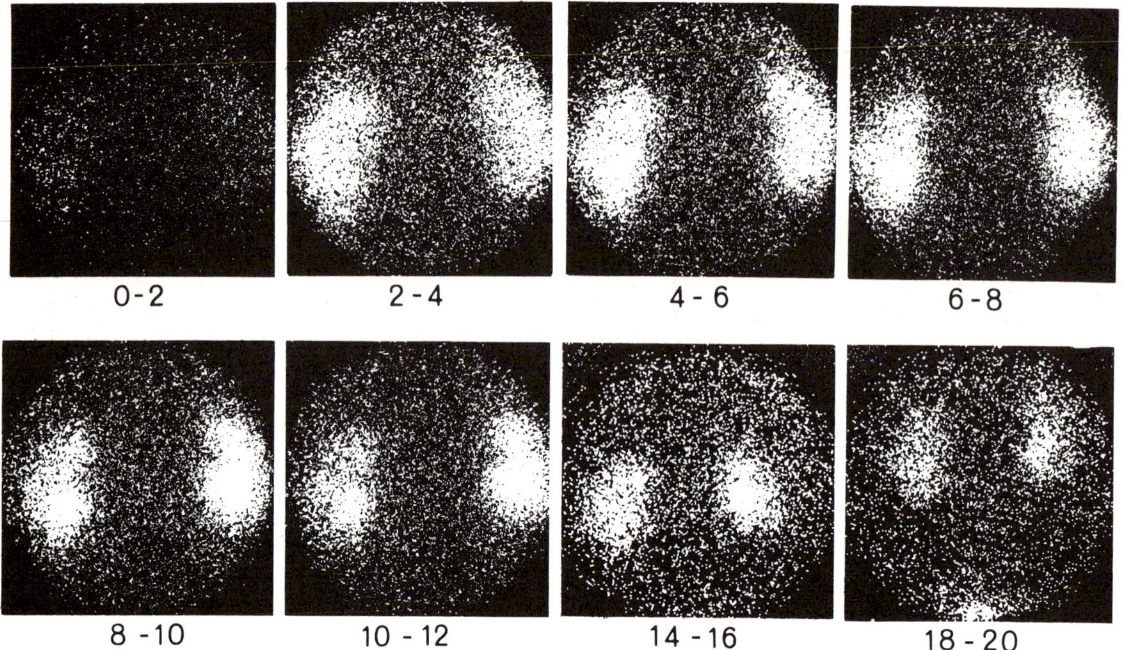

Figure 11-2 *Effect of contrast material on renal scanning. Delayed and decreased uptake of I 131 orthohippuric acid seen at two minutes suggests bilateral tubular dysfunction. However, it results from impaired tubular trapping related to presence of contrast material injected earlier in the day for intravenous pyelography, which was cancelled because of hypersensitivity reaction.*

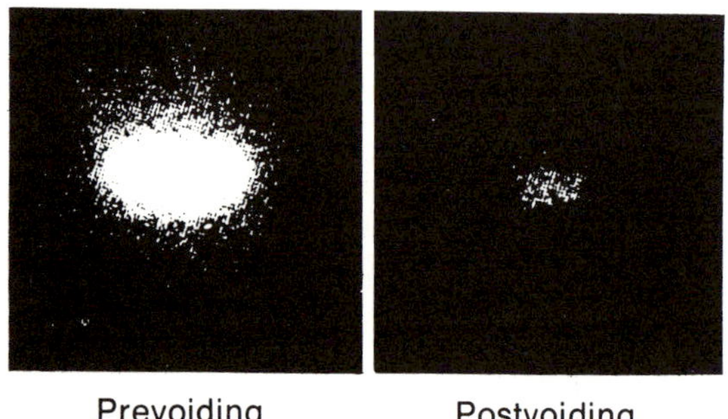

Figure 11-3 *Pre- and postvoiding scintiphotographs made during study with orthohippuric acid I 131, showing no significant residual urine in bladder.*

tape is played back, cursors can be placed over selected areas of interest over the kidneys. As the end of the procedure pre- and postvoiding scintiphotographs of the bladder are made to detect residual urine (Fig 11-3).

TC 99M PERTECHNETATE

This is a freely diffusible ion and the methods of its excretion are not fully understood. Its use allows visualization of the area at the level of the abdominal aorta and evaluation of blood flow to a specific lesion previously detected by I 131 orthohippuric acid or Hg 197 chlormerodrin scanning.[11]

A 10- to 15-mCi dose is injected rapidly in a bolus at the level of the antecubital vein. With the patient lying prone, the detector head of the camera is placed over the kidneys (previously localized by Hg 197 chlormerodrin study) and scintiphotographs are taken at two- or three-second intervals.

Indications

MORPHOLOGIC EVALUATION

The Hg 197 chlormerodrin scan shows kidney size and location and indicates the presence of focal renal lesions. Although the nuclear technique is simple and adequately displays functioning renal parenchyma, roentgenography utilizing contrast material provides better resolution. However, when kidney morphology cannot be adequately visualized by conventional roentgenography (owing, for example, to overlapping gas, fecal material, adjacent organs, or to obesity, or the presence of a plaster cast) Hg 197 chlormerodrin scanning can provide the information needed. Scanning is the method of choice for the patient who is allergic to contrast materials and for the patient with multiple myeloma suspected of having renal disease.

Evaluation of kidney size is helpful in determing whether renal failure is due to chronic or acute renal disease. Demonstration of markedly small kidneys suggests chronic renal disease.

> Demonstration of markedly small kidneys suggests chronic renal disease.

In the patient whose renal function is so impaired that adequate visualization of the kidneys is not possible by conventional roentgenography, scanning allows kidney localization so that biopsy can be done.[14]

EVALUATION OF SPACE-OCCUPYING LESIONS

Scanning can reveal a renal lesion that has produced little or no calyceal distortion and is therefore not delineated by roentgenography.[8] Scanning can distinguish between a fetal lobulation and a space-occupying lesion, both of which appear roentgenographically as a nonspecific renal bulge. If the bulge exhibits normal uptake of Hg 197 chlormerodrin or I 131 orthohippuric acid, fetal lobulation is confirmed. If radionuclide uptake within the bulge is reduced, infarct, tumor, cyst, or carbuncle of the kidney should be considered (Fig 11-4). These can be further differentiated by perfusion study using Tc 99m pertechnetate. Cyst, carbuncle, and infarct are visualized as relatively avascular areas, whereas a hypernephroma usually is well perfused; however, perfusion study findings may be equivocal. The rare functioning tubular cell adenoma has been reported to

Conditions Detected by Renal Scanning

- Abnormal location of kidney
- Abnormal size and shape of kidney
- Space-occupying renal lesion
- Renal infarction
- Renal trauma
- Renal vascular hypertension
- Renal outlet obstruction
- Transplant rejection
- Vesicoureteral reflux

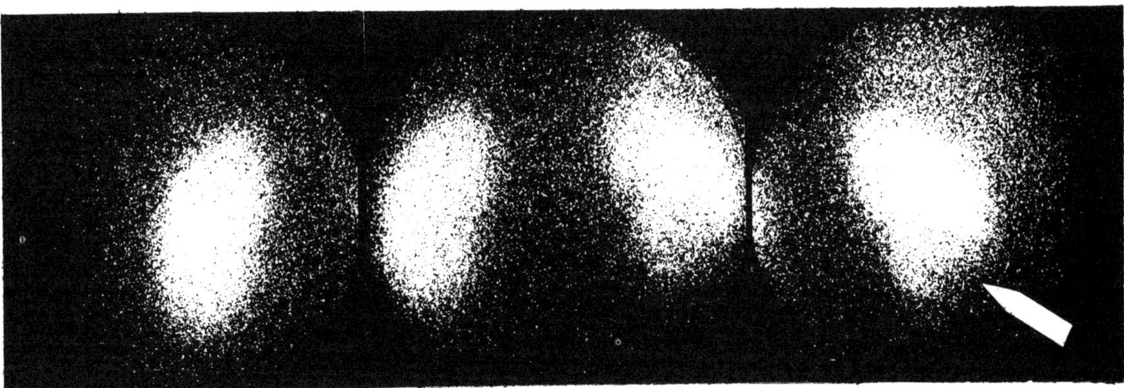

Figure 11-4 *Necrotic tumor of kidney (verified at surgery) demonstrated by chlormerodrin Hg 197 scan as region of decreased radioactivity in lower pole of right kidney.*

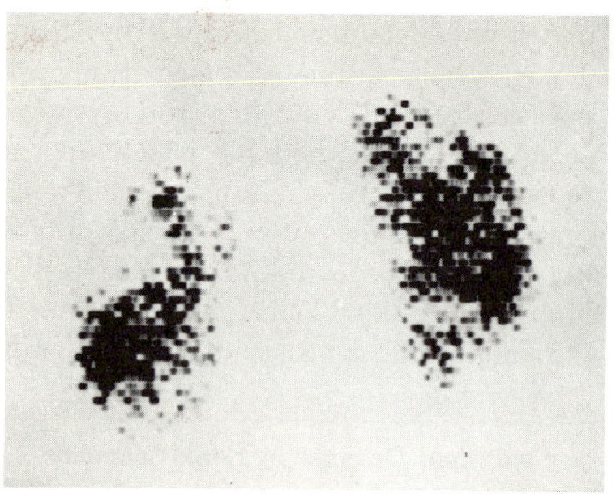

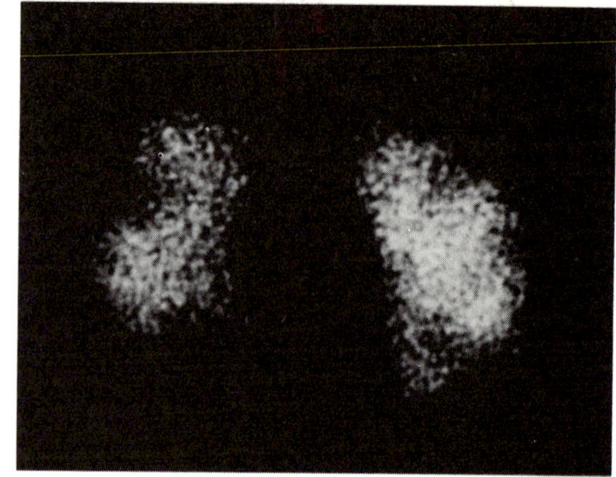

Figure 11-5 *Polycystic disease of the kidney visualized by rectilinear and Anger scintillation camera studies.*

show a focal increase of radionuclide concentration.

In polycystic disease scanning can detect the cysts before the kidney is enlarged and even when intravenous pyelography has failed because of impaired renal function (Fig 11-5). In a patient in whom pyelography has demonstrated a single lesion, scanning may reveal the multiple additional defects that would strengthen a diagnosis of multicystic disease of the kidney.[7] Scanning may not reveal lesions smaller than 2 cm located on the surface of the kidney and causing little displacement of the surrounding functioning renal tissue.

DETECTION OF HORSESHOE AND CROSS-FUSED ECTOPIC KIDNEYS

Horseshoe and cross-fused ectopic kidneys are readily detected by scanning, and parenchymal fusion can be distinguished from a ligamentous attachment. The study should be done with the patient supine and the detector head of the camera placed anteriorly over the abdomen to prevent absorption of gamma emission by the vertebral columns.

DETECTION OF INFARCTION

Scanning can readily detect renal infarction and allows a preliminary diagnosis prior to arteriography. Infarction should be suspected when intravenous pyelography demonstrates a normal renal outline and calyceal system and scanning shows a focal segmental loss of Hg 197 chlormerodrin or I 131 orthohippuric acid uptake. These findings, together with reduced perfusion to the area demonstrated by the rapid bolus Tc 99m pertechnetate flow study, suggest infarction of that segment.[3]

EVALUATION OF TRAUMA

Renal scanning readily demonstrates the extent of physiologic damage and serves as a useful screening test for patients who need further study. Its diagnostic accuracy appears at least equal to that of arteriography. In one reported series, arteriography showed no evidence of renal damage in patients whose renal scans were normal. Severe injury that disrupted the kidneys was detected equally well by renal scanning and by arteriography. Moderate trauma, consisting of intrarenal hemorrhage

> **Scanning is as accurate as arteriography in evaluating renal trauma.**

and necrosis without lacerations extending through the capsule, was delineated more accurately by scanning than by arteriography.[15]

In the patient with moderate injury, functional changes and anatomic distortions can be monitored by scanning, and the resolution or persistence of trauma-induced renal lesions can be evaluated. This is important since hypertension and infection may develop following trauma.

Following biopsy, focal abnormalities can be evaluated and biopsy-induced arteriovenous fistula can be demonstrated by Tc 99m pertechnetate flow study.

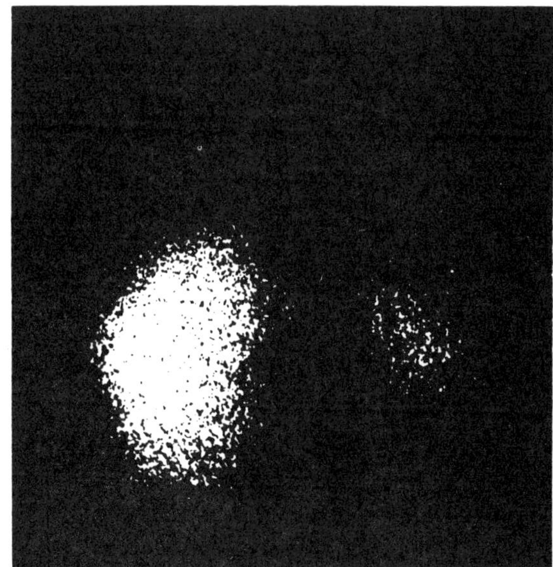

Figure 11-6 *Renal vascular hypertension. Chlormerodrin Hg 197 scan shows reduced radioactivity over right kidney and marked atrophy.*

DETECTION OF RENOVASCULAR HYPERTENSION

Renography with I 131 orthohippuric acid is commonly utilized to screen for renal vascular hypertension. The histogram changes suggesting this diagnosis are delay in the peak of the curve together with impairment of the second and third phases. Results have varied widely, and although some investigators report 90% to 100% accuracy, others report a significantly high rate of false-positive and false-negative results.[6,9] Technical factors may be responsible for the errors, since the detector can seldom be placed symmetrically over each

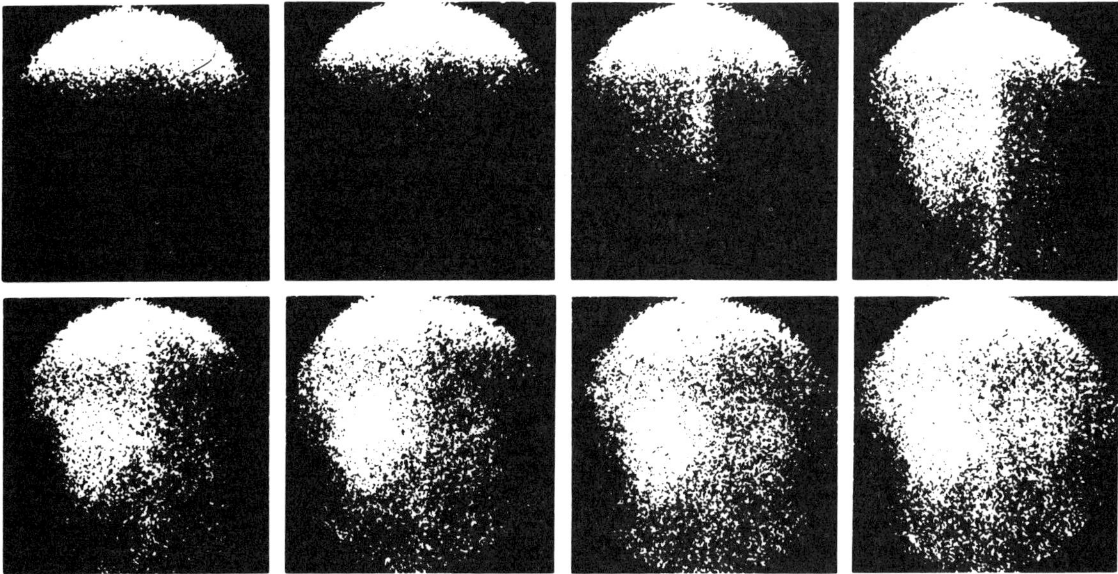

Figure 11-7 *Renal vascular hypertension. Perfusion study with pertechnetate Tc 99m (sequential scintiphotographs taken at two-second intervals) shows radioactivity in abdominal aorta with subsequent normal perfusion of left kidney and delayed and decreased perfusion of right kidney.*

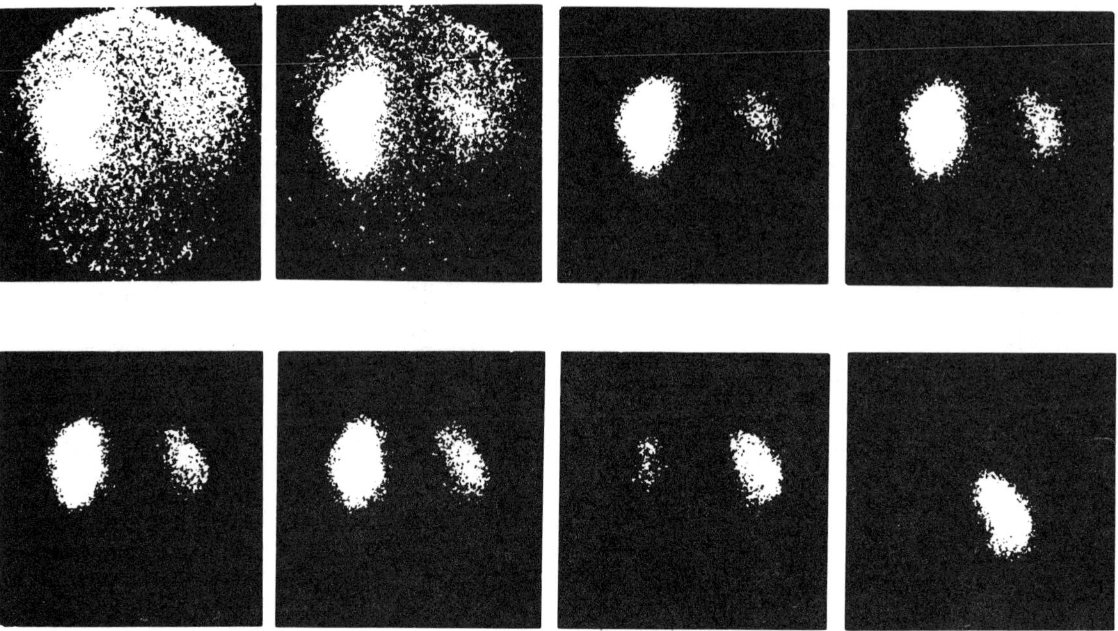

Figure 11-8 *Renal vascular hypertension. Study using I 131 orthohippuric acid shows normal radioactivity in the left kidney and delayed uptake in right kidney.*

kidney and the patient's state of hydration cannot always be controlled. Excessive hydration producing a high renal flow rate (over 7 ml per minute) can mask abnormalities typical of renovascular hypertension (producing a false-negative result), whereas dehydration accentuates these abnormalities (producing a false-positive result). In addition, interpretive criteria vary.

Triple scanning provides a more reliable index of renovascular hypertension (Figs 11-6 through 11-8). The Tc 99m pertechnetate study adequately shows the asymmetrical perfusion pattern associated with renal vascular disease.

In addition, such characteristic features as the unilateral small kidney and the delayed transit, concentration, and excretion in the affected kidney can readily be visualized in the Hg 197 chlormerodrin scan or I 131 orthohippuric acid study. Histograms constructed from data obtained in the orthohippuric acid study provide additional information.

DETECTION OF OUTLET OBSTRUCTION

The orthohippuric acid scan in conjunction with the derived time-activity histogram provides a sensitive index of even minimal outlet obstruction at all levels of the collecting system (Fig 11-9).

Scanning is more reliable than intravenous pyelography for evaluating the functional results of surgery to repair outlet obstruction.

In a patient with long-standing obstruction the question of residual kidney function may be of great clinical importance. Evidence of even slight function may allow conservative therapy that will be rewarded with substantial improvement. Scanning is sufficiently sensitive to detect even such slight function. It is more reliable than in-

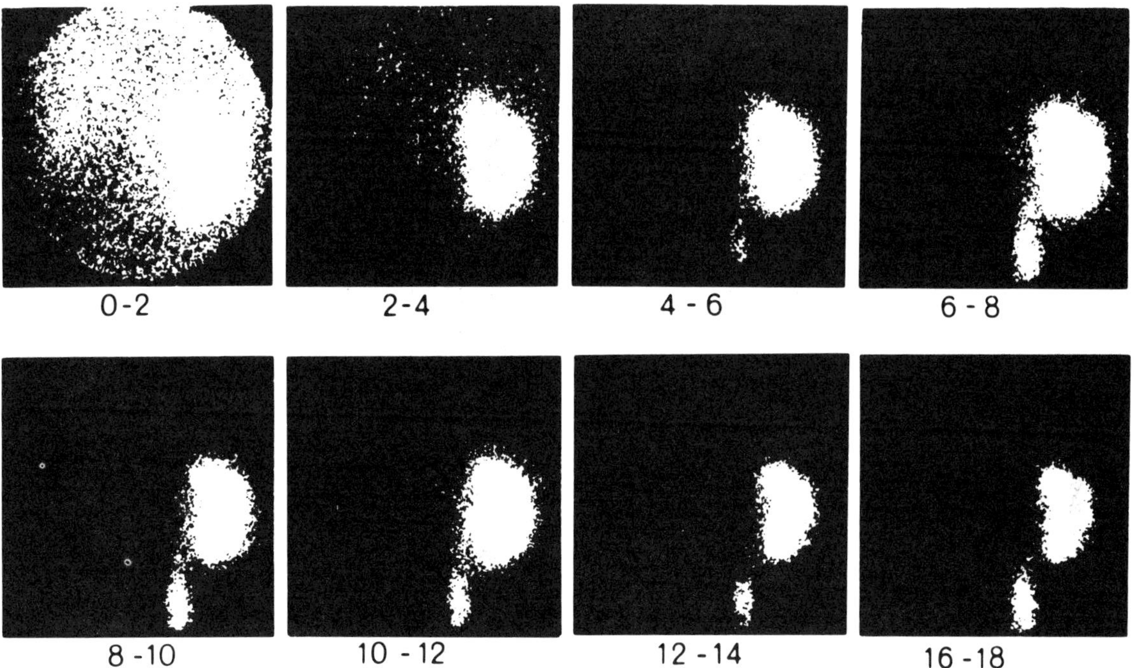

Figure 11-9 *Renal outlet obstruction. I 131 orthohippuric acid scan shows nonfunctioning left kidney and right kidney with ureteric obstruction and hydroureter.*

travenous pyelography for evaluating the results of reconstructive surgery for outlet obstruction. In the patient with an ileal conduit scanning offers a simple, nontraumatic, easily repeatable method of reevaluation. It can be performed at frequent intervals even in a young patient for whom the radiation exposure from conventional roentgenography would be undesirable. Such frequent monitoring is mandatory because these patients are at increased risk for such complications as calculus formation, ureteral stricture, and obstruction.[12,13]

For the patient with renal failure, scanning offers a useful method of differentiating obstruction from prerenal and renal causes of uremia.

EVALUATION OF TRANSPLANTS

Oliguria following renal transplant may be related to rejection, vascular thrombosis, acute tubular necrosis, or outlet obstruction and extravasation. Retrograde pyelography introduces a risk of infection in a patient already immunosuppressed, while arteriography is associated with a substantial risk of morbidity. Renal scanning is highly useful in the evaluation of such a patient.[4]

Transplant rejection is shown by reduced perfusion on the Tc 99m pertechnetate study and decreased tubular function evidenced by delayed excretion associated with a motheaten appearance of the kidney on the orthohippuric acid study (Figs 11-10 and 11-11). Response to therapy is demonstrated when the perfusion pattern and tubular function revert towards normal. A progressive increase in the disappearance time of I 131 orthohippuric acid from the blood also suggests transplant rejection.

Acute tubular necrosis associated with renal transplant usually occurs when a cadaver kidney has been utilized and the blood pressure or oxygenation to the dying donor was not adequately maintained. The technetium flow study is usually normal; the residual effects of tubular necrosis are evidenced on the orthohippuric acid study

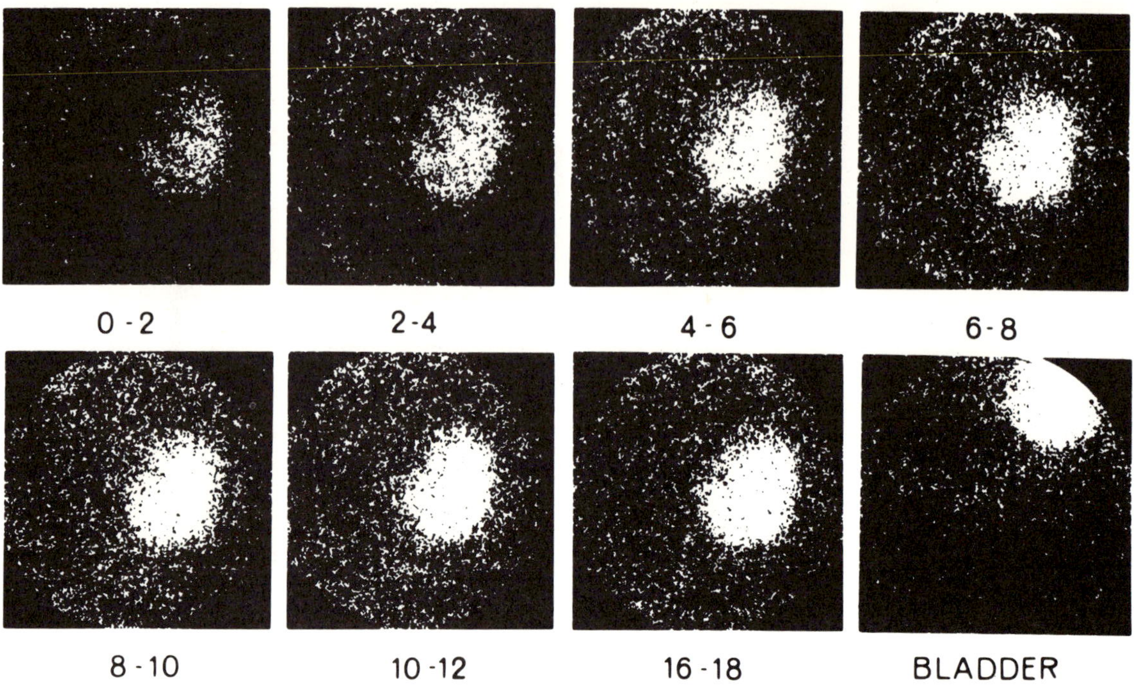

Figure 11-10 *Renal transplant rejection I 131 orthohippuric acid study shows decreased perfusion associated with decreased tubular function as evidenced by delayed uptake of radioactivity, motheaten appearance of kidney, and delayed excretion of radioactivity into bladder.*

as decreased function and delayed appearance of the tracer in the bladder.

DETECTION OF VESICOURETERAL REFLUX

Vesicoureteral reflux can be demonstrated at the completion of scanning with I 131 orthohippuric acid if sufficient radioactivity is allowed to accumulate in the bladder. With the camera placed anteriorly over the bladder, a scintiphotograph is taken with the patient at rest and another is taken with the patient straining. Vesicoureteral reflux may be noted in the second photograph.

A better method involves filling the urinary bladder, via catheter, with Tc 99m pertechnetate and 50 to 500 ml of normal saline. A scintiphotograph is then taken so that the dome of the bladder and ureters are in view (Fig 11-12). This method is

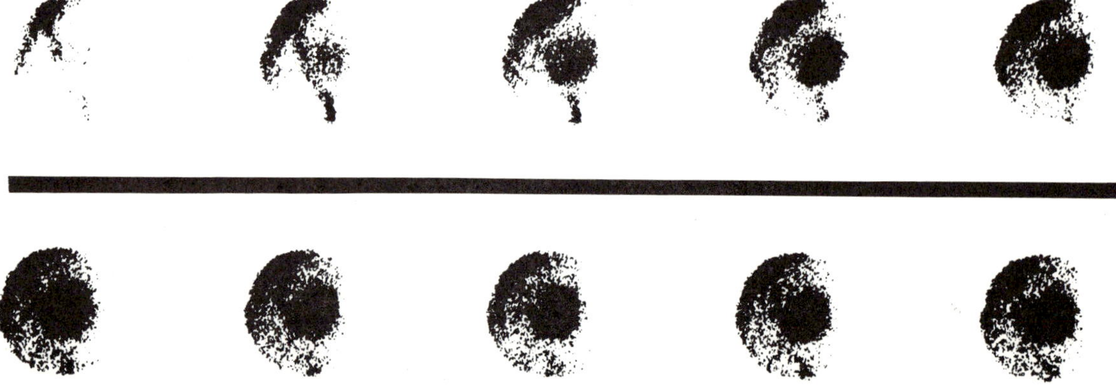

Figure 11-11 *Renal transplant rejection. Perfusion study with Tc 99m pertechnetate shows delayed and decreased perfusion of kidney during early phase of study.*

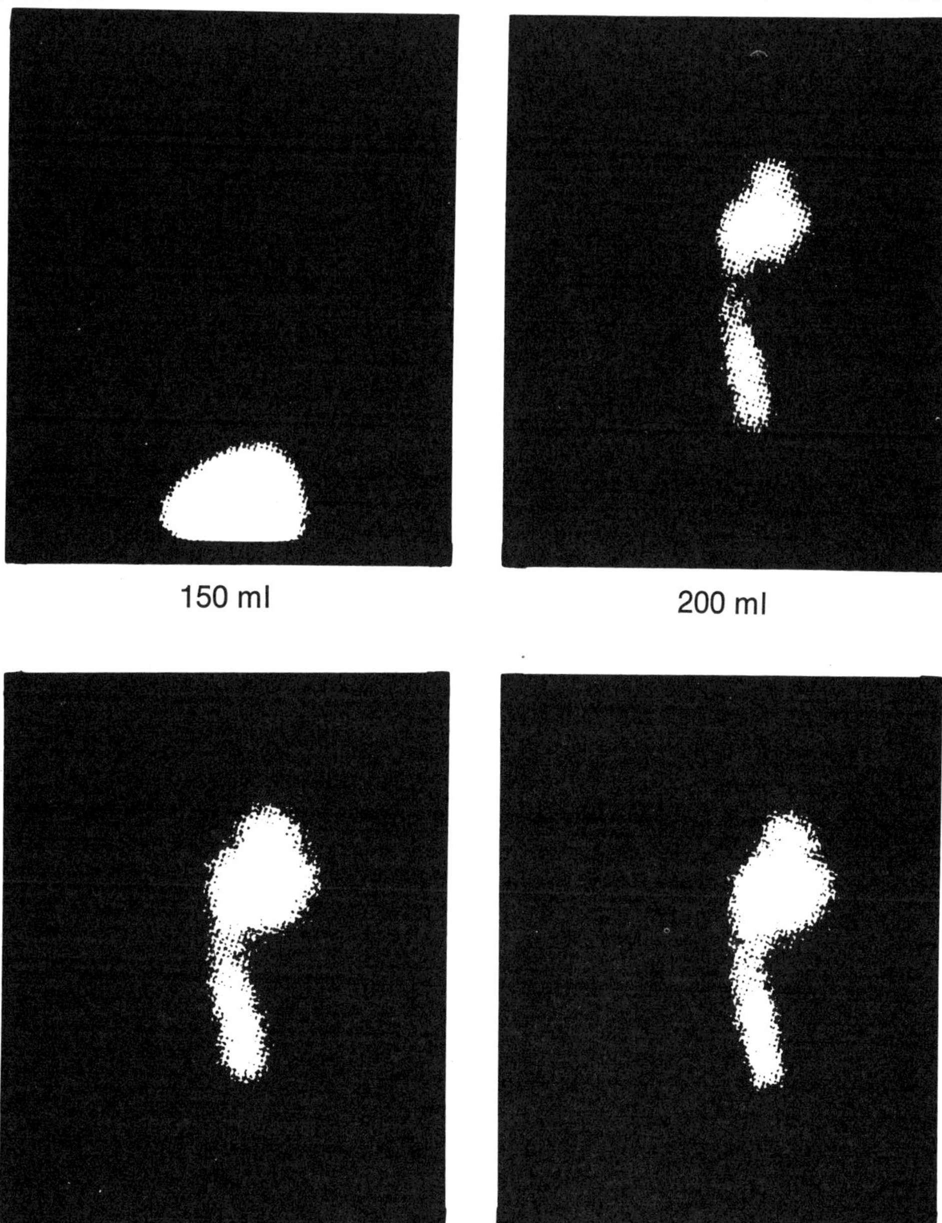

Figure 11-12 *Vesicoureteral reflux demonstrated by instillation of Tc 99m pertechnetate and normal saline into urinary bladder.*

more sensitive than routine roentgenographic techniques and exposes the patient to 50 or 100 times less radiation.[2]

Conclusion

Scintigraphy plays an important role in the management of a variety of urinary tract disorders both in adults and in children and contributes significantly to the physician's diagnostic armamentrarium. Often it serves not only as a useful screening method, but also as the only useful diagnostic study. The procedures are simple and rapidly performed. Often they supply information otherwise available only from a more hazardous procedure.

References

1. Caplan GE, Hartman HR, Young R, et al: "Hot" renal tumor: Scanning and angiographic characteristics of a solid renal tubular adenoma. *Radiology* **91**:991, 1968.
2. Conway JJ, King LR, Belman AB, et al: Detection of vesicoureteral reflux with radionuclide cystography. *Am J Roentgenol Radium Ther Nucl Med* **115**:720–727, 1972.
3. Freeman LM, Chien-Hsing Meng, Richter MW, et al: Patency of major renal vascular pathways demonstrated by rapid blood flow scintiphotography. *J Urol* **105**:473–481, 1971.
4. Hayes M, Moore TC, Taplin GV: Radionuclides procedures in predicting early renal transplant rejection. *Radiology* **103**:627–631, 1972.
5. Hosain F, Reba RC, Wagner HN Jr: Visualization of renal structure and function with chelated radionuclides. *Radiology* **93**:1135–1138, 1969.
6. Keane JM, Schlegel JU: Use of scintillation camera system for screening of hypertensive patients. *J Urol* **108**:12–14, 1972.
7. MacEwen DW, Rosenthall L: Assessment of excretory urography and radioisotopic renal scanning in diseases of the kidneys. *Radiology* **86**:1010, 1966.
8. Morris JG, Coorey GJ, Dick R, et al: The diagnosis of renal tumors by radioisotope scanning. *J Urol* **97**:40–55, 1967.
9. Quinones JD, Varma V, Macal O: Radionuclide and pyelographic tests in screening for renovascular hypertension. *Arch Intern Med* **129**:570–577, 1972.
10. Raynaud C. Ricard S, Karam Y, et al: Use of renal uptake of ^{197}Hg as a method for testing functional value of each kidney. *J Nucl Med* **11**:125–133, 1970.
11. Rosenthall L: Radiopertechnetate renography with gamma ray scintillation camera. *Can Med Assoc J* **105**:467–471, 1971.
12. Schlegel JU, Bakule PT: A diagnostic approach in detecting renal and urinary tract disease. *J Urol* **104**:2–10, 1970.
13. Shuler SE, Meckstroth GR, Maxfield WS: Scintillation camera in pediatric renal disease. *Am J Dis Child* **120**:115–121, 1970.
14. Tully RJ, Stack VJ, Hoffer PB, et al: Renal scan prior to renal biopsy–A method of renal localization. *J Nucl Med* **13**:544–547, 1972.
15. Woodruff JH, Cockett ATK, Cannon R, et al: Radiologic aspects of renal trauma with the emphasis on arteriography and renal scanning. *J Urol* **97**:184–188, 1967.

Intravenously injected radioactive tracers allow calculation of blood volume; estimation of red cell survival time, production rate, and metabolism; and identification of pernicious anemia. External imaging enables visualization of red cell production sites and detection of marrow tumors.

12
The Hematopoietic System

Morton B. Weinstein

Blood tests of varying complexity, discomfort, cost, and value have been developed that utilize radionuclides. This chapter reviews some of the more commonly employed procedures, stressing the pitfalls as well as the clinically useful information that can be gained. For the sake of this discussion, the tests are divided into three categories: in vitro procedures for determining blood volume, red cell survival time, and ferrokinetics and for identifying pernicious anemia; imaging procedures for visualization of the bone marrow, spleen, lymph nodes, etc; and procedures for evaluation of red cell metabolism.

In Vitro Procedures

Calculation of Blood Volume

The increase and decrease of the various formed elements of the blood correspond quite accurately to a variety of disease states. For example, infection is accompanied by an increase in the number of white blood cells; polycythemia rubra vera is characterized by an increase in red cell mass and plasma volume. Thus, while quantitation of the formed elements of the blood is seldom diagnostic by itself, it supplies important information which, taken with other clinical and laboratory findings, enables diagnosis.

The standard method of quantitation is, of course, the acutal counting of red cells, white cells, and platelets in a sample of blood from a peripheral vessel. Though simple and convenient, this technique does not accurately reflect the proportions of formed elements in blood throughout the entire body. Peripheral blood is not representative of blood in every part of the body.[1,7] This is illustrated by the difference in hematocrit values of blood samples drawn from different body areas (Table 12-1).[5] Clearly, a blood volume measurement calculated from the hematocrit value of peripheral venous blood is subject to large error. Similarly, it is well established that the white cells in the peripheral blood

Table 12-1. Hematocrit at Different Sites

Sample from	Hematocrit (%)
Large peripheral vein	45
Artery	50
Capillary	30
Splenic vein	70
Pulmonary vein	35
Hepatic vein	40

reflect less than half the white cells in the body.

The use of radioactive tracers allows a more accurate determination. Although no single tracer distributes itself equally within the plasma compartment and the formed element compartment of the peripheral blood, iodine 131 provides a fairly accurate measurement of the plasma compartment and chromium 51 gives a good measurement of red cell mass. Both together—the dual-isotope technique—give a reliable indication of total blood volume.[8]

The dual-isotope technique gives a reliable indication of total blood volume.

DETERMINATION OF PLASMA VOLUME

Radioactive iodine (^{131}I) is readily bound to protein molecules, and this characteristic is the basis for its use in determining plasma volume. Human serum albumin labeled with iodine 131 is injected into the patient. Twenty minutes later a sample of the patient's blood is drawn, the amount of radioactivity present (postequilibrium activity) is determined, and plasma volume is calculated on the basis of the dilution principle. The dilution principle states that if a known volume with a known amount of radioactivity is injected into a longer volume, the equilibration concentration of activity will be relative to the size of the larger volume. Thus, where A_1 is the known activity, V_1 is the known injected volume, A_2 is the activity postequilibration, and V_2 is the unknown (plasma) volume.

$$A_1 V_1 = A_2 V_2$$

$$V_2 = \frac{A_1 V_1}{A_2}$$

Blood volume is determined from a chart that correlates plasma volume and the measured peripheral vein hematocrit.

$$\text{Hematocrit} = \frac{\text{RBC mass} \times 100}{\text{Blood volume}}$$

The chances for error are many. Despite the various correction factors that have been developed, peripheral vein hematocrit correlates with true body hematocrit only by ± 30%. Another source of error is the variability of exit of the HSA I 131 from the intravascular compartment into the interstitial compartment. In a normal individual less than 50% of the original activity is found at 24 to 48 hours. In patients observed immediately after surgery, the 20-minute equilibration volume is sometimes calculated as more than 9000 ml of plasma —clearly an indication that large amounts of albumin are being lost into the traumatized surgical area.

DETERMINATION OF RED CELL MASS

Since in the normal individual the red cells constitute the major portion of the formed element compartment,[10] determination of red cell mass gives a fair indication of the volume of that compartment. Radioactive diisopropyl fluorophosphate (DFP 32) and radioactive sodium chromate (sodium chromate Cr 51) have been used to label red cells so they can be counted.

Today, DFP 32 is rarely used because the well counters employed in most laboratories have sodium iodide crystals which cannot count the beta emissions of ^{32}P. Sodium chromate Cr 51 is the label commonly used. Its physical half-life of 27.8 days makes it easy to maintain in the laboratory, and about 9% of its deexitations are associated with a 320-kev photon.

The hexavalent chromium passes rapidly through the intact red cell and binds to the beta chain of globin. Binding is efficient at room temperature, but incubation at 37°C shortens the process to 10 to 15 minutes. With binding, the +6 state is reduced to +3; any unbound chromium is chemically reduced by the addition of 50 mg of ascorbic acid.

Unfortunately, in vivo binding of ^{51}Cr to the intact red cell is not entirely irreversible.[9,16] In the first 24 hours after injection into the patient, approximately 5% of the radioactivity is lost. In addition, about 1% is elicited from the cells every 24 hours. These loss rates must be taken into consideration when red cell mass is quantitated.

Like plasma volume, red cell mass is quantitated on the basis of the dilution principle according to the formula,

$$V_2 = \frac{A_1 V_1}{A_2}$$

only here V_2, the unknown volume, is red cell mass. Blood volume is calculated from red cell mass and hematocrit by the formula

$$\text{Hematocrit} = \frac{\text{RBC mass} \times 100}{\text{Blood volume}}$$

Here again errors are likely. Hematocrit measurement from peripheral venous blood is not a reliable index of true body hematocrit, as explained above. Technical errors—in pipetting, counting, or injecting—distort the results. A common error is inadvertent injection of part of a sample into subcutaneous tissue instead of into a peripheral vein; this results in a low recovered activity count from the sample drawn from the patient, and calculations indicate an inordinately large blood volume. Another source of error is related to the recent fad of self-administration of vitamin C. A high blood level of ascorbic acid causes immediate reduction of the ^{51}Cr and prevents it from binding to the patient's red cells. Whereas normally almost 100% of 100 μCi of sodium chromate Cr 51 binds to the 30-ml sample of the patient's blood, only about 10% to 15% binds to the sample when ascorbic acid level is high. When the sample is recovered 20 to 30 minutes after injection, plasma ^{51}Cr activity exceeds whole blood ^{51}Cr activity, making calculations impossible in a dual-isotope examination.

Inadvertent injection of part of the radioactive sample into subcutaneous tissue instead of a peripheral vein is a common error that produces a falsely low recovered activity count and an inordinately large calculated blood volume.

Estimation of Red Cell Survival Time

Labeling of red cells with sodium chromate Cr 51 also allows estimation of red cell survival time. Following tracer injection, daily blood samples are taken and residual red cell radioactivity is measured. When cell death and elution of ^{51}Cr are taken into account, normal red cell survival is about 26 to 30 days. This corresponds with a known mean cell life of 120 days.

Shortened red cell survival has obvious clinical significance. It reflects either an abnormality in the patient's erythrocytes or some mechanism of cell destruction extrinsic to the erythrocytes. The distinction can be made by examining the fate of labeled donor cells in the patient and of labeled patient cells in a recipient. For example, labeled red cells from a normal donor survive normally in a patient with hereditary spherocytosis; labeled cells from such a patient have a shortened survival time in a normal recipient but a normal

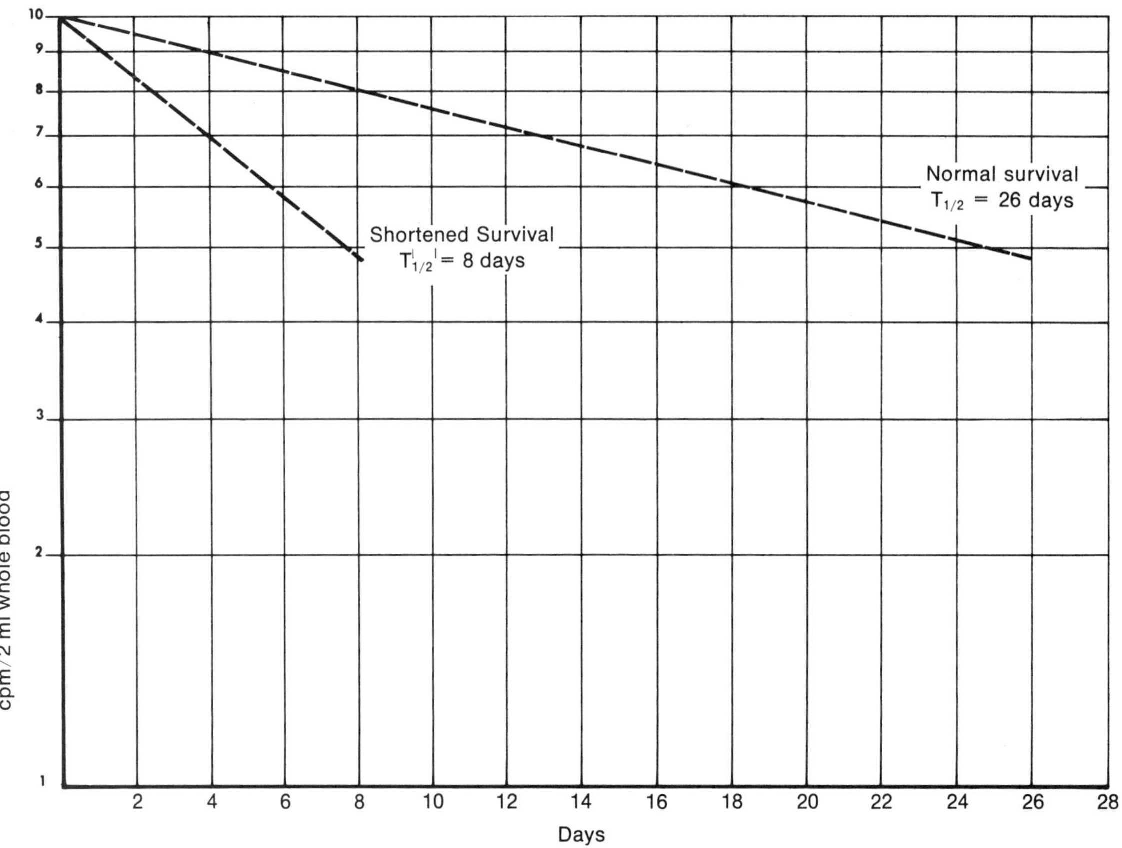

Figure 12-1 *Definition of intrinsic red cell abnormaity by ⁵¹Cr survival study. Normal cells from normal donor survive normally in patient with hereditary spherocytosis, but defective cells from such a patient have shortened survival time in a normal recipient.*

survival time in a splenectomized recipient (Fig 12-1).

^{51}Cr study can detect shortened red cell survival that is not reflected by hemoglobin or hematocrit determinations in peripheral blood samples owing to the bone marrow's ability to increase red cell production seven- to tenfold. For example, compensated hemolytic anemia may be suggested by peripheral blood and bone marrow smears, but can be documented only by demonstration of significantly shortened survival of chromium-labeled red cells.

> ^{51}Cr study can detect shortened red cell survival not reflected by hemoglobin or hematocrit determinations on peripheral blood samples.

The chief sources of error in survival determinations are the presuppositions that for every red cell destroyed a new red cell is produced and that this production rate is constant in a given patient. The assumptions may be quite incorrect: A patient's red cell production may suddenly cease or may suddenly increase tenfold. Failure to produce a new cell for a destroyed cell gives a falsely long red cell survival time. Sudden increase in cell production dilutes the tagged cells and suggests a falsely short red cell survival time.

Estimation of Red Cell Production

Red cell production is a formidable activity. The erythropoietic system routinely produces 6 billion cells per hour and can increase this output tenfold under stress or discontinue production instantaneously. Radioactive iron, especially iron 59, has been extensively employed to study erythropoietic activity in terms of ferrokinetics.[3,6,12,17]

The principle and the performance of the ferrokinetic study can be summarized briefly. A 70-kg man is estimated to have a blood volume of approximately 5000 ml. His red cell mass is approximately 2000 ml and his venous hematocrit 44.5%. His hemoglobin mass can be calculated as 666 gm. Since the iron content per gram of hemoglobin is 3.38 mg, this man has a circulating iron mass in hemoglobin of 2.2 gm. Since red cell destruction per day is approximately 1/120 of the red cell mass, or 0.83%, this man makes approximately 6 gm of hemoglobin daily, which requires approximately 20 mg of iron. Serum iron concentration in a normal individual is approximately 100 μg/100ml, which renders the transferrin one-third saturated. The plasma iron must be in a dynamic state if its total content is but 2.5 mg and the marrow requires 20 mg/24 hours. The total plasma iron must be removed and replenished seven to ten times daily if the individual is to remain in the steady state.

Serial plasma samples can be counted to determine the disappearance of radio-

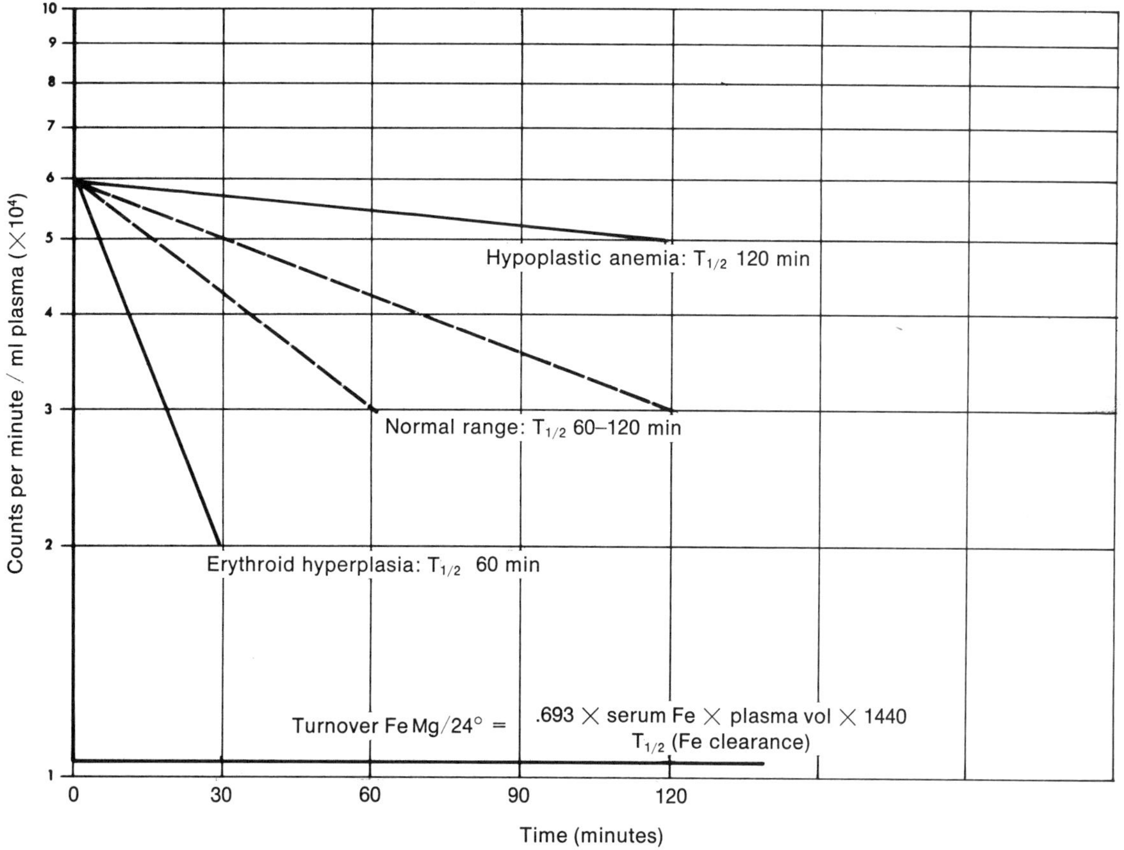

Figure 12-2 *Plasma clearance of transferrin Fe 59. Normally one half of radioactivity clears plasma in first two hours after intravenous injection. Hyperplastic disorder hastens clearance; aplasia delays clearance. Serum iron content also affects clearance.*

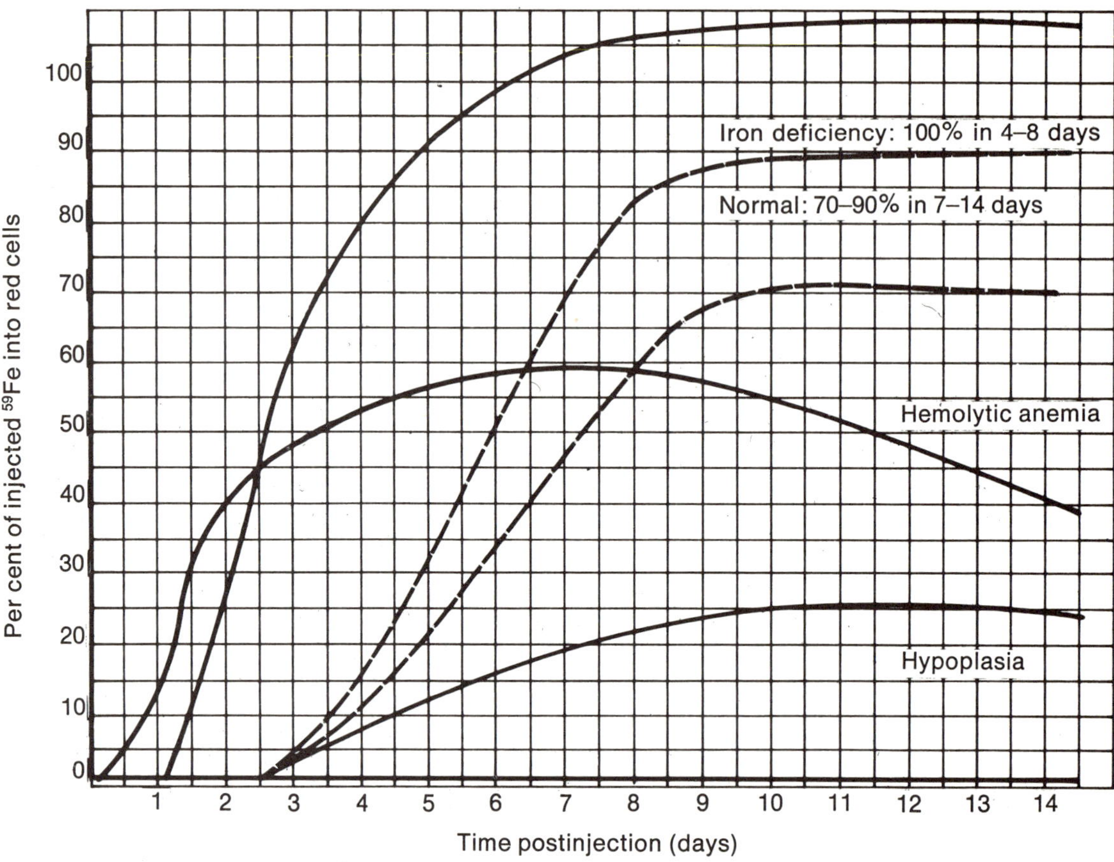

Figure 12-3 *Effect of various hematologic abnormalities on rate of appearance and persistence of* ^{59}Fe *in circulating red cells.*

activity following an intravenous injection of iron 59 bound to normal plasma (transferrin). In the normal individual one half of the radioactivity disappears within 60 to 120 minutes. This tracer dose of 10 μCi of ^{59}Fe does not interfere with the movement of the milligram quantities of stable iron from the plasma to the bone marrow. Very slow disappearance of ^{59}Fe is associated with very high serum iron content and with aplastic anemia resulting in very small bone marrow iron requirement; the two conditions cannot be differentiated on this basis. Very rapid clearance of radioactivity from the plasma usually reflects hyperplasia of the patient's erythropoietic marrow (Fig 12-2).

In a normal individual between 70% and 100% of this administered radioactivity appears in the circulating red cell mass by 7 to 14 days after the intravenous administration. There is a short period during which most of the radioactivity is found in the marrow, but it quickly reappears in peripheral red cell hemoglobin (Fig 12-3). This circulating ^{59}Fe in peripheral red cells persists for the life span of that red cell (approximately 120 days) and there is a subtle decrease in radioactivity at that time with a second cycling of the iron from the senescent red cell.

Ferrokinetic study is basically an investigative procedure and is only occasionally used to obtain data directly applicable to care of the patient. One such occasion is use of the percentage incorporation of iron into the peripheral red cell mass, as well as the half-time clearance from the plasma, to determine the site of erythropoiesis. At times this is of critical importance in a patient with splenic extramedullary hematopoiesis. Generally, however, splenic erythropoiesis is ineffectual, and the enlarging spleen destroys more cells each day than it produces.

Estimation of Platelet Survival Time

Chromium 51 and DFP 32 can bind to white cells and to platelets. White cell studies have found limited clinical application owing to the difficulty in separation and the difficulty of examining white cell function in a patient with significant leukopenia. Platelets, however, have been extensively investigated, and platelet survival studies have been reported in normal persons, in patients with decreased production, and patients with increased destruction. In idiopathic thrombocytopenic purpura, a disease that causes rapid immunologic destruction of a patient's platelets, the severity of this destruction as well as its response to various chemotherapeutic agents can be defined with serial platelet survival studies.

The Schilling Test

The Schilling test employs orally administered radioactive cobalt to differentiate pernicious anemia from other megaloblastic anemias. Pernicious anemia results from reduced ability to absorb vitamin B_{12} from the gastrointestinal tract owing to failure of gastric mucosal secretion of intrinsic factor. Other megaloblastic anemias are also characterized by deficient body content of vitamin B_{12}, but the deficiency is related not to lack of intrinsic factor, but to such other causes as deficient B_{12} intake, blind loop syndrome, gastrectomy, infestation of the gut with certain bacteria or worms, and disease of the absorptive site in the distal portion of the bowel.[4]

The Schilling test employs orally administered radioactive cobalt to differentiate pernicious anemia from other megaloblastic anemias.

Radioimmunoassay defines the serum level of vitamin B_{12} and can thus identify megaloblastic anemia,[11] but pernicious anemia can be diagnosed only on the basis of defective intestinal absorption that is corrected by administration of intrinsic factor.

The Schilling test relies on the principle that a person with normal gastric intrinsic factor absorbs from the intestine most of an orally administered dose of vitamin B_{12} labeled with radioactive cobalt.[13] This normal person subsequently excretes in his urine more than 8% of this absorbed vitamin B_{12} following a flushing dose (1 mg) of nonlabled vitamin B_{12} given parenterally within 60 minutes of the oral dose. A patient lacking intrinsic factor does not absorb the orally administered labeled vitamin B_{12} and does not excrete it following the flushing dose. His conversion to the normal pattern when the test is repeated with administration of intrinsic factor is diagnostic of pernicious anemia (Table 12-2).

External Imaging

The separation of technetium 99m from molybdenum 99 gave nuclear medicine its most versatile radionuclide. Imaging procedures for brain, blood pool, bone, bone marrow, liver, spleen, and kidneys are among its many applications. In hematology ^{99m}Tc is most often used to visualize sites of red cell production and to detect invasive tumor of the marrow.

Identification of Red Cell Production Sites

A normal adult possesses approximately 2.5 kg of bone marrow about 40% of which

Table 12-2. Urinary Excretion of Orally Administered Vitamin B_{12} Co 57 in Normal Persons and in Patients with Pernicious Anemia and Malabsorption Syndrome*

Condition	Excretion (% of oral dose)	
	Without intrinsic factor	With intrinsic factor
Normal	15–40	15–40
Pernicious anemia	0–7	10–20
Malabsorption syndrome	0–3	0–3

* 24-Hour urine collection after oral administration of 0.5 μg = 0.5 μCi vitamin B_{12} Co 57 and intramuscular administration of 1 mg vitamin B_{12}.

is fatty marrow. Functioning red marrow is confined to the axial skeleton—sternum, vertebrae, ribs, pelvis, scapula, proximal humerus, and proximal femur. This so-called red marrow contains more white cells than red cells. The reticuloendothelial component of the marrow concentrates a certain amount of intravenously administered sulfur colloid Tc 99m. When hemolysis or excessive blood loss triggers accelerated red cell production, normal production sites become hyperplastic and the red marrow extends into the fatty marrow. In addition, extramedullary hematopoiesis may occur—in lungs, liver, or spleen. This increased production is difficult to quantitate, but qualitative images can be obtained of the total body reticuloendothelial system. In general, erythroid hyperplastic states are associated with a marked increased uptake of radioactive colloid in normal sites as well as extension into abnormal sites.[14,15] However, a variety of diseases that affect the erythron do not disturb the reticuloendothelial system, and in these cases the correlation fails. Myeofibrosis and myeloid metaplasia are almost always associated with decreased colloid concentration in axial skeletal marrow with extention into peripheral marrow sites. Excessive hepatic and splenic uptake of radioactivity and enlargement of these organs are also characteristic of myelofibrosis and myeloid metaplasia.

Recent observations suggest the indium chloride 111, administered intravenously, defines the erythron more reliably than does sulfur colloid Tc 99m.

Detection of Marrow Tumor

Tumor involvement of bone marrow as defined by scanning the reticuloendothelial system has not been very successful in our laboratory. We have found that the polyphosphate Tc 99m bone scan or the gallium 67 tumor scan is often more rewarding. Some of the shortcomings of reticuloendothelial system scanning relate to particle size, which markedly affects radionuclide distribution. In addition, care must be taken that no free label is present because free label does not find its way into the reticuloendothelial system but accumulates in a variety of organs. Instrument setting must be precise, and comparable areas must be examined for total time, not total cumulative counts.

Evaluation of Red Cell Metabolism

Erythropoiesis is a dynamic process resulting in the formation of hemoglobin-containing biconcave discs and the circulation of these cells in the intravascular compartment. The cells function primarily in the exchange of oxygen and carbon dioxide at a cellular level. The kinetic function of the entire system is rather well defined with chromium 51 tagging, but the biochemical function of cellular enzymes and the intracellular synthesis of hemoglobin require more complex investigative procedures. Many of these procedures have been performed using radionuclides.[2] The availability of tritium and carbon 14 have enabled the biochemist to synthesize a large number of precursors and substrates which have been used to analyze biochemical pathways within the red cell. Hemoglobin synthesis has been extensively evaluated by noting the incorporation of labeled glycine into heme and tracing subsequent catabolic pathways by recovery of carbon-labeled degradation products. Recent studies in immunohematology have followed the response of the lymphocyte from normal and abnormal patients after exposure to various antigenic materials. Tritiated thymidine incorporation into stimulated cells can be evaluated.

Future Prospects

The development of the medical cyclotron heralds a new era of investigative procedures with radioactive pharmaceuticals. These facilities make available to the clinician and basic scientist a variety of short-lived gamma-emitting radionuclides whose potential use is limited only by the imagination of the investigator. Short-lived carbon 11, oxygen 15, and nitrogen 13 available in millicurie quantities can be incorporated into a large number of molecules which can then be used to study a variety of hematologic disease processes.

Colloidal materials can be synthesized with these short-lived radionuclides to improve definition of the reticuloendothelial system, liver, and the spleen. Iron 52, readily produced in the cyclotron, can enable quantitative imaging of iron distribution and kinetics. Many of these short-lived materials can aid in the evaluation of the distribution and toxicity of many of the drugs used to treat patients with hematologic diseases.

References

1. Albert SN: *Blood Volume and Extracellular Fluid Volume.* Springfield, Ill, Thomas, 1971.
2. Barnham BF: The chemistry of the porphyrins. *Semin Hematol* **5**:296, 1968.
3. Bothwell TH, Finch CA: The intestine in iron metabolism. *Am J Digest Dis* **2**:145, 1957.
4. Castle WB: Factors involved in the absorption of vitamin B_{12}. *Gastroenterology* **37**:377, 1955.
5. Chaplun H, et al: The body venous hematocrit range. *J Clin Invest* **32**:1309, 1953.
6. Conrad ME, Brosby WH: Intestinal mucosal mechanisms controlling iron absorption. *Blood* **22**:406, 1963.
7. Ebert RV, et al: Response of normal subjects to acute blood loss. *Arch Intern Med* **65**:578, 1941.
8. Gillett DJ, Halmagye DFS: A simple method of dual label of blood volume measurement. *Am Surg* **166**:48, 1967.
9. Gray, SJ, Sterling K: The tagging of red cells and plasma proteins with radioactive chromium. *J Clin Invest* **29**:1604, 1950.
10. Harris JW, Kellermeyer RW: *The Red Cell.* Cambridge, Mass, Harvard University Press, 1970.
11. Herbert V: Diagnostic and non-diagnostic values of measurement of serum vitamin B_{12} binding protein. *Blood* **32**:305, 1968.
12. Huff RL, et al: Ferrokinetics in normal persons and in patients having various erythropoietic disorders. *J Clin Invest* **30**:1512, 1951.
13. Schilling RF, et al: Intrinsic factor studies. *J Lab Clin Med* **45**:926, 1955.
14. Van Dyke D: Difference in destruction of erythropoietic and reticuloendothelial marrow in hematologic diseases. *Blood* **30**:364, 1967.
15. Van Dyke D, Anger HO: Patterns of marrow hypertrophy and atrophy in man. *J Nucl Med* **6**:109, 1965.
16. Weinstein MB, Smoak WM: Technical difficulties in ^{99m}Tc labeling of erythrocytes. *J Nucl Med* **11**:411, 1970.
17. Weintraub LR, Weinstein MB, Huser HS: Absorption of hemoglobin iron: The role of a heme-splitting substance in the intestinal mucosa. *J Clin Invest* **47**:531, 1968.

^{111}Indium and ^{67}Gallium concentrate nonspecificity in tumors that can then be localized by total body scanning. Positive scans draw attention to pathological areas, though negative scans do not exclude the possibility of disease.

13 Tumor Localization

Morton B. Weinstein and Eugene B. Rosenberg

In view of the great variety of clinical manifestations of neoplastic disease and the equally great variety of morphologic diseases called cancer, it is not surprising that no single diagnostic procedure can identify all cancers. Injection of a radioactive tracer and subsequent external imaging is one cancer-detection procedure. It can provide valuable clinical data, and it is a noninvasive, harmless method.

Organ Scanning

The types of radioactive agents ordinarily used for tumor localization depend on the organ suspected of harboring the neoplasm. A space-occupying lesion in the liver usually can be visualized with sulfur colloid Tc 99m, though a tumor smaller than 2 cm in diameter may be missed unless it lies on the periphery of the liver. Thyroid cancer that produces physiologic dysfunction of the gland can be defined with sodium pertechnetate Tc 99m. This is a familiar proedure to most laboratories today, and the scintigram of the thyroid was one of the first widely applied diagnostic procedures in nuclear medicine. Metastatic or primary carcinoma of the bone usually causes an osseous reaction in the form of the deposition of calcium and phosphorus that can be defined with strontium 85, fluorine 18, and technetium 99m. Exquisite sensitivity of bone scans have been clearly shown to reflect bone metastasis prior to the time that they are visualized on routine x-ray studies. Precursor requirements such as amino acids for the synthesis of protein form the basis of the use of radioactive amino acid analog such as selenomethionine.

Pancreatic carcinoma is less active and can be defined with abdominal scanning after the administration of this selenomethionine Se 75. Disruption of the blood-brain barrier allows a variety of radioactive chemicals to pass from the blood into the area of the lesion, and scanning with sodium pertechnetate Tc 99m allows detection of primary as well as metastatic brain tumors.

Total-Body Scanning

In addition to the organ related radiopharmaceuticals, two radioactive isotopes —^{111}indium and ^{67}gallium—concentrate in tumors, which can thus be localized by means of total-body scanning. The mechanism responsible for their accumulation in tumors is currently unknown. The initial observation that tumors concentrate gallium 72 was made by chance during the performance of a bone scan. The boneseeking quality of a positively charged (3+) ion was predictable, but the concurrent concentration in adjacent soft tissue tumor masses was totally unexpected. The gallium 72 studies were followed by investigations with gallium 67 both in experimental animals and in man. Attempts to define the normal and abnormal distribution of this radiopharmaceutical are well documented.[1-5,7-12,14]

Principles and Procedures

For scanning purposes 35–45 μCi/kg of ^{67}Ga or ^{111}In is given in either the citrate or the chloride form. Indium possesses slightly more favorable radiation characteristics than gallium. In animal experiments ^{111}In-chloride showed the greatest total-body retention and the highest tumor/muscle ratio.[13]

We have examined more than 300 patients with gallium 67 and more than 200 with indium 111. Some of the latter group had previously been studied with gallium. In all patients, the radioactive compound was injected intravenously as a bolus. No patient suffered immediate or delayed adverse effects, and none complained of discomfort related to the site of injections, even though subcutaneous infiltration was not uncommon.

Following intravenous injection, both indium and gallium rapidly became associated with serum proteins. Half-time clearance from the blood is about ten hours. Scanning is delayed until 48 hours after injection to allow time for reduction of blood radioactivity, which would interfere with scan interpretation.

Because gallium normally tends to accumulate in the gut, the patient is prepared with a laxative on the night preceding the examination and an enema on the day of the study. Despite these precautions, gallium sometimes concentrates in the gut to such an extent that scan interpretation is impossible in the abdominal region. This is a major disadvantage of gallium as an abdominal-tumor-localizing agent.

Indium concentration in the gut is normally minimal, and the patient need not be prepared.

Scan Evaluation

Evaluation of the total-body scan is based on the distribution of radioactivity outside normal sites of accumulation as well as on markedly asymmetrical concentration within normal sites of accumulation.

Following injection of ^{67}Ga-chloride, the contour of the colon is normally visualized. The liver also is visualized, and sometimes a small amount of radioactivity can be noted in the left upper quadrant. This is assumed to represent the spleen but may represent splenic flexure of colon in some cases. A large amount of radioactivity in the left upper quadrant is distinctly abnormal and frequently reflects splenic involvement by a neoplastic disease such as Hodgkin's. A variable amount of radioactivity is normally noted in the bony structures of the pelvis and sacrum. The testes and the penis are usually seen and in the female the mucosa of the vagina is at times well defined. Following ^{111}In-chloride, the retroperitoneal region is normally clear and bone uptake of radioactivity is confined to the functioning narrow space.

A large amount of radioactivity in the left upper quadrant following ^{67}Ga injection is distinctly abnormal and suggests splenic involvement by a neoplastic disease.

A variety of nonneoplastic diseases can

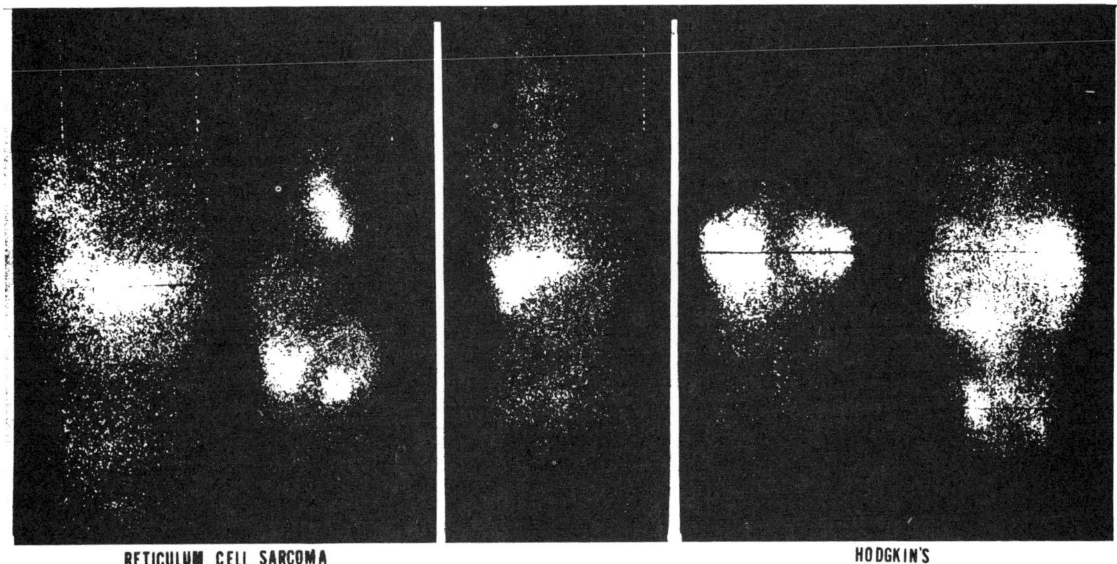

Figure 13-1 *Lymphoma defined by total-body chloride Ga 67 scans. Central scan, taken seven years after irradiation cure of Hodgkin's disease, constitutes normal control. Other scans show abnormal uptake of gallium 67 in lung, mediastinum, abdomen, and spleen.*

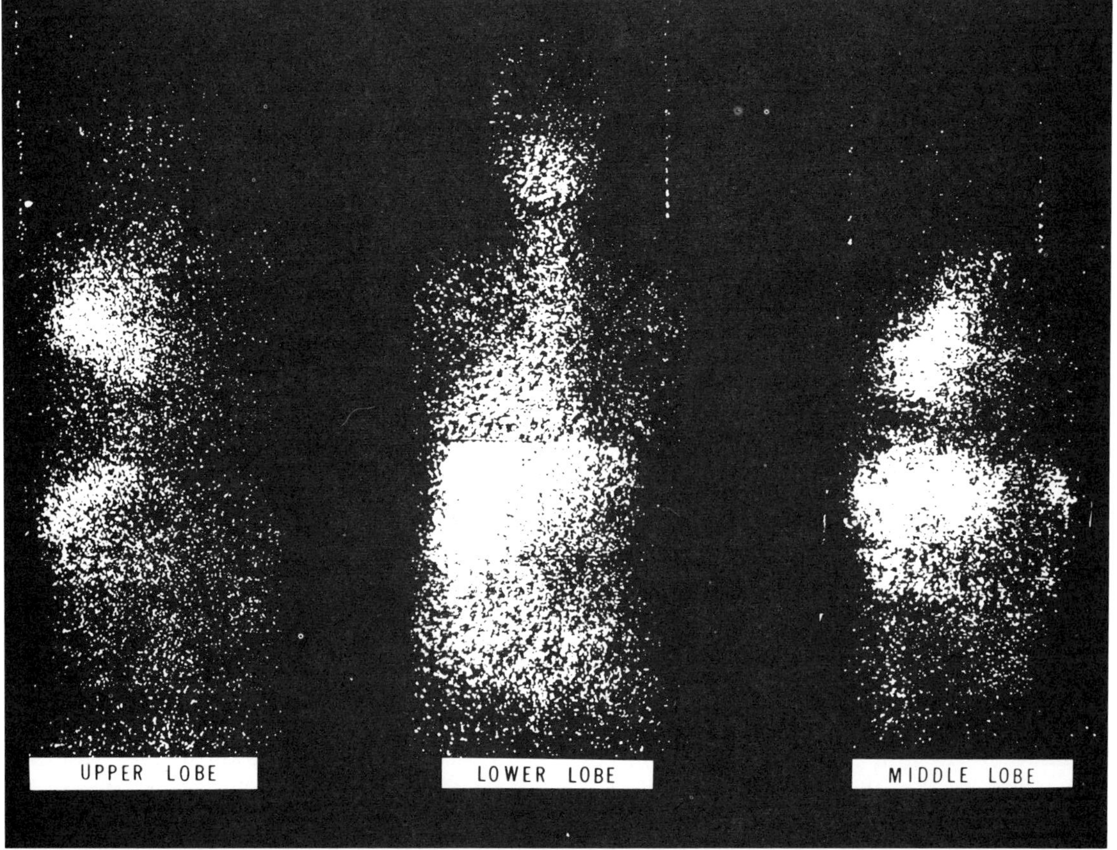

Figure 13-2 *Carcinoma of upper, lower, and middle lobe of the lung, defined with chloride Ga 67 scan. Uptake of radioactivity by liver and abdominal organs is variable.*

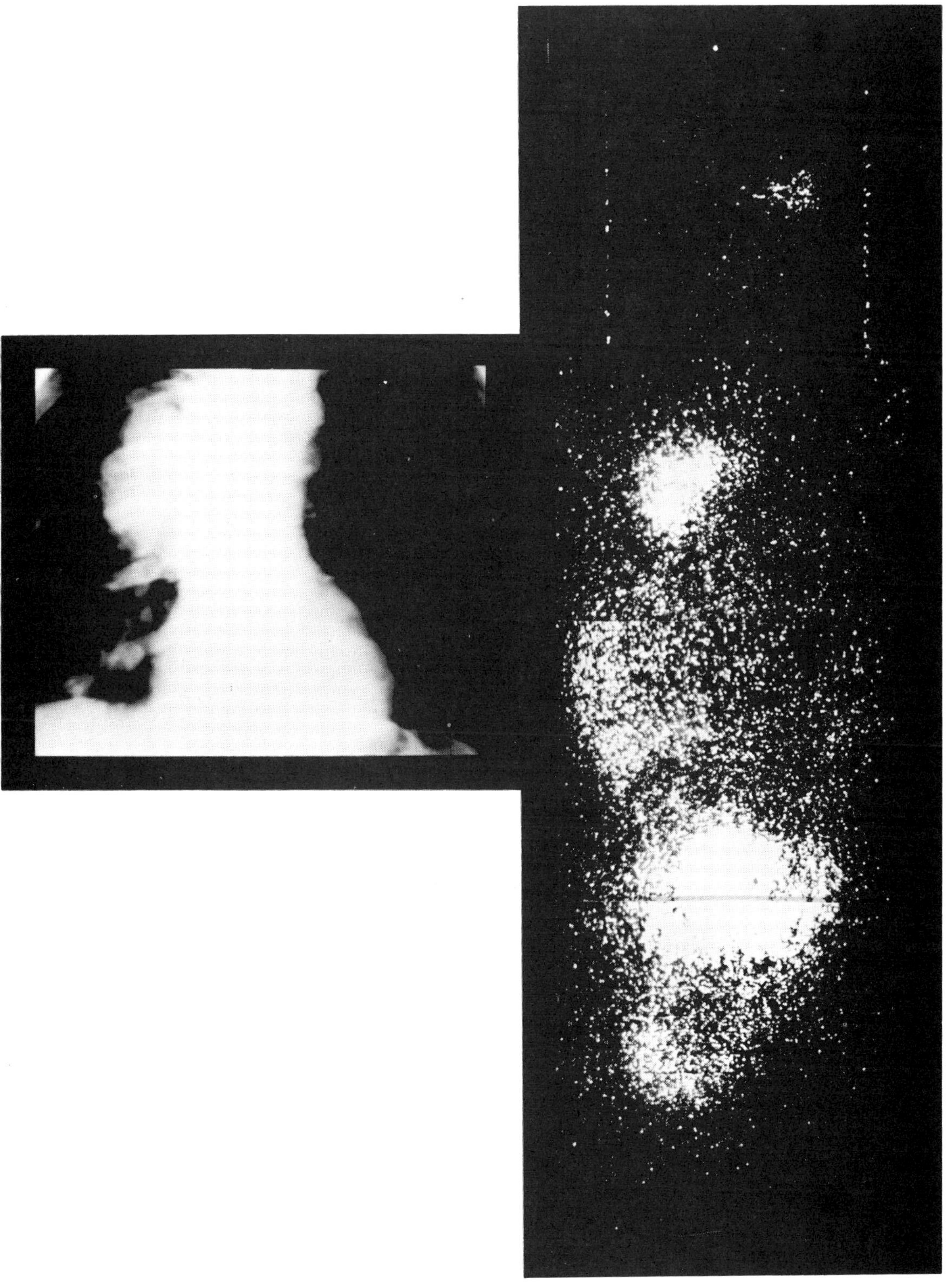

Figure 13-3 *Neuroblastoma seen on chest roentgenogram and defined by chloride Ga 67 scan. Exophytic skull lesion and abdominal and pelvic masses seen here were proved at postmortem examination to be neuroblastoma.*

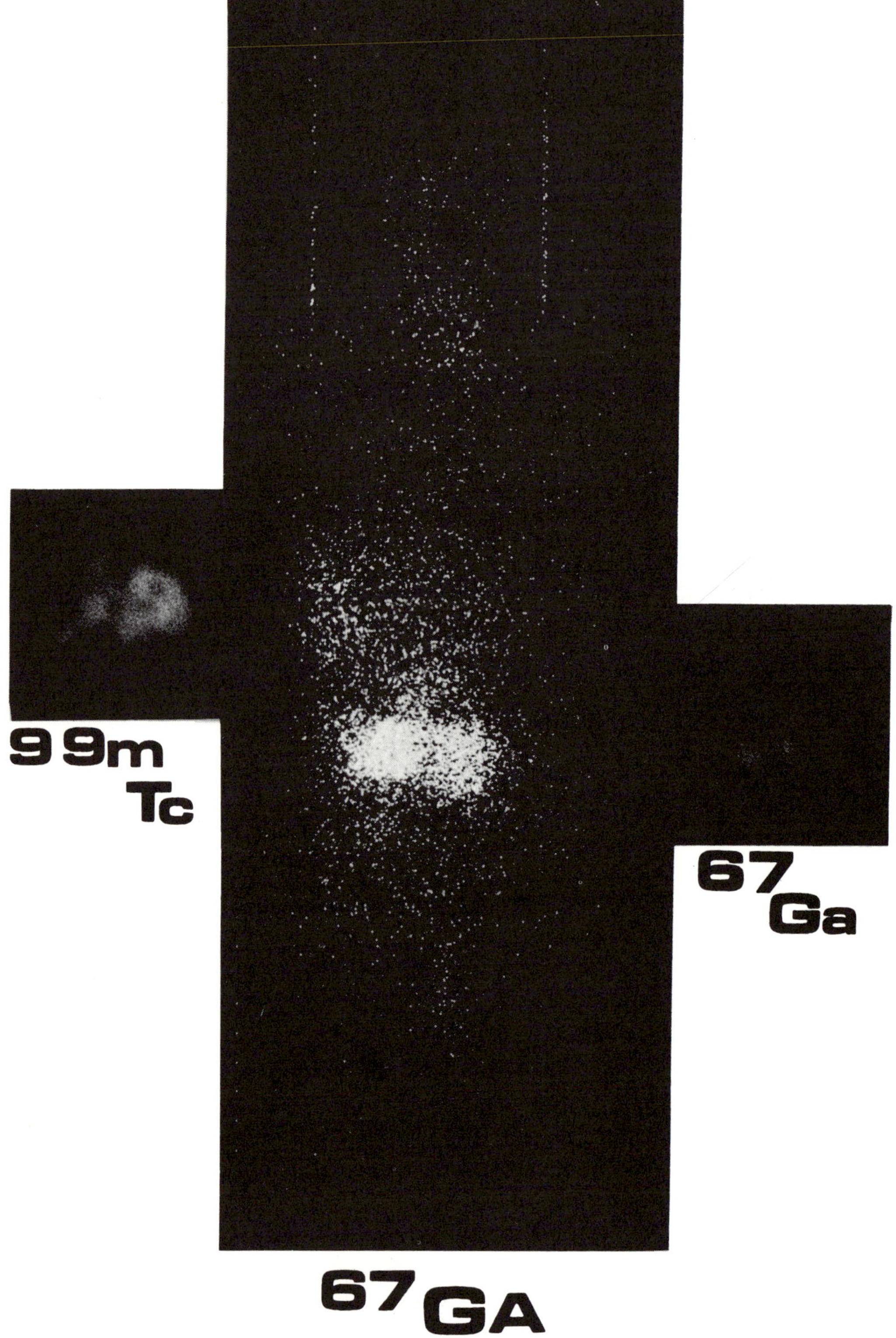

Figure 13-4 *Leiomyosarcoma in abdomen. The multiple space-occupying lesions in the liver demonstrated by sulfur colloid Tc 99m scan fail to concentrate gallium 67 as well as normal liver tissue.*

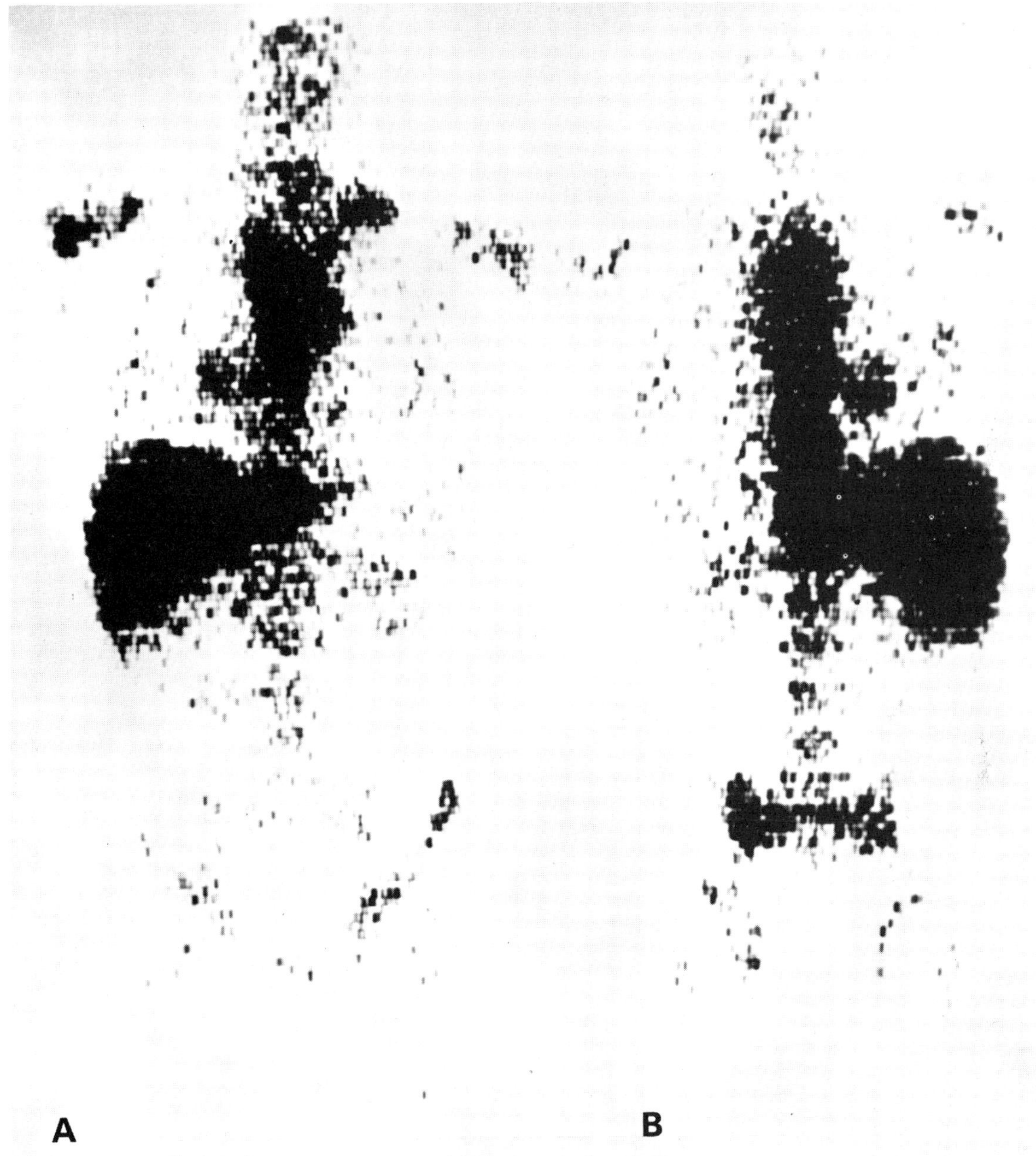

Figure 13-5 *Multiple lung, mediastinal, and neck tumors demonstrated by rectilinear anterior* (A) and *posterior* (B) *scans using* ^{111}In.

modify the distribution of gallium and indium. In patients with renal disease who have long been maintained by hemodialysis, distribution of gallium is modified from normal. Very little radioactivity is noted outside the bony structures and the liver is poorly seen. Such patients frequently develop secondary hyperparathyroidism, and the increase in bone metabolism associated with this disorder accounts for the increased gallium concentration in bone. Patients with osteomyelitis show a marked increase in gallium concentration at the site of infection. Sarcoidosis with hilar adenopathy and Paget's disease are also associated with avid concentration of gallium.

Tumors are manifested as abnormal concentrations of radioactivity. Figures 13-1 through 13-4 show chloride Ga 67 scans indicative of various malignant lesions. Of particular interest is the role of scanning in identifying malignant lymphoma. The method is not at present entirely reliable. Not all lesions in a given patient are visualized, and tumors recovered at postmortem vary widely in amount of radioactivity they contain per gram of tissue (Table 13-1). Tumors of the same histologic type are visualized in some patients but not in others.

Figures 13-5 through 13-7 show tumors localized by abnormal concentration of ^{111}In-chloride. Since indium is normally taken up by the bone marrow, erythron destruction (by radiation or drugs) or replacement (by tumor) appears on scanning as decreased radioactivity compared with the opposite normal side. The same lesion would be visualized with ^{67}Ga as an area of increased radioactivity. Scanning with ^{99m}Tc-sulfur-colloid would show the reticuloendothelial system in the affected area to be intact.

Neither indium nor gallium detects all neoplastic lesions (Fig 13-8), and both agents sometimes concentrate in nonneoplastic lesions (Fig 13-9).

Conclusion

The chief advantage of total-body scanning for tumor localization is its harmlessness: The procedure is not associated with morbidity or mortality. It is also rapid and frequently provides clinically useful information, such as suspected sites of disease which can be easily biopsied. A cooperative study under the auspices of the Oak Ridge

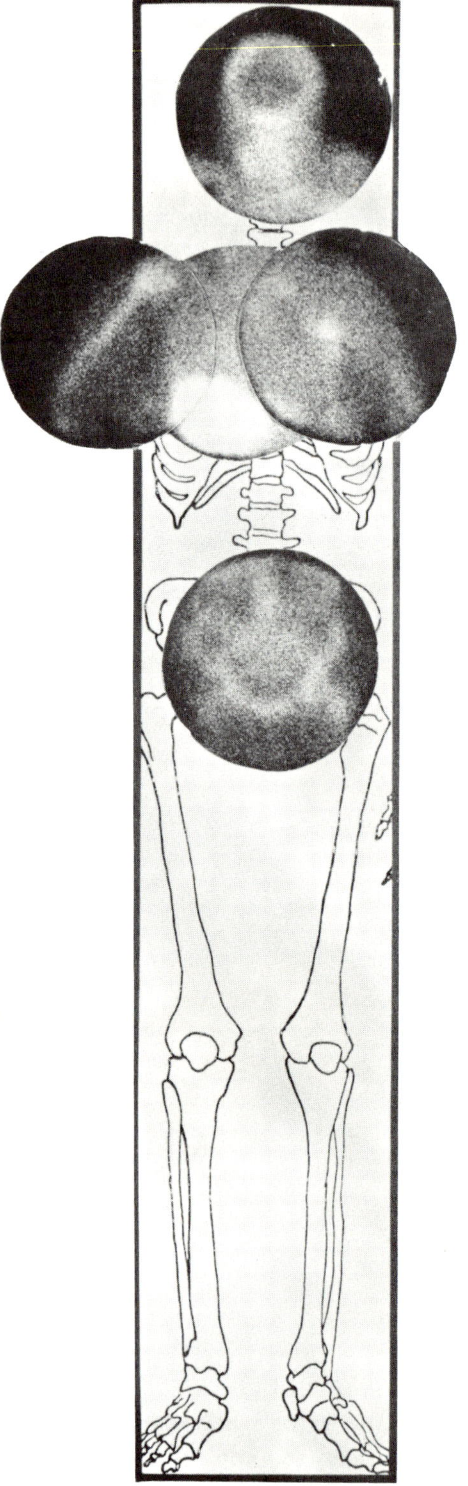

Figure 13-6 *Metastatic carcinoma from left breast to left axilla demonstrated with chloride In 111 scan. Marrow of left humerus has been affected by radiation therapy.*

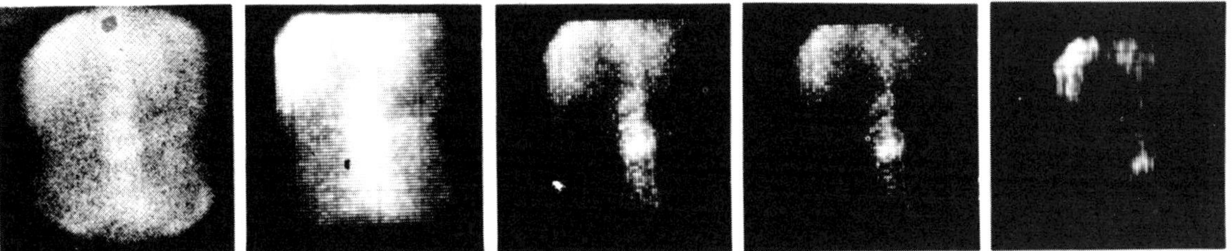

Figure 13-7 *Vertebral body metastasis depicted by digital processing of analog image obtained with chloride In 111.*

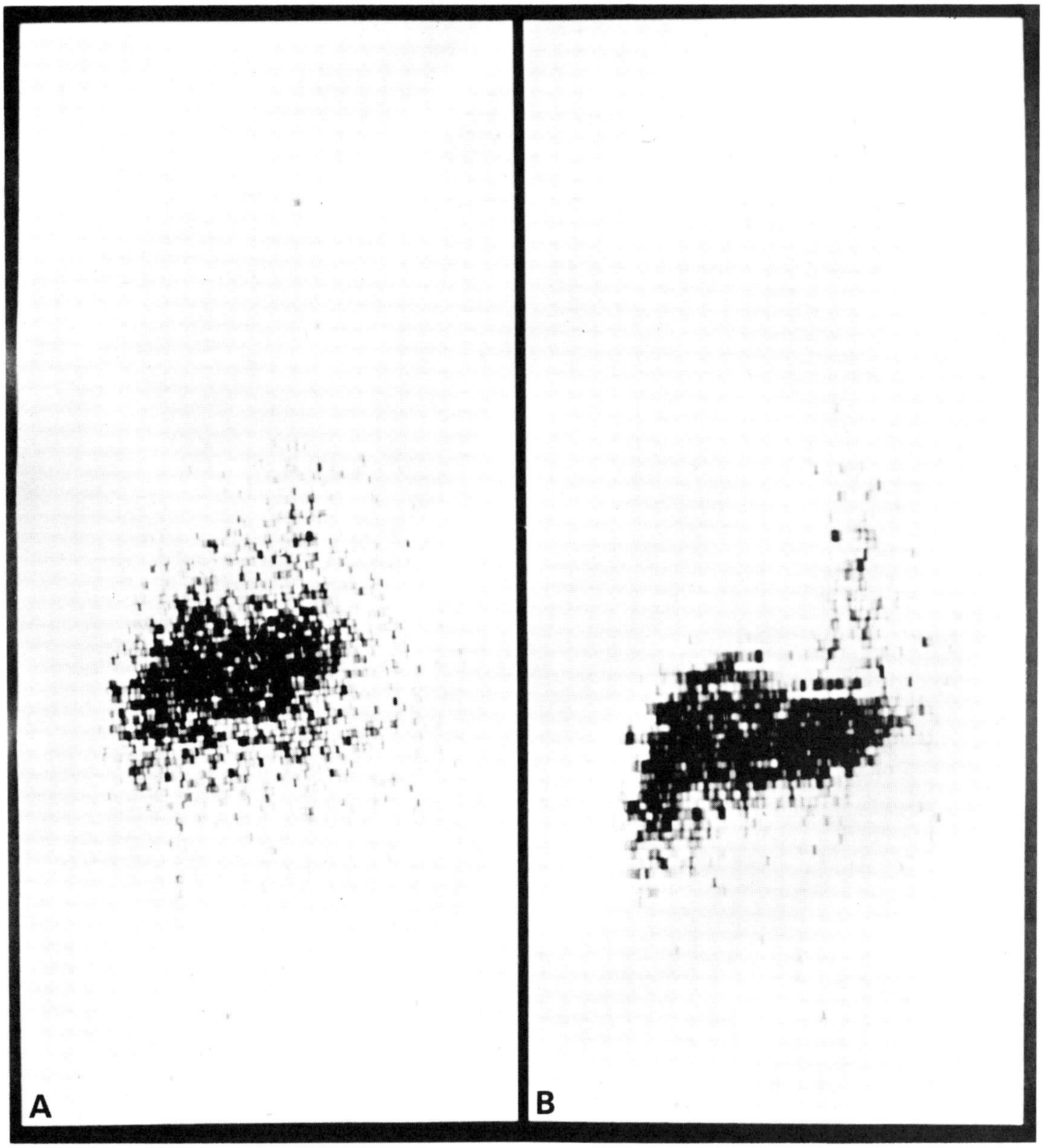

Figure 13-8 *Large, palpable left supraclavicular and cervical adenopathy not defined by scanning with chloride Ga 67* (A) *or chloride In 111* (B).

Table 13-1. Variability of Gallium Uptake by Four Neoplastic Lesions in Humans

Tumor	Uptake (counts/gm) Min	Av	Max	Tumor/muscle ratio
Poorly differentiated hepatocellular carcinoma	3,429	5,536	8,267	0.76
Adenocarcinoma of lung	15,596	30,904	41,304	3.30
Histiocytic lymphoma (reticulum cell sarcoma)	2,575	16,812	48,562	159.00
Squamous cell carcinoma of lung	8,552	18,151	38,828	52.00

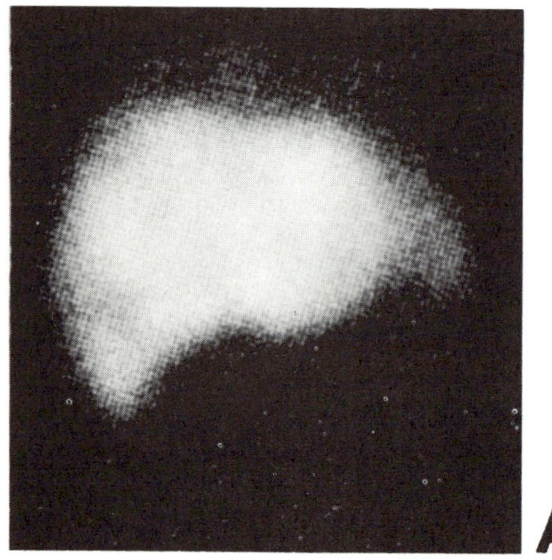
A

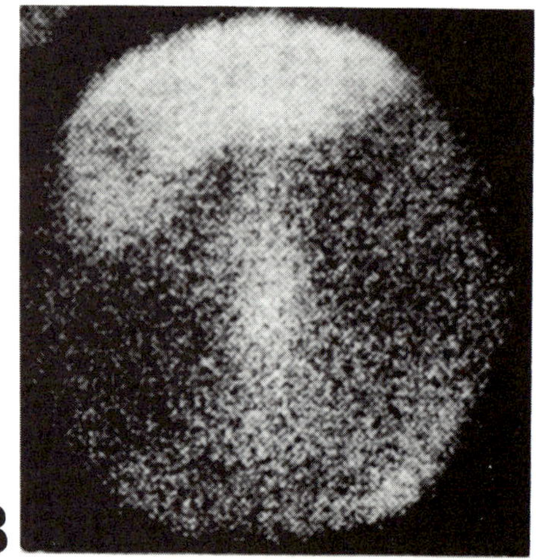
B

Figure 13-9 *Multiple filling defects in liver demonstrated by scanning with sulfur colloid Tc 99m* (A) *and chloride In 111* (B).

Associated Universities will shortly present the results of over 2000 examinations in 14 university centers. This study will attempt to answer specific questions relative to the type of tumors seen, size and location of lesions, and the effect of previous treatment on the positivity of scans. It is anticipated that this large computer data bank of ^{67}Ga studies will serve as a basis of comparison for other tumor localizing radiopharmaceuticals.

References

1. Andrews GA, Root SW, Interman HD: Study of gallium-67. *Radiology* **61**:570–588, 1953.
2. Bruner HD, Hayes RL, Perkinson JD: Preliminary data on Ga-67. *Radiology* **61**:102, 1953.
3. Dudley HC, Imirie GW, Istock JT: Depositions of radiogallium (Ga-72) in proliferating tissues. *Radiology* **55**:571–588, 1950.
4. Dudley HC, Maddox GE: Deposition of radiogallium (Ga-72) in skeletal tissue. *J Pharmacol Exp Ther* **96**:224–227, 1949.

5. Edwards CL, Hayes RL: Tumor scanning with Ga-67 citrate. *J Nucl Med* **10**:103–105, 1969.
6. Glatstein E, Tnueblood HW, Enright LP, et al: Surgical staging of abdominal involvement in unselected patients with Hodgkin's disease. *Radiology* **97**:425, 1970.
7. Hayes RL, Byrd BL, Carlton JE, et al: Factor affecting the localization of ^{67}Ga in animal tumors. *J Nucl Med* **11**:324, 1970.
8. Hayes RL, Nelson B, Swartzenruber DC, et al: Gallium-67 localization in rat and mouse tumors. *Science* **167**:289–290, 1970.
9. Higasi T, Ikemoto S, Nakayama Y, et al: Diagnosis of malignant tumor with ^{67}G-citrate. *Jap J Nucl Med* **6**:217–226, 1969.
10. Langhammer H, Glaubitt G, Grebe SF, et al: ^{67}Ga for tumor scanning. *J Nucl Med* 13:25–30, 1972.
11. Lavender JP, Barker JR, et al: Gallium-67 citrate scanning in neoplastic and inflammatory lesions. *Br J Radiol* **44**:361–366, 1971.
12. Mulry CWC, Dudley HC: Studies of radiogallium as diagnostic agent in bone tumors. *J Lab Clin Invest* **37**:239–252, 1951.
13. Weinstein MB: ^{67}Gallium and ^{111}Indium concentration in R2788 lymphosarcoma (rodent). Unpublished data.
14. Winchell HS, Sanchez PD, Watanabe CK, et al: Visualization of tumors in humans using ^{67}Ga citrate and the Anger whole-body scanner, scintillation camera, and tomographic scanner. *J Nucl Med* **11**:459–466, 1970.

Radioisotopic techniques allow detection and quantitation of circulating antigens associated with tumor cells, providing potentially valuable tools for early cancer detection.

14
Detection of Human Tumor-Associated Antigens

Eugene B. Rosenberg, Patricia M. Smith and Morton B. Weinstein

Gold's investigations in 1965 demonstrated that human tumor cells possess unique antigens. Carcinoembryonic antigen (CEA) is a glycoprotein present in adenocarcinomas of the entodermally derived digestive tract epithelium. When this antigen was detected in the blood of patients with adenocarcinoma, its potential as a diagnostic test for cancer was recognized.[2] Other circulating tumor-associated antigens, identified, include alpha fetoprotein (AFP), gamma fetoprotein (GFP), fetal sulfoglyprotein antigen (FSA), and T-globulin.[5] Their characteristics are presented in Table 14-1.

Tumor-associated antigens have also been detected on cells of patients with melanoma, Burkitt's lymphoma, leukemia, Wilms' tumor, sarcoma, and neuroblastoma. The presence of these antigenic markers on human tumor cells, but not on normal cells, affords an opportunity to interpret clinical events that parallel changing concentrations of circulating tumor antigens. The existence of human tumor-associated antigens provides a rational basis for immunotherapy of human cancers.

Tumor-Associated Antigens

- Carcinoembryonic antigen (CEA)
- Alpha fetoprotein (AFP)
- Gamma fetoprotein (GFP)
- Fetal sulfoglycoprotein antigen (FSA)
- T globulin

Methods

Human tumor-associated antigens induce both humoral and cellular immune responses. These immune responses, in turn, can be utilized in assays for detection and quantitation of the tumor-associated antigens. For example, antibodies to tumor-associated antigens are used in radioimmunoassays for precise quantitation of concentrations of circulating tumor antigens, and lymphocyte responses to tumor-associated antigens can be measured by lymphocyte transformation studies and the lymphocyte cytotoxicity reaction.

The most sensitive techniques to detect and quantitate human tumor-associated antigens utilize radioisotopes. Table 14-2 outlines the currently available nuclear procedures for detecting and quantitating

Table 14-1. Characteristics of Circulating Tumor-Associated Antigens

Characteristic	AFP	CEA	FSA	T Globulin	GFP
Molecular weight	70,000	200,000	?	160,000	?
Electrophoretic mobility	Alpha 1	Beta	Alpha 2	Alpha	Gamma
Fetal expression	Yes	Yes	?	?	Yes
Circulating antibody	No	Yes	?	Yes	Yes
Glycoprotein	Yes	Yes	Yes	Yes (globulin)	Yes
Tumor association	Mostly hepatoma	Mainly colonic carcinoma; also other tumors and inflamatory conditions	Mainly stomach cancer	Wide variety of tumors	Wide variety of tumors

human tumor-associated antigens. In theory most radionuclides can be used in these assays, but in practice the iodine isotopes have been employed because they bind to proteins like CEA. Tritiated thymidine has been valuable because it is incorporated into DNA; ^{51}Cr because it is incorporated into viable cells. CEA can be quantitated with a radioimmunoassay employing three isotopes (^{125}I, ^{131}I, ^{22}Na) and two antibodies. AFP can be measured by a radioimmunoassay utilizing a single antibody and a single isotope (^{125}I). Leukemia-associated antigens can be detected (1) by lymphocyte transformation studies that use tritiated thymidine as a measure of blastogenic transformation and (2) by the lymphocyte cytotoxicity test, which is a sensitive indicator of cell-mediated immunity. In this test, leukemc blast cells are labeled with ^{51}Cr and the destruction of these leukemic blast cells by sensitized lymphocytes is measured by the chromium released from cells into supernate fluids.

The first assays for human tumor antigens used antibodies produced by laboratory animals following the injection of human tumor cells. Gold, for example, immunized

Table 14-2. Radioisotopic Techniques for Detection of Human Tumor-Associated Antigens

Tumor-associated antigen	Radioisotopic technique	Radionuclide
CEA	Radioimmunoassay	^{125}I, ^{131}I, ^{22}Na
AFP	Radioimmunoassay	^{125}I
Leukemia-associated antigen	Lymphocyte transformation	Thymidine H^3
Leukemia-associated antigen	Lymphocyte cytotoxicity	^{51}Cr

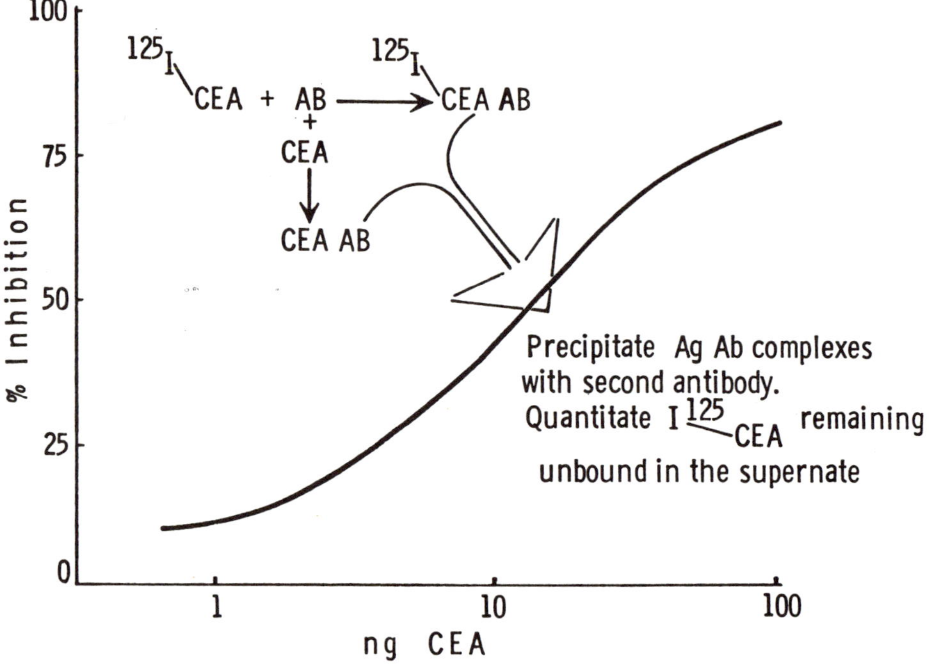

Figure 14-1 *Use of radioimmunoassay to quantitate circulating CEA. Radioactive CEA and unlabeled CEA compete for antibody-binding site. Increasing concentrations of unlabeled CEA progressively inhibit binding of labeled CEA. Inhibition curve shown was obtained by addition of increasing amounts of unlabeled CEA to a constant amount of CEA I 125.*

rabbits with human colon tumor cells and obtained antibodies to these tumor cells. In early work, CEA was detected using these specific antibodies in immunodiffusion tests. The presence of a tumor-associated antigen was indicated by a visible precipitin band between wells containing the test sample and the specific antisera. Immunodiffusion tests can detect AFP, GFP, T globulin, and FSA. However, they provide only a qualitative determination of whether or not the tumor-associated antigen is present. They lack the quantitative precision of the radioimmunoassay. We anticipate that radioimmunoassays will soon be developed for precise measurement of GFP, T globulin, FSP, and other yet-to-be-defined tumor-associated antigens. Certain of these tumor-associated antigens are believed to exist in normal tissues in amounts so small they can be detected only with radioimmunoassays.

Radioimmunoassay for CEA

The test is based on the competition of labeled and unlabeled antigens for specific antibodies. The binding of labeled antigen to antibody is inversely proportional to the amount of unlabeled antigen present. Figure 14-1 illustrates the competition between radioactive CEA and unlabeled CEA for an antibody-binding site; the curve indicates the increasing inhibition of binding of radioactive CEA in the presence of increasing amounts of unlabeled CEA.

During the past eight years, five different assays for CEA have been developed (Table 14-3). They utilize different methods of separating antigen from antigen-antibody complexes, have different normal values, and require different amounts of sample and time for completion of the assay. In our laboratory we initially used immunodifusion and countercurrent elec-

Table 14-3. Characteristics of the CEA Radioimmunoassays

Assay	Extraction	Precipitation	Requirements	Normal values (ng)
Gold	1 M PCA	$(NH_4)_2 SO_2$	10 ml serum 5 days	2.5
Hansen	0.6 M PCA	Zirconyl-PO_4 gel	2 ml plasma 3 days	2.5
Todd	None	Antibody to IgG	0.4 ml serum or plasma 1 day	12.0
Langer	0.6 M PCA	Hemagglutination	5 ml serum 1 day	5.0
Go	None	Zirconyl-PO_4	0.2 ml plasma 1 day	2.0

trophoresis to measure CEA levels. Because these assays lacked reproducibility, were insensitive, and yielded only qualitative information, we have adopted Todd's double-antibody, triple-isotope radioimmunoassay for measurement of CEA. This method is rapid, has internal standard controls, and can be performed in a single tube. It is readily adaptable to the rapid assay of large numbers of samples and to computer calculation of results.

TODD'S PROCEDURE

Todd's radioimmunoassay for CEA is based on a technique originated by Berson and Yalow, that was routinely used to measure small amounts of insulin. In the double-antibody radioimmunoassay, the antigen-antibody complex is precipitated by a second antibody directed against the immunoglobulins of the species engendering the first antibody. Thus, goat anti-CEA bodies are allowed to equilibrate with labeled and unlabeled CEA. All the goat antibodies to CEA are precipitated by the addition of horse antibodies to goat IgG. The quantity of CEA not bound by the goat anti-CEA antibody is measured by counting the amount of radioactivity remaining in the supernate after precipitation of all antigen-antibody complexes.

Todd has improved this technique by adding two more isotopes, ^{22}Na and ^{131}I.[1] ^{22}Na serves as a volume marker, allowing rapid sample processing and eliminating errors related to inadvertent loss of precipitate during pipetting. ^{131}I provides an internal control to check that the appropriate conditions for the assay are achieved for each sample.

CLINICAL USE

Todd's assay was used in a large clinical study of patients with colonic carcinoma and detected CEA in 67% of these patients. This proportion is comparable to the results obtained with Hansen's and Gold's radioimmunoassays. The proportion of positive results reflects the clinical characteristics of the patient population more than the sensitivity of the assay. Patients with small colonic tumors (Duke A lesions) have low CEA levels; patients with extensive metastatic spread of colonic carcinoma (Duke C lesions) have higher CEA levels. A positive result with the CEA assay is

> The CEA assay can detect recurrent metastatic colonic carcinoma.

more often associated with advanced disease. The CEA assay can detect recurrent metastatic colonic carcinoma and helps distinguish localized from metastatic tumors in preoperative evaluation. The assay suggests completeness of resection in postoperative patients and may provide a rational basis for reexploration in patients with suspected residual or recurrent tumors.

Quantitation of circulating levels of CEA is a reliable means of monitoring the clinical course of patients with carcinoma of the colon. The CEA level falls dramatically following surgery and rises following spread of disease with metastasis to the liver.

Radioimmunoassay for AFP

The tumor-associated antigen AFP appears in the serum of over 70% of patients with hepatoma. Very few false-positive results are associated with the assay, and a positive AFP result strongly suggests the presence of a hepatoma or of another tumor. Other tumors which are rarely associated with elevated levels of circulating alpha fetoprotein include testicular neoplasm, gastric carcinoma, and childhood tumors from a wide variety of organs.

> A positive AFP result strongly suggests hepatoma.

A single-antibody radioimmunoassay for AFP has recently been developed,[6] which is similar in principle to the CEA procedure described above but utilizes a single isotope (I^{125}) and a single antibody against AFP. Deletion of AFP in amniotic fluid is proving to be a useful test for the early detection of prenatal congenital anomalies.

Lymphocyte Transformation Assay

In the presence of a foreign antigen, human lymphocytes are stimulated to undergo blastogenic transformation. Lymphocyte transformation reactions have recently been used to detect foreign antigens on tumor cells from patients with cancer that are not present on normal cells from the same patients.

PROCEDURE

This assay, which utilizes tritiated thymidine to measure incorporation of a nuclide into DNA, is illustrated in Figure 14-2. Blastogenic transformation does not follow incubation of lymphocytes with cells that possess normal tissue antigens (Fig 14-3*A*). However, incubation of lymphocytes with tumor cells and the recognition of foreign tumor-associated antigens by host lymphocytes lead to blastogenic transformation with active DNA synthesis and rapid incorporation of tritiated thymidine (Fig 14-3*B*). To determine whether lymphocytes have undergone blastogenic transformation, cells are harvested after standard incubation times and assayed for tritiated thymidine content. High concentration of tritiated thymidine in lymphocytes is a direct measure of blastogenic response and an indirect measure of a foreign tumor-associated antigen.[3]

CLINICAL USES

In addition to its role in cancer detection, lymphocyte transformation study allows evaluation of donor-recipient transplant compatibility and assessment of immune competence.

The assay is performed routinely, using lymphocytes of potential donors and recipients, before kidney and bone marrow

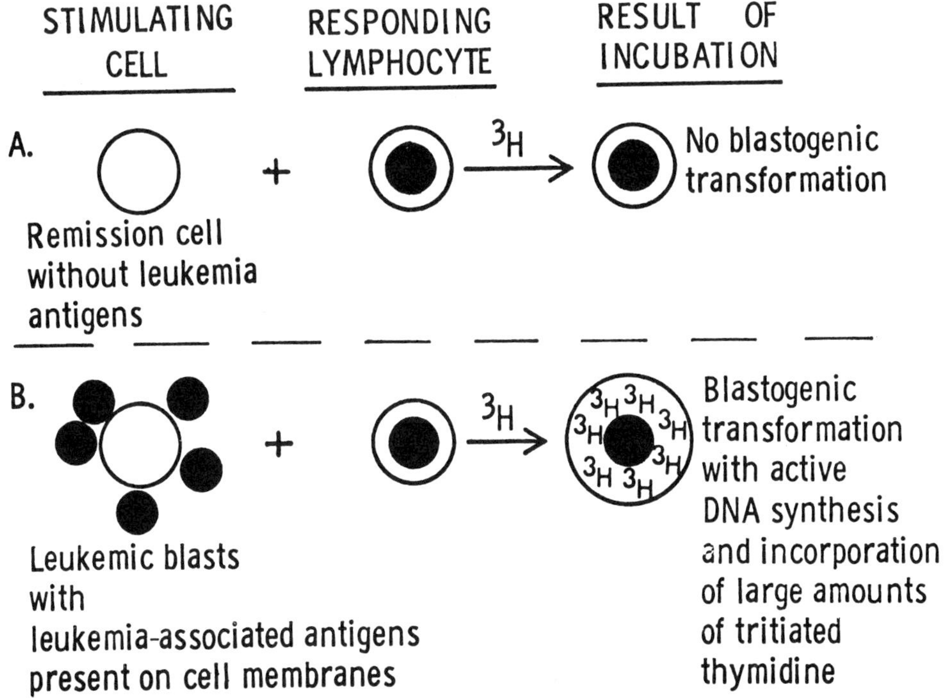

Figure 14-2 *Detection of leukemia-associated antigens by means of lymphocyte transformation study.* A. *No blastogenic transformation in response to normal stimulating cells after five days' incubation.* B. *Blastogenic transformation in response to leukemia-associated antigen after five days' incubation.*

transplants. A compatible mixed lymphocyte reaction is associated with better transplant results. An incompatible mixed lymphocyte reaction indicates that donor and recipient cells are not matched and that the transplant should be attempted only for compelling reasons.

A second use for this assay system is to test for immune competence of lymphocytes. This is of particular importance to patients who are immunodeficient and to those who have cancer. Normal lymphocytes undergo blast transformation in the presence of phytohemagglutinin (PHA), a universal mitogen. Lymphocytes derived from immunodeficient patients are incapable of responding to this mitogen. Thus, a low PHA response indicates abnormal lymphocyte function and constitutes a measure of immune deficiency. Since immune integrity, as measured by the response of lymphocytes to PHA, correlates well with the prognosis of cancer patients, the assay will be used more frequently in the future. This assay also supplies a gauge of the immune reactivity of cancer patients being treated with immunotherapy.

Lymphocyte Cytotoxicity Assay

While lymphocyte transformation is an accurate measure of the afferent limb of the immune response, it does not reflect the efferent limb of the immune response. Following blastogenic transformation a clone of sensitized lymphocytes is produced. Lymphocytes are directly capable of destroying other cells which bear antigens to which the lymphocytes are sensitized. In addition, these sensitized lymphocytes can specifically combine with antigen and release a variety of soluble proteins including lymphotoxin, lymphokinin, chemotactic factor, migration-inhibition factor (MIF), macrophage-aggregating factor (MAE), and interferon. The effectiveness of the

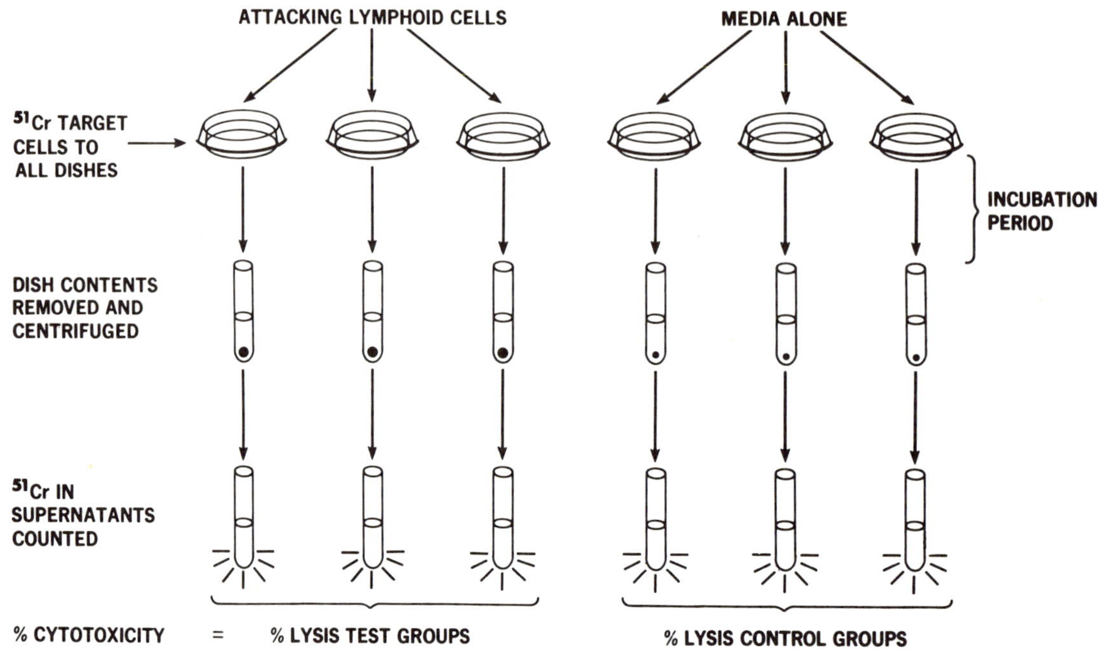

Figure 14-3 *^{51}Cr-release assay for quantitation of lymphocyte cytotoxicity to tumor antigens.*

efferent limb of the immune response can be estimated by quantitating the release of soluble proteins or by quantitating direct lymphocyte cytotoxicity.

Lymphocyte cytotoxicity to cells bearing tumor antigens can be quantitated with a ^{51}Cr-release assay, a sensitive indicator of cell-mediated immunity to tumor antigens. In this assay, target cells are labeled with ^{51}Cr and then incubated in the presence of lymphocytes. Cell destruction is quantitated by the amount of ^{51}Cr released from target cells into supernates (Fig 14-3). This assay is useful in defining leukemia-associated antigens. Recent studies indicate that sensitized lymphocytes from patients with leukemia actively destroy leukemic blasts which have leukemia-associated antigens. However, these sensitized lymphocytes do not damage remission leukemic lymphocytes which do not bear leukemia-associated antigens. Similar ^{51}Cr-release studies of identical twins, one twin with leukemia and the other normal, show the presence of leukemia-associated antigens on cells of the leukemic twin, but not on cells of the normal twin.[4]

Lymphocytes sensitized to leukemia-associated antigens do not destroy remission lymphocytes from leukemia patients lacking these antigens. In contrast, these sensitized lymphocytes actively destroy leukemia blasts possessing leukemia-associated antigens. The amount of destruction of these blast cells is related to the amount of ^{51}Cr released into the supernate.

While the lymphocyte cytotoxicity assay has been most successfully employed in the study of leukemia-associated antigens, new evidence suggests that lymphocytes from patients with a wide variety of cancers are sensitized to their own tumor antigens. Thus the ^{51}Cr-release lymphocyte cytotoxicity assay has great potential for further studies of other human tumor antigens.

Anticipated Progress

Much has been achieved in the past eight years and rapid further development is anticipated. Such distinct tumor antigens as GFP, FSA, and T globulin have been defined with Ouchterlony immunodiffusion tests. At present these antigens can be detected only qualitatively, but methods for their precise quantitation by radioimmunoassay cannot be far off.

The next logical step beyond in vitro detection of tumor antigens is in vivo detection and quantitation of tumor antigens. Gold and others have shown that specific antibodies will react with tumor antigens, whether the antigens are in serum contained in a test tube or on cells fixed to a slide. These antibodies can be conjugated with fluorescein dyes for detection of tumor antigens with fluorescent antibody studies. Antibodies can also be conjugated with ferritin for antigen detection with electron microscopy. In the future conjugation of specific antibodies with radionuclides will probably enable tumor localization by scanning in vivo. Potentially, neoplastic diseases will be treated by a radionuclide bound to an antibody specific for tumor and delivered, owing to the great specificity of antibodies, directly to the tumor and not to surrounding normal tissues.

References

1. Egan ML, Lautenschleger JT, Coligan JE, et al: Radioimmune assay of carcinoembryonic antigen. *Immunochemistry* **9**:289, 1972.
2. Gold P: Tumor specific antigen in GI cancer. *Hosp Practice* **7**:79, 1972.
3. Levanthal BG, Halterman RH, Rosenberg EB, et al: Immune reactivity of leukemia patients to autologous blast cells. *Cancer Res* **32**:1820, 1972.
4. Rosenberg EB, Herberman RB, Levine PH, et al: Lymphocyte cytotoxicity reactions to leukemia associated antigens in identical twins. *Int J Cancer* **9**:648, 1972.
5. Stillman A, Zamcheck N: Recent advances in immunologic diagnosis of digestive tract cancer. *Digest Dis* **15**:1003, 1970.
6. Waldman TA, McIntire KR: Serum alpha fetoprotein levels in patients with ataxia telangiectasia. *Lancet* **2**:1112, 1972.

Radioimmunoassay allows nanogram and picogram quantities of hormones, enzymes, pharmaceuticals, and chemicals to be measured in the blood. It facilitates diagnosis of pituitary, pancreatic, and gastrointestinal disorders and of anemia, hepatitis, and digitalis misuse.

15 Radioimmunoassay

Fuad S. Ashkar and Albert V. Heal

Principles and Techniques

Radioimmunoassay (RIA) was first introduced in 1959 when Berson and Yalow reported the measurement of insulin in plasma by this method. In 1960 Unger and associates reported the use of RIA to measure glucagon, and in the same year Herbert, employing the RIA principle, demonstrated the use of intrinsic factor for the assay of vitamin B_{12}. The latter method, known as competitive protein binding (CPB), is a more general term than RIA. The basic difference between the two methods is that in RIA the substance which reacts with the substrate is a specific antibody, whereas in CPB the substance is a protein, not necessarily an antibody.

Since the late 1950s, refinement of the RIA procedure has made possible the quantitation of low concentrations of hormones in the blood, facilitating diagnosis and treatment of various diseases. At present, the majority of known peptide hormones in the body fluids can be measured by RIA.

RIA is based on the competition for binding sites on a specific antibody by its radioactively labeled antigen and unlabeled antigen. Thus three substances are necessary for the reaction: unlabeled antigen, radioactively labeled antigen, and a specific antibody.

Three substances are needed for RIA: unlabeled antigen, labeled antigen, and a specific antibody.

The Antigen

Any substance that can stimulate an antibody response and react specifically with that antibody is an antigen. Most antigenic substances are proteins; some are carbohydrates. In order for substances to be antigenic, it must have a molecular weight of at least 10,000. Certain substances, such as digoxin, are unable to stimulate an antibody response owing to their small size. These substances, called haptens, can

Antigen: A substance that can stimulate an antibody response and react specifically with that antibody
Labeled antigen: A purified standard antigen with a radioactive isotope introduced into the molecule
Antibody: A substance produced in response to an antigen

stimulate antibody production if they are conjugated to high-molecular-weight proteins. Therefore, it is now theoretically possible to stimulate antibody production with any substance. Since antigens have many and different types of reaction sites, different antibodies can be produced for the same antigen.

The "standard" antigen used in the assay to generate the standard curve must be highly purified to prevent crossover reactions due to similarly structured antigen. The standard must also be available in sufficient quantity.

The Labeled Antigen

The labeled antigen is simply the purified standard antigen with a radioactive isotope introduced into the molecule. The radioactive label may be ^{125}I, ^{131}I, ^{57}Co, tritium, etc. depending on what antigen is to be labeled and which label can be introduced into the molecule. The isotope of choice is ^{125}I for three reasons: 1) high isotopic abundance, 2) high counting efficiency, and 3) long half-life.

The smaller the quantity of labeled antigen, the greater the sensitivity of the assay since the other components of the test may be correspondingly reduced. The count rate of the final products is the only limiting factor. If the specific activity of the antigen is increased smaller quantities may be used. Here the limiting factors are chemical degradation and instability, which may accompany high specific activity.

The concentration of labeled antigen is held constant throughout the assay.

The Antibody

An antibody is a substance produced in response to an antigen. It is produced by animal immunization to an antigen and may be specific for that antigen or may react with structurally similar antigens and have various reaction energies and rates. In RIA the most essential property of an antibody is its specificity for a particular antigen. Unfortunately, most antibodies have a long incubation period. However, they are quite stable and highly sensitive, and can be prepared for virtually any substance.

The concentration of antibody used in RIA is usually that amount of antibody necessary to bind 30% to 70% of the labeled antigen when only labeled antigen is present. This predetermined concentration of antibody is held constant throughout the procedure.

The Assay

As previously mentioned, three substances must be combined in an assay tube. Fixed concentrations of labeled antigen and antibody are placed in the assay tubes, plus either varying concentrations of standard (for the generation of the standard curve) or a known volume of the patient's plasma (Fig 15-1). In most cases special preparation of the plasma is unnecessary. The assay tubes are allowed to incubate for a time that depends on the antigen-antibody reaction rate. The reaction that occurs (Fig 15-1) is simply a competition for antibody by the labeled and unlabeled antigen. The quantity of labeled antigen-antibody complex formed is inversely proportional to the quantity of standard or patient's antigen present. That is, the more standard or patient's antigen present, the less labeled antigen-antibody complex formed. Therefore, most RIAs are indirect. The reaction rate depends on the pH of the solution and the incubation temperature. Each antigen-antibody reaction has its own pH values and incubation temperatures for maximum reaction rates.

Separation

After incubation the amount of free and bound antigen must be determined. First, they must be separated. In the past several

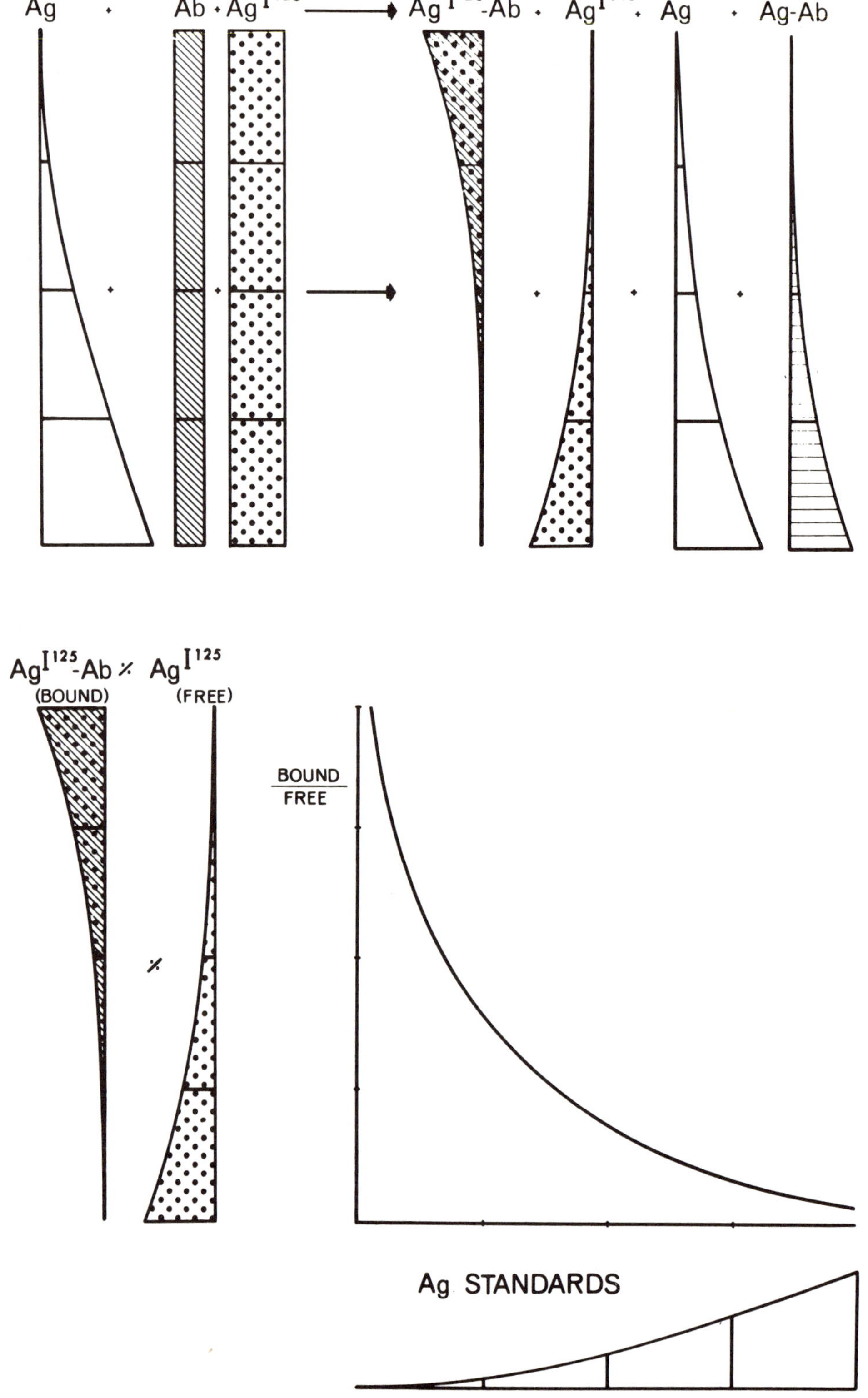

Figure 15-1 *RIA principle and standard curve derivation. Ag: antigen; Ab: antibody; AgI¹²⁵: labeled antigen; Ag¹²⁵I–Ab: labeled antigen antibody complex; Ag–Ab: unlabeled antigen antibody complex.*

methods have been used—chromatography, electrophoresis, filtration, dialysis, ammonium sulfate precipitation, among others. At present, two basic methods are employed: liquid- and solid-phase separation.

In the liquid-phase method the reaction is exposed to a suspension of dextran-coated charcoal, resin, or similar substance which will adsorb the free antigen. The mixture is centrifuged, and the supernatant, which contains the antigen-antibody complex, can be separated from the residue which contains the free antigen.

In the solid-phase method the antibody is bound to a particle such as Sephadex or to the sides of a polyethylene tube. The antigen binds to the antibody, which is already attached to the separation system. The tubes are centrifuged (Sephadex) or washed out (antibody-coated tubes) to separate free from bound antigen.

Data Derivation

The supernatant and residue are counted for radioactivity by gamma or liquid scintillation, depending on the isotope used. A ratio of the bound antigen to the free antigen is then calculated by dividing the supernatant counts by the residue counts. A standard curve is constructed by plotting the concentration of standard on the ordinate against the bound/free ratio on the abscissa and joining the points. A typical standard curve is shown in Figure 15-1.

Other variations of the standard curve are possible, such as plotting concentration of standard against percent bound (supernatant count divided by total activity added) or percent unbound (residue count divided by activity added). In the case of solid-phase separation, the percent bound must be plotted since the antigen-antibody complex is bound to the Sephadex or a tube, which is counted.

To determine the patient's antigen value, the same calculations are performed as on the standards. The bound/free ratio is then found on the abscissa. A line is drawn to the curve and down to the ordinate, where the patient's antigen level is determined.

Special Applications

RIA is the most sensitive of all diagnostic tests (determinations in the picogram range) and is highly reproducible. Usually basal hormone levels are measured, and often these are not very useful to the physician since separation between normal and abnormal values is poor. The use of provocative stimulation or suppression techniques makes the separation of normal from abnormal more dramatic.

A special application of the RIA method is the assay for Australian antigen (hepatitis-associated antigen). Control or patient antigen reacts with antibody which is bound to the sides of tubes. Labeled antibody is then allowed to bind to other reaction sites on the antigen. The result is an antibody-antigen-antibody complex bound to the tube. This is then counted.

Determination of antibodies in plasma is another special application of RIA which can be performed by a slight change in the procedure.

Table 15-1 lists the RIAs used in our laboratory and outlines their characteristics.

Clinical Applications

Despite its newness, radioimmunoassay is already beginning to show its potential as a clinically valuable procedure. It is precise, specific, easily available, rapid, and economical; in addition it spares the patient exposure to radioactivity. By enabling measurement of nanogram and picogram quantities of hormones, enzymes, pharmaceuticals, and chemicals, RAI facilitates the diagnosis of pituitary diseases, pancreatic

Table 15-1. Characteristics of Some Common RIAs

Substance	Label	Method of separation	Type of separation
Digoxin	^{125}I	Dextran-charcoal	Liquid phase
Gastrin	^{125}I	Resin	Liquid phase
ACTH	^{125}I	Charcoal	Liquid phase
Angiotensin I	^{125}I	Charcoal	Liquid phase
Insulin	^{125}I	Sephadex	Solid phase
Vitamin B_{12}*	^{57}Co	Sephadex	Solid phase
Growth hormone	^{125}I	Antibody-coated tubes	Solid phase
Hepatitis-associated antigen	^{125}I	Antibody-coated tubes	Solid phase
Morphine	^{125}I	Ammonium sulfate	Precipitation
Carcinoembryonic antigen	^{125}I	Double antibody	Precipitation

* Not RIA, but CPB; uses intrinsic factor instead of an antibody.

diseases, gastrointestinal diseases, anemia, hepatitis, and digitalis misuse (Table 15-2).

Pituitary Disorders

Measurement of human growth hormone (HGH) simplifies the diagnosis of growth disorders due to pituitary gland dysfunction. Although normal levels range from 0 to 4 mμg/ml, normal and abnormal values can be easily separated by the use of stimulation or suppression tests. Hypoglycemia induced by insulin or tolbutamide, as well as the use of arginine and glucagon, raise HGH levels in the normal but not in the dwarf whose small size results from HGH deficiency. Hyperglycemia induced by glucose intake suppresses HGH levels in the normal but not in gigantism or acromegaly.

Diabetes and Hypoglycemia

Insulin (IRI) measurement enhances understanding of the abnormalities of carbohydrate metabolism. The assay facilitates separation of normals from early diabetics and diagnosis of functioning islet cell tumor. Following glucose or tolbutamide stimulation, normals can be further separated from patients with borderline dysfunction.

Hypertension

Reversible hypertensive states are a clinically challenging problem. Their diagnosis is considerably aided by the determination of plasma renin activity or angiotensin I levels. Renin is a proteolytic enzyme released by the kidney under certain blood pressure or volume stimuli. It acts on a substrate protein in plasma to release a physiologically inactive decapeptide, angiotensin I, which is converted in the pulmonary circulation to an octapeptide, angiotensin II. This is a highly effective pressor agent and a major stimulus to the

Conditions Detectable by RIA

- Pituitary disorders
- Diabetes
- Hypertension
- Digitalis misuse
- Peptic ulcer
- Megaloblastic anemia
- Hepatitis

Table 15-2. Clinical Applications of RIA

Substance	RIA indications	Normal range	Stimulation: Test	Stimulation: Results	Suppression: Test	Suppression: Results	Pitfalls
Insulin (IRI)	Hyperglycemia Hypoglycemia Diabetes Obesity	Mean: 26 μU/ml	Glucose	Increases level 3–4 times			Limited clinical use
Somatotropin (HGH)	Acromegaly Gigantism Dwarfism	0–4.5 mμg/ml	Hypoglycemia Insulin Tolbutamide Glucagon Arginine	Normal: increases level 2–5 times Pituitary dwarfs: no increase	Hyper-glycemia	Normal: suppresses Acromegaly, gigantism: no suppression	
Angiotensin I	Hypertension	1–4 pg	Diuretic intake	Increases level	Excessive salt intake	Depresses levels	
Gastrin	Peptic ulcer Zollinger-Ellison syndrome Anemia	0–300 pg/ml	Food Hypoglycemia	Increases level 2–3 times			Most ulcer patients have normal values
Digoxin	Therapy Intoxication Digitalization	0.8–2.1 ng/ml					
Vitamin B_{12}	Anemia Malabsorption Peptic ulcer	300–1000 pg/ml					Technical problems
Australian antigen	Blood donation Blood receipt Jaundice Liver disease	0					Guinea pig contact gives positive reaction

release of aldosterone even at subpressor levels.

Variations of salt intake, diuretic use, and measurement of plasma renin activity can separate normals from patients with renal vascular disease or patients with adrenal tumors producing primary hyperaldosteronism. Since plasma renin activity is influenced by any change in plasma volume resulting from diuretic therapy, a low-salt diet, upright posture, dehydration, pregnancy, or the use of oral contraceptives, these variables should be controlled when the test is being performed.

Digitalis Levels in Cardiac Disease

Digoxin is assayed for the purpose of monitoring digoxin levels in patients medicated with digitalis preparatons for heart failure and cardiac arrhythmias. The controversy concerning the potency of this medication, the lack of accurate history of dosage in patients with digitalis intoxication, and the use of digoxin in patients exhibiting fluctuations of renal function and gastrointestinal abnormalities make the assay desirable clinically. Nontoxic digoxin levels range between 0 and 3 ng/ml; levels ranging between 1.5 and 8 ng/ml are observed in overdosed patients.

Peptic Ulcer

Gastrin was the first enteric hormone to be isolated, synthesized, and assayed. Fasting levels in the normal population range between 0 and 300 pg/ml. These levels increase following food ingestion, insulin hypoglycemia, alcohol ingestion, and vagus nerve stimulation. Pernicious anemia and achlorhydria are associated with elevated gastrin levels. Peptic ulcer patients have a higher mean gastrin level than the normal population, but this finding is not very helpful because overlap between the two levels is great. Gastrin is also elevated in the Zollinger-Ellison syndrome, and the hormone produced by the pancreatic tumor responsible for the syndrome is identical to the natural hormone.

Megaloblastic Anemias

Measurement of the serum vitamin B_{12} level is the single definitive test for the diagnosis of vitamin B_{12} deficiency. This deficiency causes maturation failure in the erythropoietic process and results from defective absorption of vitamin B_{12} due either to the absence of intrinsic factor or to malabsorptive disease of the gastrointestinal tract.

The normal range is 300 to 1000 pg/ml; levels below 300 pg are consistent with vitamin B_{12} deficiency. The assay can differentiate the causes of the deficiency as being either megaloblastic anemia or folate deficiency.

Hepatitis

A simple, yet extremely sensitive RIA procedure makes it possible to detect hepatitis-associated antigen by a solid-phase technique that yields a yes-no answer. This procedure, when compared with several standard methods for measuring hepatitis-associated antigen, surpassed all other methods in sensitivity. The test has revolutionized blood-banking techniques and has considerably lowered the incidence of hepatitis.

References

1. *Angiotensin I Immutope Kit: Diagnostic Reagent.* New Brunswick, NJ, Squibb (monograph), 1971.
2. Ashkar FS: Clinical Usefulness and Reliability of Commercially Available Radioimmunoassay Kits. Presented at 11th Annual Meeting, Southeastern Chapter, Society of Nuclear Medicine, Cincinnati, Ohio, Oct 28, 1970.
3. Ashkar FS: In Vitro Techniques in Endocrinology.

In *Continuing Education Lectures*. Atlanta, Southeastern Chapter, Society of Nuclear Medicine, 1971, chap 23.

4. Ashkar FS: Radioimmunoassay in Gastroenterology. In Gilson AJ, Smoak WM (eds). *Hematopoietic and Gastrointestinal Investigations with Radionuclides*. Springfield, Ill, Thomas, 1972.
5. Beller GA, Smith TW, Ablmann, WH, et al: Digitalis intoxication: A prospective clinical study with serum level correlations. *N Engl J Med* **284**:989, 1971.
6. Berson SA, Yalow RS: General principles of radioimmunoassay. *Clin Chim Acta* **22**:51, 1968.
7. Berson SA, Yalow RS, Glick SM, et al: Immunoassay of protein and peptide hormones. *Metabolism* **13**:1135, 1964.
8. Catt KJ: Insulin and glucose homeostasis. *Lancet* **2**:352, 1970.
9. Haber E, Koerner T, Page LB, et al: Application of a radioimmunoassay of angiotensin I to the physiological measurement of plasma renin activity in normal human subjects. *J Clin Endocrinol Metab* **29**:1348, 1969.
10. *HGH-125 Immusay, HGH Immunoassay Kit*. North Chicago, Abbott Radiopharmaceuticals (monograph), 1970.
11. Hunter WM, Greenwood FC: Preparation of iodine-131 labeled human growth hormone of high specific activity. *Nature (Lond)* **194**:495, 1962.
12. Kofman S (ed): *Radioimmunoassay, Ausria: Programmed Learning Course on Australian Antigen*. North Chicago, Abbott Laboratories Press, 1971.
13. Kofman S (ed): *Radioimmunoassay: Programmed Learning Course on Radioimmunoassay*. North Chicago, Abbott Laboratories Press, 1971.
14. *Phadebas B_{12} Test*. Piscataway, NJ, Pharmacia (monograph), 1972.
15. Smith TW, Haber E: Measurement of clinical blood levels of digoxin by radioimmunoassay. *J Clin Invest* **48**:78, 1969.

Radionuclides have an important role in treating hyperthyroidism and thyroid carcinoma, a limited role in treating polycythemia vera. They aid control of recurrent pleural and peritoneal effusion resulting from malignant disease.

16
Radioisotope Therapy

Fuad S. Ashkar

Hyperthyroidism

Diagnosis

Hyperthyroidism can usually be diagnosed easily on the basis of clinical evaluation and the results of thyroid function tests, especially 24-hour radioactive iodine uptake and total serum thyroxine level. The disorder should be suspected in any patient who manifests cardiac arrhythmias, weight loss without obvious cause, bulging of the eyes, weakness, widening of the pulse pressure, unexplained nervousness or apathy, and edema.

Two types of hyperthyroidism are recognized: Graves's disease (diffuse toxic goiter) and Plummer's disease (toxic nodular goiter). Graves's disease is an autoimmune condition manifested by thyrotoxicosis, diffuse enlargement of the thyroid gland, exophthalmos, and abnormal serum level of LATS (long-acting thyroid stimulator). Plummer's disease, a less common form of hyperthyroidism, occurs in elderly persons and is characterized by the presence of one or more functioning autonomous thyroid nodules, lack of true exophthalmos, and absence of LATS. In contrast to the overt hypermetabolism associated with Graves's disease, patients with Plummer's disease display apathy and disturbances of cardiac rhythm.

Table 16-1. Treatment of Severe Hyperthyroidism

Reduction of rate of thyroid hormone release
- Antithyroid drugs
  - Tapazole® (10 mg four times daily)
  - PTU (100 mg four times daily)
- Stable iodine
  - SSKI (10 drops daily)

Blocking peripheral effects of thyroid hormone
- Adrenergic blocking agents
  - Reserpine (0.25 mg three times daily)
  - Guanethidine (10–25 mg four times daily)
  - Propranolol (80 mg daily)
  - Corticosteroids (when indicated)

Supportive and corrective measures

Sedation and rest
- High caloric intake (3000 cal, multiple feedings)
- Multivitamins
- Digitalis, diuretics, oxygen (when indicated)
- Avoid surgery, exertion, stress

Definitive therapy
- ^{131}I (preferred)
- Surgery (when indicated only)

Treatment

Once hyperthyroidism is diagnosed, treatment should be instituted promptly to prevent the complications of chronic untreated disease and the precipitation of thyroid

Table 16-2. Treatment of Thyroid Storm

Supportive and corrective measures
  Rest and sedation (as indicated)
  Fluid replacement
  Cooling mattress
  Oxygen, digitalis, diuretics (as indicated)
  Antibiotics (when indicated)
Blocking thyroid hormone release and effects
  Thiourea drugs (minor role)
  Sodium iodide (2 gm IV daily)
  Corticosteroids (cortisone, 600 mg IV daily or its equivalent)
  Adrenergic blocking agents
    Reserpine (3–12 mg IM or IV daily, or 0.07–0. 3 mg/kg body weight daily)
    Guanethidine (40–100 mg daily, or 1–2 mg/kg body weight daily)
    Propranolol (80 mg daily)
Reduction of hormone level in blood
  Blood exchange
  Plasmapheresis (5–10 units per day)
Definitive therapy at later date with radioactive iodine

storm. For early hyperthyroidism, of either the Graves or the Plummer type, radioactive iodine is the treatment of choice for all but pregnant or lactating patients. If hyperthyroidism is severe and advanced, or if thyroid storm has occurred, the gland hypersecretion must be controlled and the complications relieved by medical means before definitive treatment with radioactive iodine is begun (Tables 16-1 and 16-2).

Treatment with radioactive iodine, even when prolonged, has never been shown to have a carcinogenic or teratogenic effect.

IODINE 131

^{131}I administration is the initial treatment of choice in adults (except in pregnant or lactating women) with Graves's disease or Plummer's disease.

In Graves's disease, treatment is aimed at suppressing secretion of excessive amounts of thyroid hormone. If successful, the derangement driving the thyroid to uncontrolled secretory activity seems to abate, and in months or years the gland is able to reestablish a normal homeostatic relation with the pituitary and to supply the body with physiologic amounts of thyroid hormone.

Since the average range of the beta particles in tissue is 0.5 mm, there is no significant extrathyroid radiation. Only two reports exist of possible injury to parathyroid glands or other perithyroid tissues. On these occasions salivary gland amylase was noted to be depressed temporarily after radioactive iodine administrating atropine along with the ^{131}I to decrease iodine accumulation in the salivary glands.

The preferred method of treatment is a single dose of ^{131}I designed to deliver 80μCi/gm of thyroid tissue to the gland at 24 hours.

$$D\ (\mu\text{Ci}) = \frac{(80\ \mu\text{Ci/gm})\ (\text{gm wt of gland})}{\text{24-hr radioiodine uptake}}$$

For a gland heavier than 50 gm, the dose for that part of the gland over 50 gm should be cut to 40μCi/gm. Another method is to give a fixed dose of ^{131}I ranging from 5 to 7 mCi regardless of gland weight. A third method calculates the dose by the formula $D(\text{mCi}) = 2N + 1$, where N represents the number of times the thyroid gland is enlarged.

Reevaluation should take place two to three months after the first dose, and the decision to re-treat should be based on clinical, not laboratory, findings.

Agreement about the role of ^{131}I therapy in Plummer's disease is lacking. Dose calculation is less accurate than for Graves's disease, because the iodine uptake is irregularly distributed and low-uptake nodules receive little or no radiation. Gland size is difficult to estimate because of its irregular shape and the presence of retrotracheal and substernal extensions. Recurrence is more likely than in Graves's disease. Hamburger et al suggest treating "small glands" with 8 mCi retained in the gland and the largest glands with up to 20 mCi retention, with administered doses of 20 to 50 mCi.[6]

POSTTHERAPY HYPOTHYROIDISM

Hypothyroidism is very common after ^{131}I therapy for Graves's disease, less common after therapy for Plummer's disease. It occurs most frequently one year after therapy, and it exists ten years after therapy in 60% of patients. Among its several causes

> Hypothyroidism is common after ^{131}I therapy for Graves's disease; less common after therapy for Plummer's disease.

are the direct effect of ^{131}I radiation on the thyroid cell nucleus, the occurrence of a thyroid-destructive autoimmune process after therapy, the onset of fibrosis in the gland, and the posible coexistence of mild chronic thyroiditis with the hyperthyroidism that results in total gland destruction.

IODINE 125

In recent years ^{125}I has been used for the treatment of hyperthyroidism in hopes of reducing the incidence of posttherapy hypothyroidism. ^{125}I has a longer half-life than ^{131}I and a different radiation effect on the thyroid cell that spares the nucleus from intense irradiation. In theory this should reduce the incidence of hypothyroidism, but clinical experience has been disappointing and inconclusive. The currently used dose is 200μCi of ^{125}I in a single ingestion.

Thyroid Carcinoma

Thyroid carcinoma is not rare and is more common in patients with goiter than in the normal population. It has been reported in association with 4% to 17% of nontoxic multinodular goiter, 9% to 33% of solitary nodules, 2.5% of toxic goiters, and 0.9% of patients undergoing thyroidectomy for thyrotoxicosis. Almost 50% of thyroid nodules in children are malignant; however, thyroid carcinoma most commonly develops in the fifth and sixth decades of life.

X-ray therapy to nonthyroid head and neck lesions has been stressed by many authors as a possible cause of thyroid carcinoma, but lately it has been shown that chronic stimulation with endogenous thyrotropin and the long-acting thyroid stimulator causes increased mitosis in animal thyroid and may explain the increased incidence of thyroid carcinoma in goiters and following thyroidectomy for hyperthyroidism.

Diagnosis

The diagnosis of thyroid carcinoma is challenging, since no dramatic symptoms are associated with the lesion initially. The most initial finding is a lump in the thyroid, but enlarged cervical lymph nodes, bone pain, pathologic fracture, cough, dyspnea, hemoptysis may be early signs. Neurologic deficits are occasionally encountered, but they occur late in the disease.

The following clinical findings suggest thyroid carcinoma:

- History of head and neck irradiation in childhood
- Male patient under 40 years
- Sudden painless growth of gland
- Firm or hard nodule in gland
- Single nodule in normal gland
- Fixation of gland to trachea or skin

- Presence of local or distant metastasis
- Lack of change in size after thyroid hormone intake
- Recurrent laryngeal nerve paralysis

Histologic Types

Three histologic types of thyroid carcinoma are recognized:

- Papillary carcinoma. About 62% of all carcinomas of the thyroid are of this type. Roughly, half of these tumors are thyrotropin-dependent, are multifocal, and metastasize primarily through lymphatics.
- Follicular carcinoma. About 20% of all thyroid carcinomas are of this type. It is slow-growing, well-differentiated, and thyrotropin-dependent and metastasizes primarily to bones and lungs.
- Undifferentiated carcinoma. About 18% are of this type, which include medullary tumors. Undifferentiated carcinomas are solid, highly malignant, and rapidly growing tumors that are not thyrotropin-dependent.

Treatment

Depending on its histologic type, carcinoma of the thyroid is treated by surgery or by a combination of surgery and radiotherapy.

Carminoma of the thyroid is treated by surgery or a combination of surgery and radioisotope therapy. Results are best following combination therapy.

SURGERY

What constitutes *adequate surgery for thyroid carcinoma* is debatable, but most thyroidologists agree that in papillary carcinoma the extent of surgery depends on the size of the neoplasm and its lymphatic spread. Radical neck surgery is still done in some centers when lymph node metastasis is present, and conservative total thyroidectomy is recommended because of the multifocal nature of the tumor.

Follicular carcinoma develops slowly, and surgery limited to the involved lobe and isthmus is adequate in most cases. However, since this tumor is thyrotropin-dependent, part of the second lobe is usually removed, without injuring the recurrent laryngeal nerve and the parathyroid glands, because this facilitates further treatment with ^{131}I.

In the undifferentiated thyroid carcinomas (the tumors found in older age groups), tumor spread is usually extensive, and surgery is indicated only for airway maintenance.

COMBINATION THERAPY

Recent work by Beierwaltes and coworkers[8] has shown beyond any doubt that the death rate from thyroid carcinoma is significantly decreased by the use of ^{131}I therapy concomitantly with surgical treatment of the disease. Sodium iodide I 131 is effective in controlling well-differentiated carcinoma or carcinoma with thyrotropin-dependence. Unfortunately, few of these carcinomas concentrate ^{131}I initially (only 10% of follicular carcinomas concentrate ^{131}I on initial scans). However, following thyroidectomy, most folicular carcinomas and their metastases, and half of the papillary carcinomas, do concentrate ^{131}I.

Following surgery, all thyroid- and iodine-containing medications are withheld from the patient. Six weeks later, if scanning shows ^{131}I concentration in the neck or other sites, a therapeutic dose of sodium iodide I 131 (50 to 100 mCi) is given in

Table 16-3. Management of Thyroid Carcinoma

Partial or total thyroidectomy as indicated

Withholding of iodine and thyroid medications for six weeks

Scanning for ^{131}I concentration in neck or metastasis

Ablation of all iodine-concentrating areas with ^{131}I (50–100 mCi)

Repetition of above until all ^{131}I uptake disappears and the patient becomes myxedematous

Thyroid replacement between ^{131}I ablations

Restudy of patient yearly for first five years and every five years thereafter

Techniques for Inducing Iodine Concentration

Thyroidectomy
Thyrotropin injection (10 U, *USP*, for one to six days)
Antithyroid drug withdrawal with rebound rise in ^{131}I uptake
Low-iodine diet with diuretics for four days with or without TSH

the hospital and the patient is isolated until the body count falls below 30 mCi. The regimen is outlined in Table 16-3. Scanning is repeated every three months for a year and then annually, and repeated doses of ^{131}I are given until the patient is completely myxedematous and all scintigraphic evidence of ^{131}I uptake by the body has disappeared. (Doses should not exceed 500 mCi in patients under 30 years and 800 mCi in older patients, to avoid bone marrow damage.)

All patients should receive thyroid replacement folowing therapy (Cytomel is preferred because of its fast disappearance time). At yearly intervals for five years and at five-year intervals following that, thyroid medication is discontinued for six weeks and thyroid studies are repeated.

CONVERSION METHODS

A significant number of carcinomas with metastases can be induced to concentrate ^{131}I after surgical removal of the thyroid gland. However, if that is unsuccessful, other conversion maneuvers should be employed. Serial injections of thyrotropin (10 U *USP* daily for one to six days) improve concentration of ^{131}I in thyrotropin-dependent tumors and in so doing deliver a good ablative dose of radiation to the tumor.

Antithyroid drug therapy, utilizing the rebound phenomenon, sometimes enhances ^{131}I concentration by thyroid tumor.

The use of new potent diuretics (Lasix or Edicrine) and a low-iodine diet for four days causes a drop in serum iodine level so that a transient iodine deficiency state prevails. The tumors and metastases are iodine-starved and are thus induced to concentrate ^{131}I. After the above regimen, ^{131}I therapy is effective in more than 50% of previously untreatable cases.

Survival and Prognosis

Survival and prognosis in thyroid carcinoma are influenced by the histologic type of the tumor, the extent of the disease, and the therapy applied. All patients with undifferentiated carcinoma, young or adult, will die in five years. The five-year survival in follicular carcinoma is better than 60% and in papillary carcinoma is better than 70%. These survival rates have been greatly improved by the new tumor-conversion techniques that enhance the results of ^{131}I therapy in previously resistant cases. Today the five-year survival rate is at least 20% higher than the above recorded statistics.

Polycythemia Vera

Polycythemia vera is a chronic hematologic disorder characterized by increased proliferative activity of erythroid, myeloid, megakaryocytic, and fibroblastic cell lines. An absolute increase in the red cell mass can be determined only by direct measurement using ^{51}Cr-labled autologous erythrocytes. The presence of a compensatory erythrocytosis secondary to tissue hypoxia must be ruled out by the demonstration of a normal arterial oxygen concentration (in the absence of an abnormal hemoglobin with increased oxygen affinity or diminished oxygen-carrying capacity).

After confirmation of the disease process, 3 to 5 mCi of radioactive phosphate is injected intravenously. The patient is reevaluated after 10 to 12 weeks and this dose is repeated if his clinical status and laboratory data so indicate. A single course of therapy may induce a remission lasting several years. The ^{32}P dose probably should not exceed 6 mCi during any six-month period. Treatment with ^{32}P should not be used if the platelet count is less than 15,000, reticulocytes less than 0.2%, or the blood cell count less than 3000. An 11% incidence of acute leukemia in ^{32}P-treated patients has considerably limited the usefulness of this therapy.

Intracavitary Use of Radioactive Colloids

Control of recurrent effusions in the pleural and peritoneal cavities that result from malignant disease presents a serious and difficult problem. Colloidal gold Au 198 was initially chosen because it emits both beta and gamma radiation. The beta radiation provides the therapy and the gamma radiation allows determination of the spatial distribution of the radioactive colloid. A major difficulty is the exposure risk to the personnel administering the colloidal gold Au 198. Chromic phosphate P 32, which has also been used, lacks penetrating gamma rays and poses far less risk of exposure.

The colloids act by fibrosis of the mesothelium and small blood vessels and destruction of the free tumor cells in the fluid and the tumor seedings along the pleura. The total dose used for each treatment is from 35 to 75 mCi of gold Au 198 and 10 mCi of chronic phosphate P 32. Repeated treatment is seldom required, but the dose may be repeated after four weeks if the fluid reaccumulates to a significant degree.

Intraperitoneal use of these two radionuclides is essentially the same as intrapleural use, except that the average dose may be up to twice that used in the pleura.

References

1. Ashkar FS: Thyroid storm: How to detect and treat this emergency. *Consultant* **11**:49, 1971.
2. Ashkar FS: A better outlook in thyroid cancer. *Consultant* **12**:148, 1972.
3. Ashkar FS, Katims RB, Smoak WM, et al: Thyroid storm treatment with blood exchange and plasmapheresis. *JAMA* **214**:1275, 1970.
4. Burke G, Silverstein GE: Hypothyroidism after treatment with sodium iodide I^{131}. *JAMA* **201**: 1051, 1969.
5. Franko J, Coppler M, Kovaleski B: Propranolol and I^{131} in the treatment of diffuse thyroid hyperplasia with hyperthyroidism. *J Nucl Med* **11**:219, 1970.
6. Hamburger JI, Kadian G, Rossini HW: Why not radioactive iodine therapy for toxic nodular goiter? *Arch Intern Med* **119**:75, 1967.
7. Silver S: *Radioactive Nuclides in Medicine and Biology*. Philadelphia, Lea & Febiger, 1968.
8. Varma VM, Beierwaltes WH, Nofal MM, et al: Treatment of thyroid cancer. *JAMA* **214**:1437, 1970.

Glossary and Appendix Tables

Sharad Amtey

Words Used in Nuclear Medicine

Absorption

A homogeneous or monoenergetic beam of x- or gamma rays in passing through matter loses energy at a rate which can be described by the exponential equation

$$I_t = I_0 e^{-\mu t}$$

where t is the thickness of the sheet of matter and μ the linear absorption coefficient for the particular photon energy in the particular matter. A half-thickness or half-value layer bears the same relation to the absorption coefficient as does the half-period to the decay constant for a radioactive nuclide:

$$\text{half-thickness} = (0.603)/\text{linear absorption coefficient}$$

Frequently, instead of the linear absorption coefficient (absorption per unit thickness), the mass absorption coefficient (absorption per unit mass) is used. This is μ/ρ, the linear absorption coefficient divided by the density of that particular matter. The absorption coefficient μ/ρ is made up of three parts: the photoelectric (τ/ρ), Compton (σ/ρ), and pair (κ/ρ) (if the energy is sufficiently great).

$$\mu/\rho = \tau/\rho + \sigma/\rho + \kappa/\rho$$

In case of absorption of beta radiation, a value usually desired is the *range* or the thickness of filter necessary to stop all the particles.

Acceleration

Velocity is the rate of change of distance with respect to time, and acceleration is the rate of change of velocity with respect to time. Thus, acceleration is an increment of velocity divided by the increment of time in which that change in velocity took place.

Accelerators

Accelerators are designed to supply the high-energy particles which can serve as the projectiles for nuclear scattering and disintegration or can be used for the production of high-energy x-rays. During the acceleration process, energy is imparted to electrically charged particles or ions by the force exerted upon them when they are placed in an electric field. Present-day accelerators have been designed mainly for the acceleration of the very lightest atoms and of electrons. Accelerators can be divided into two groups: cyclic and linear. In the cyclic accelerator, the particles travel in circular orbits and make multiple traversals of the accelerating field. In the linear accelerator, the acceleration occurs along a line. The cyclotron is an example of a cyclic accelerator designed primarily to accelerate positively charged particles such as protons, deuterons, and alpha particles.

Activation Analysis

Activation analysis utilizes the nuclear properties of elements for their quantitation, rather than properties dependent upon the number and configuration of orbital electrons. In neutron activiation analysis, a sample containing the element (or elements) in question is exposed to a neutron flux so that a fraction of the nuclei present absorbs neutrons and forms a new, unstable radioisotope which can be identified by the resultant particulate and/or electromagnetic radiations emitted. Although absolute measurements can be made and the number of atoms present can be calculated, it is easier and usually more accurate to relate the induced radioactivity in an unknown sample to the induced radioactivity in a measured standard of the same element.

Activity

If N represents the number of radioactive atoms present at any instant, $-dN/dt$ represents the decrease in this number during a very short time. This decrease is a fixed percentage of all the atoms present. Thus $dN/dt = -\lambda N$ where λ is the decay constant or the fraction transformed per unit time. In practical work with radioactive nuclides, a quantity called activity (A) is usually measured and this is proportional to the number of disintegrations per unit time. Thus,

$$A = c\lambda N$$

where c is a constant of proportionality and its value depends on the nature and efficiency of the measuring and recording instruments, and on the geometric arrangement of sample and detector. The unit of activity is *curie* (Ci), which is 3.7×10^{10} disintegrations per second.

ADP (Automatic data processing)

Data processing performed largely by automatic means, ie, by a system of electronic or electrical machines which require little human assistance or intervention.

Alpha Particle

The nucleus of the helium atom consisting of two protons and two neutrons is called alpha (α) particle. It lacks orbital electrons and therefore is positively charged. Because of its relatively heavy mass (compared with that of electron or proton) and double positive charge, the alpha particle has tremendous ionizing power, but because of its size, little penetration.

Ampere

The motion of a charge is called a current. The unit of current is ampere (amp) which is defined as flow of 1 coulomb (C) per second where coulomb is the unit of electric charge. The charge on an electron is 1.602×10^{-19} C. Thus, when the current is 1 amp, approximately 625×10^{16} electrons are flowing per second. If the flow was of protons, the same number of protons would be required for 1 amp current since the charge on a proton is of opposite sign but same magnitude as the charge on an electron.

Amplifier

Amplifiers are used to increase the size or the amplitude of the electrical pulse from a radiation detector. Amplifiers whose output pulse height is directly proportional to the imput pulse height are called linear amplifiers. The amplification factor, the frequency range of linear operation, and the stability of the output are some of the factors to be considered in designing an amplifier. These requirements for an amplifier depend upon the radiation detector.

Analog Computer

A computer that operates on data represented in the form of continuously variable physical quantities (eg, voltage or angular position) by performing physical processes on the data.

Analyzers

A radiation detector produces pulses which are proportional in height to the amount of energy absorbed in the detector. To sort these pulses according to their height, an electronic device is used and is called an analyzer. A single-channel analyzer is a combination of two discriminators and an anticoincidence circuit. This type of analyzer can select pulses between only one predetermined range. The multichannel analyzer can select pulses between many predetermined ranges.

Annihilation Radiation
The positron emitted in a positron β decay first loses its kinetic energy by collisions with other atoms and then combines with an atomic electron. The two annihilate each other with the disappearance of their equal and opposite charges and of their total inert mass. The product of this annihilation is the so-called annihilation radiation and consists of two gamma rays each of exactly 0.511 mev energy emitted in exactly opposite directions.

Anti-Coincidence Circuit
A circuit which gives output pulse only when one of its two input pulse sources registers a pulse. If both the input sources register pulses simultaneously, there will be no output pulse from the anticoincidence circuit.

***ASCII* (American Standard Code for Information Interchange)**
A seven-bit USA standard code adopted to facilitate the interchange of data among various types of data-processing and data-communications equipment.

Atomic Mass Unit
Atomic masses are specified in terms of the atomic mass unit, which is 1/12 of the mass of an atom of ^{12}C.

Atomic Number
The atomic number of an atom is the number of protons in its nucleus.

Attenuation
Photons are attenuated in matter through primarily three interactions: the photoelectric interaction, the Compton interaction, and, at sufficient energies, the pair production. The attenuation follows an exponential law and the photons do not have a definite range. However, the penetrating power of photons can be described in terms of their mean free path, which is the reciprocal of the linear attenuation coefficient.

Auger Electron
Electrons emitted by an excited atom as an alternative process to characteristic x-ray emission are called Augur electrons.

Autofluoroscope
The autofluoroscope consists of a scintillator mosaic with a coincidence system and suitable readout equipment.

Average Life
The average life of a radionuclide is the reciprocal of its decay constant, whereas the half-period or half-life of the radionuclide is 0.693 times the reciprocal of its decay constant. Thus the average life is always greater than the half-life.

Background Radiation
Any Geiger counter or scintillation counter will show a small counting rate even when no radioactive source is placed near it. This background count which arises from the cosmic rays, natural radioactivity in the surroundings, and other remote sources of radiation in the laboratory, is said to be due to background radiation.

Backscatter
As a narrow beam of beta particles (or photons) penetrates matter, some of the particles (or photons) are scattered away from the original path. Some of them undergo very wide angular deflections, so that the path is essentially reversed; this is called backscatter.

Barn
In describing the yield of nuclear reactions the concept of nuclear cross sections is used. The unit of these cross sections is barn and is equal to 10^{-24} sq cm.

Beta (β) Particles
The negatively charged particles discovered initially in the radioactive decay were re-

fered to as beta particles in contrast to the heavier, positively charged alpha particles and massless and chargeless particles called photons or gamma rays. Beta particles are actually electrons, identical with those from other sources such as heated filaments and atomic orbits. They do not reside inside the atomic nucleus but are ejected in the nuclear transformations when neutrons are transformed into protons.

Binary Numbers

The number system with a radix of 2. For example, the binary numeral 1101 means

$$(1\times2^3)+(1\times2^2)+(0\times2^1)+(1\times2^0)$$

which is equivalent to decimal 13. The decimal system has a radix of 10. Therefore the decimal numeral 1101 means

$$(1\times10^3)+(1\times10^2)+(0\times10^1)+(1\times10^0)$$

In the binary number system only two numerals are necessary, 0 and 1. In the decimal number system ten numerals are necessary, 0 through 9. The binary number system is widely used in digital computers because most computer components (vacuum tubes, transitors, flipflops, and magnetic cores) are essentially binary in that they have only two stable states.

Binding Energy

In Bohr's atomic model the negative leectrons orbit around the central massive positively charged nuclues. The orbital electrons occupy certain definite quantum orbits only. The energy with which an electron is bound to the atom depends upon the orbit it occupies and is called its binding energy. The electrons in the inner orbit are more tightly bound than those in the outer orbit. The electrons' binding energy is not to be confused with nuclear binding energy. The measured mass of a nucleus is always less than the sum of the masses of its constituent nucleons. The difference between the two represents the loss of mass in consolidating the nucleons into the nucleus. Its energy equivalent is called the binding energy of the nucleus.

Biologic Half-Life

The decrease of radioactive material from any organ is due to two factors: physical decay of the radionuclide and physiologic elimination. This elimination follows an exponential law in many cases. However, the decay rate could be different from the physical decay rate. The biologic decay coefficient is equal to the product of 0.693 and the reciprocal of the biologic half-life.

Bit

A binary digit; a digit (0 or 1) in the representation of a number in binary notation.

Bremsstrahlung

Bremsstrahlung (braking radiation) is the radiation emitted by fast-traveling charged particles when they are slowed down. Such a radiation is emited, for example, when an electron of either sign passes near an atomic nucleus.

Buffer

A storage device used to compensate for differences in the rates of flow of data or in the times of occurrence of events when transmitting data from one device to another.

Bug

A mistake in the design of a program or a computer system, or an equipment fault.

Byte

A group of adjacent bits operated on as a unit and usually shorter than a word. In a number of current computer systems, this term stands specifically for a group of eight adjacent bits that can represent one alphanumeric character or two decimal digits.

Carrier

A particular radioactive sample may consist entirely of a radioactive nuclide or it may contain stable isotopes of the same element. In the first case, the radioactive material is said to be carrier-free. In the second, if the stable and radioactive isotopes are in the same chemical form, it is said to be with carrier.

***Cathode Ray Tube* (CRT)**
An electronic vacuum tube containing a screen on which information can be displayed.

***Central Processing Unit* (CPU)**
The unit of a computer system that includes the circuits which control the interpretation and execution of instructions.

Characteristic Radiation
Electromagnetic radiation released during electron transitions is termed characteristic radiation because the photon energies are characteristic of differences in binding energies of electrons in a specific atom.

Coincidence Circuit
A circuit that counts only those pulses which occur simultaneously with some other pulse.

Collimator
A collimator is usually needed to define the tissue region from which the photons are being accepted by the imaging device. The scanners use a focusing type collimator, ie, a collimator which looks at a finely defined region at a particular instant. The scintillation camera uses a single pinhole, parallel-hole multichannel, or diverging multichannel collimator. It is usually made of lead, but other materials as well as many other designs have been tried for specific purposes.

Compton Scattering
During a Compton interaction, part of the energy of an incident photon is transferred to a loosely bound or free electron within the attenuating medium. Gamma and x-ray protons with energy between 30 kev and 30 mev interact in soft tissue predominantly by Compton scattering.

Conversion Electron
Internal conversion is an alternate process to gamma emission for the deexcitation of an excited nucleus. These two processes are competitive. The nucleus interacts with the orbital electron which is ejected with kinetic energy equal to the energy released by the nucleus, reduced by the binding energy of the electron.

Cosmic Rays
The origin of primary cosmic rays has been and still is the object of much study and conjecture. These high-energy protons and other heavier particles strike the earth's atmosphere and trigger many reactions. Of the total gonadal dose per year resulting from background radiation, 25% is due to cosmic rays.

Cow
When a radioactive nuclide has a daughter of shorter life, it is often possible to separate the two, mechanically or chemically. The supply of the parent can be maintained and the daughter periodically removed or "milked" from it. Such a system is know as a "cow." In the ^{99}Mo—^{99m}Tc combination, the separation is achieved by means of a chemical solution poured over the "cow," dissolving the technetium but not affecting the molybdenum.

Dead Time
The time interval immediately following the occurrence of a pulse, during which the counter is insensitive and does not respond to ionizing (or scintillating) events, is called the dead time of the counter. The dead time puts an upper limit on the counting rate which can be measured accurately.

The true counting rate is related to the observed counting rate by the formula

(true counting rate—observed counting rate) = true counting rate × observed counting rate × dead time

Digital Computer
A computer is a machine for performing complex processes on information without manual intervention. Digital computers represent numerical quantities by discrete electrical states which can be manipulated logically and hence arithmetically. In contrast to this, analog computers perform this function by directly measuring continuous physical quantities such as electrical voltages.

Discriminator
The discriminator passes on to the counting circuit only pulses which exceed a certain predetermined threshold value.

Dose
For all radiation the absorbed dose unit is the rad, which is 100 ergs absorbed per gram of any absorber. Dose rates from radioactive sources can be determined with suitable instruments or can be calculated when certain basic data about the nuclides are available.

Effective Half-Life
The effective half-life of a radionuclide is always less than either its physical or biologic half-life. In dose calculation the use of physical half-life gives the maximum dose; the effective half-life, which is result of physical decay as well as physiologic elimination, should be used in dose calculations.

Efficiency
Counting efficiency in a narrow sense is the number of counts registered by the detector per 100 events reaching the counter or entering its sensitive volume. In a broader sense, the efficiency is the number of counts registered by the counting device per 100 disintegrations occurring in the radioactive sample under observation. However, the sensitivity of an instrument should be measured in terms of the counting rate per unit of radioactive material (eg, counts per minute per microcurie).

Film Badge
Film badges consisting of calibrated dental films mounted in special holders are routinely used for personnel monitoring. Film badges, though they provide only crude estimates of radiation dosage, are generally accepted medicolegally.

Fission
Fission is a nuclear reaction in which an external neutron interacts with a heavy nucleus; the latter splits into two parts of intermediate atomic mass and releases more than one neutron, on the average. Under suitable circumstances the reaction can be made to be self-sustaining. Such a chain reaction takes place in a fisson bomb and in a nuclear reactor.

Fluorescence
Inorganic crystals which luminesce are often called phosphors. Their luminescence in most cases originates from impurities or imperfections. When the crystal absorbs energy, eg, in the form of x-rays, the energy leads to the excitation of the lattice. The deexcitation can be prompt (10^{-10} seconds) and is then called fluorescence; The color of light emitted depends upon the chemical composition of the material and on the type of impurity.

***Fortran* (Formula Translator)**
A procedure-oriented language designed to facilitate the preparation of computer programs that perform mathematical computations.

Fusion
A nuclear reaction in which very light nuclei coalesce to produce heavier nuclei with release of neutrons and enormous amounts of energy.

FWHM **(full width at half maximum)**
The photopeak representing the absorption of a fixed gamma-ray energy is not a sharp spike in the pulse-height spectrum. The efficiency of various processes involved in producing the final output pulse from the photomultiplier varies from event to event resulting in a distribution in the height of the output pulse. This distribution results in the spread of the photopeak. The magnitude of this spread specifies the resolution of the system. It is stated in terms of the width of the photopeak at a count value equal to one half the count at the peak of the curve. The resolution is generally given as a percentage and is equal to 100 times the ratio of the FWHM divided by the abscissa value at the peak.

Half-Life
The time required, neglecting statistical fluctuation, for half the atoms of a radionuclide to disintegrate. Physical half-life of a radionuclide is 0.693 times the reciprocal of its disintegration constant.

Half-Value Layer
An index of photon beam radiation quality. It is the thickness of appropriate attenuating material which, when inserted in a narrow beam, reduces its intensity by half.

Hollerith Code
A widely used code for representing alphanumeric data on punched cards.

Integrated Circuit
A complete complex electronic circuit, capable of performing all the functions of a conventional circuit containing numerous discrete transistors, diodes, capacitors, and/or resistors, all of whose component parts are fabricated and assembled in a single integrated process. The resultant assembly cannot be disassembled without destroying it.

Interface
A shared boundary, eg, the boundary between two systems such as a computer and an Anger camera.

Inverse Square Law
The intensity of the radiation from a point source is inversely proportional to the square of the distance from the point source. This decrease in intensity due to increased distance results purely from geometric considerations.

I/O
The term is used in connection with data-processing equipment and refers to input/output.

Ionization
Release of an electron from an atom by ionizing radiation such as x-rays, gamma rays, and certain charged particle beams.

Isobars
Atoms having same mass number, but different atomic number.

Isomeric Transition
An excited state of nuclei of a radionuclide having an observable half-life is called an isomeric state. A transition between two isomeric states of a nucleus or from an isomeric state to the ground state is called an isomeric transition. The best known example of such a transition is

$$^{99m}\text{Tc} \rightarrow {}^{99}\text{Tc} + \gamma$$

Isotone
Atoms having the same neutron number, but different atomic number and therefore different mass number, are called isotones.

Isotopes
Atoms having the same atomic number ie, having the same number of protons in the

nucleus, but different mass number, are called isotopes. Since the number of orbital electrons depends upon the atomic number, the isotopes have the same number of orbital electrons. Thus, chemically they are same. The word isotope is incorrectly used to mean radionuclide. This should be discouraged since not all isotopes are radioactive.

K-electron Capture
This is an alternative transformation to positron emission. In positron emission the proton is transformed into a neutron with ejection of a positron and a neutrino. This transformation may also take place by nuclear capture of an electron from the inner (k) electron orbit and its amalgamation with a nuclear proton. The two processes are competitive.

Kinetic Energy
That part of the energy of a particle which is due to its motion is called its kinetic energy. The energy equivalent of the mass of the particle is called its mass energy. Thus the total energy of particle radiation consists of its mass energy plus its kinetic energy. For heavy particles such as alpha partciles, the kinetic energy is equal to half the product of the mass of the particle and the square of its velocity. However, smaller particles such as electrons increase in mass as their speed increases and this simple formula for the kinetic energy has to be modified. Energy of photons is measured in another way since they have no mass. A photon's energy is given by the product of Planck's constant and the frequency of the photon.

Lead Bricks
Storage shielding is accomplished easily by shielding the individual radioactive material containers or by constructing a small lead enclosure or box to hold all containers. These enclosures can be economically assembled out of lead bricks.

***Line Spread Function* (LSF)**
A line source is an extended distribution of radioactivity in the shape of a line of minimal diameter and length greater than but not greatly exceeding the field of view of the detector. The line sensitivity is the ratio of the counting rate measured to the photons emitted per second per unit length from a line source. A line spread function is the variation of the line sensitivity with transverse displacement of the line source at a fixed distance from the collimator. This function contains necessary information to define the sensitivity of a detector system and also expresses a measure of the spatial resolution of the system. The index of resolution of a system is defined as the width in centimeters of the system's line spread function, measured at a specific distance from the collimator, measured at the 50% response level.

***Linear Energy Transfer* (LET)**
The energy released along a track of a particle is described by the energy lost by the particle per unit length of path, usually specified in kiloelectron volts per micron of track. This is called linear energy transfer.

Liquid Scintillation
Certain organic solutions fluoresce when they are subjected to ionizing radiation. This is called liquid scintillation. It is used mostly for the measurement of low-energy bea-emtting radionuclides.

***Maximum Permissible Dose* (MPD)**
For radiation protection purposes, the maximum dose equivalent that a person or specified parts thereof shall be allowed to receive in rems in a stated period of time is specified by radiation protection agencies.

Metastable State
If the excited state of a nucleus persists for an appreciable time, ie, if it can be experimentally measured, it is said to be metastable. It is denoted by the letter *m* following the mass number in the superscript—eg, ^{99m}Tc.

***Modulation Transfer Function* (MTF)**
Spatial frequency, ν, expressed in cycles per centimeter, is a measure of the periodicity of a sinusoidal distribution of radioactivity. If the count rate recorded by the detector system is C_{max} and C_{min}, corresponding to maximum and minimum concentrations of the activity in the sinusoidal distribution, then the modulation of the distribution is said to be $(C_{max} - C_{min})/(C_{max} + C_{min})$. The MTF is the mathematical entity that expresses the ability of the detector system or any component of the system to reproduce the modulation of a planer radioactive source whose radioactivity varies inusoidally in one dimension in space. The MTF is equal to m_i/m_o where m_i is the modulation of the image and m_o is the modulation of the source which is the object imaged. Note that the MTF is a function of the spatial frequency ν.

Multiplex
To transmit two or more messages simultaneously over a single channel or other transmission facility.

Neutrino, Neutron
The atomic nucleus is made of protons and neutrons. They are together referred to as nucleons. The neutron is a neutral particle and slightly heavier than the positive particle, proton, which carries a charge equal to an electronic charge. The proton weighs 1.007825 mass units and an electron weighs 0.0005486 mass unit. The neutron weighs 1.008665 mass units. Thus the protons and neutrons are approximately 1800 times heavier than the electron. The neutron transforms into a proton during a beta-minus decay process, giving also the beta-minus particle and an antineutrino. The third particle, antineutrino, explains why the beta spectrum is a continuous spectrum, since it shares the energy of the neutron-proton mass difference with the beta-minus particle. In positron decay the proton transforms into a neutron giving beta-plus and a neutrino.

Off-Line
Pertaining to equipment or devices that are not in direct communication with the central processor of a computer system.

On-Line
Pertaining to equipment or devices that are in direct communication with the central processor of a computer system. On-line devices are usually under the direct control of the computer.

Pair Formation
The high-energy photon passing close to the field of a nucleus may interact with it with its complete transformation into a positron-negatron pair. The minimum energy of the photon required for such transformation is equal to the energy equivalent of the mass of the positron-electron pair: 1.02 mev.

Penumbra
When a collimated detector is looking at a source, the field of view can broadly be classified into three distinct regions; a region of maximum sensitivity called umbra; a region with reduced sensitivity, surrounding the umbra, called penumbra; and the region beyond penumbra where the sensitivity is minimum. The entire detector is seen by the source in the umbra region, whereas only part of the detector is seen by the source in the penumbra region.

Photoelectron
In the photoelectric effect, a photon interacts with an orbital electron and ejects it

with a kinetic energy equal to the difference of energy between the energy of the photon and the binding energy of the electron. These electrons are called photoelectrons. The photoelectric absorption is important for low-energy electrons in materials of high atomic number.

Photomultiplier Tube
A special vacuum photoelectric cell which uses secondary emission of electrons from a series of electrodes to amplify the number of electrons released from the photocathode by a light signal.

Photon
A quantum of energy of the electromagnetic field. It exhibits wave properties as well as particle properties.

Photopeak
A peak in the pulse-height spectrum which corresponds to the total energy absorption of the gamma ray.

Poisson Distribution
Poisson distribution describes all random processes whose probability of occurrence is small and constant. It applies to substantially all observations made in experimental nuclear physics. The probability P_x of observing x events when the average for a large number of tries is m events is given by the equation

$$P_x = m^x e^{-m} / x!$$

Note that the Poisson distribution can be completely characterized by only one parameter, m.

Positron
A particle of the same mass as an electron but with a positive charge.

Program
Program is used in data processing in the following four different ways: (1) a plan for solving a problem; (2) to devise a plan for solving a problem; (3) a computer routine, ie, a set of instructions arranged in proper sequence to cause a computer to perform a particular process; (4) to write a computer routine.

Radioactivity
Spontaneous transformation within the nucleus of the number of protons and neutrons or of their internal arrangement is called radioactivity. There are five types of radioactivity: alpha decay, beta decay, electron capture, isomeric transition, and spontaneous fission.

Rate Meter
The ratemeter measures the counting rate and not the individual counts. The output current of this electronic circuit is proportioned to the counting rate. This output is connected to a meter so that the counting rate at any instant can be read on its dial.

Resolution
The resolution of a detector is usually stated in terms of the full width at half-maximum (FWHM). The spatial resolution of a nuclear medicine imaging system can be defined in terms of its capability to distinguish the fine detail needed to identify small inhomogeneities in a radionuclide distribution. One parameter indicative of the system's resolution is its index of resolution, which is the width in centimeters of the system's line spread function measured at 50% response level. However, the system's modulation transfer function is a better measure of its capability to distinguish the finer details.

Scaler
An electronic instrument that counts the number of received pulses (as opposed to a ratemeter which measures the count rate) and displays the total in some suitable fashion. Most scalers have the capability of counting in two different modes: preset time (records total counts during preset

time) and preset counts (records only up to the preset number of counts and then stops counting).

Scanner
A nuclear medicine imaging device that maps the in vivo spatial distribution of radioactivity in a given area by actually moving the detector across the area in a pre-determined manner. Scan is used for the image developed by the scanner as well as the camera.

Scattering
In passing through matter, charged particles as well as photons are deflected from their original path by their interactions with matter. These are referred to as scattering processes. In nuclear medical imaging, the Compton scattering of gamma rays is of utmost concern. The window of the pulse height analyser (PHA) will usually accept a range of energies to be detected and identified as the principal gamma-ray energy. Thus, the scattered lower-energy photons which originate at a different location from the principal energy photons are given the wrong location as their point of origin. This reduces the overall resolution of the system.

Scintillation Detector
When charged particles pass through certain substances ionized and/or excited states are produced, which, during their return to the normal states, produce light flashes or scintillations. By coupling the scintillators with a photomultiplier tube, a pulse of charge can be passed to an electronic system, making counting possible.

Sensitivity
The sensitivity of a nuclear medicine imaging system is that characteristic which expresses the number of photons counted by the detection system in terms of the number of photons emitted from the radioactive source which is being imaged. System sensitivity depends on, among other things, the configuration of the radioactive source, ie, whether it is pont, line, plane, or volume source. Thus for comparing sensitivities of two systems identical source distributions and geometrics must be used.

Software
A collection of programs and routines associated with a computer which facilitate the programming and operation of the computer. This is to be distinguished from the actual physical equipment, which is called hardware.

Solid State
Pertaining to electronic components whose operation depends on the control of electric or magnetic phenomena in solids, eg, transistors, crystal diodes.

Solid-State Detector
A detector made of semiconductor material such as silicon (Si) or germanium (Ge) aded with controlled impurities. It has the advantage of good absorption for ionizing radiation and, unlike the scintillation detector, also has the simplicity of a gas detector which converts the absorbed energy directly into an electric pulse. The energy resolution of such a detector is far superior to the thallium-activated sodium iodide, NaI (Tl), scintillation detector. However, the effective atomic number of Si (Li) or Ge (Li), 14 and 32 respectively, is smaller than the effective atomic number 50 of NaI (Tl). Therefore, these solid-state detectors have lower stopping power for gamma rays compared to NaI (Tl). Also the solid-state detectors have to be cooled to liquid nitrogen temperatures for proper operation. Until solid-state detectors of larger thickness and higher effective atomic number become operational at room temperatures, their use in nuclear medical imaging is greatly limited.

Specific Activity
This can be expressed as the number of millicuries of radioactive isotope per gram of the total mixture of radioactive and stable isotopes of the same element.

Standard Deviation
The breadth of the statistical fluctuations of the individual readings about the true mean value is expressed quantitatively by the standard deviation. For a given mean value a small standard deviation gives a sharply peaked distribution. In normal distribution 68% of the individual observations should lie within the band (mean ± standard deviation).

Time Constant
This is a parameter associated with ratemeters. The longer the time constant, the more counts will the ratemeter accumulate with a given counting rate to reach its final deflection, and the slower will its pointer deflect in response to a change in radiation intensity.

Time Sharing
Time sharing is a method of operation by means of which several computer jobs are interleaved, giving the appearance of simultaneous operation. In many time-shared systems, users have individual terminals which are on-line.

Transient Equilibrium
When the daughter of a radioactive nuclide is also radioactive the quantities of different members of the series present at any given time depend upon the two decay constants. When the decay constant of the parent is less than the decay constant of the daughter, ie, when the parent's half-life is longer than that of the daughter, the ratio of the quantity of parent to that of the daughter becomes a constant. They are then said to be in equilibrium. When both parent and daughter have relatively short lives, the equilibrium is said to be transient. Such is the case of $^{99}Mo \rightarrow {}^{99m}Tc$. If the half-life of the parent is much longer than that of the daughter so that the parent does not decay appreciably over the period of study, the equilibrium reached is called secular equilibrium. Such is the case of radium → radon.

Wavelength
A wave can be characterized by any two of the following three parameters: length, frequency, and velocity. The wavelength is the distance from crest to crest. The frequency is the number of waves passing a given point per second. The velocity, which is the distance traveled in a second, is therefore given by the product of the wavelength and frequency.

Word
As used in data processing, word means a group of bits or characters treated as a unit and capable of being stored in one storage location. The number of bits and characters in a word is called word length.

Appendix Tables

Appendix Table 1. Physical Constants

Atomic mass unit	931.14 mev
Avogadro's number	6.023×10^{23} molecules/mole
Electronic charge	4.80×10^{-10} esu $= 1.602 \times 10^{-19}$ C
Electron volt	1.602×10^{-19} J $= 1.602 \times 10^{-12}$ ergs
Mass of an electron	0.51100 mev
Mass of a proton	938.26 mev
Mass of a neutron	939.55 mev
Planck's constant	6.625×10^{-27} erg-sec
Velocity of light	2.998×10^{10} cm/sec

Appendix Table 2. Units of Radioactivity

1 kilocurie (kCi)	3.7×10^{13} disintegrations/second
1 curie (Ci)	3.7×10^{10}
1 millicurie (mCi)	3.7×10^{7}
1 microcurie (μCi)	3.7×10^{4}
1 nanocurie (nCi)	3.7×10
I picocurie (pCi)	3.7×10^{-2}

Appendix Table 3. Half-Life and Mass per Microcurie of Several Useful Radionuclides

Radionuclide	Half-Line T*	AT†	μg/μCi
	Short Half-Life		
^{32}P	14.3	1.254	3.43×10^{-6}
^{51}Cr	27.8	3.88	10.6
^{59}Fe	45.1	7.28	19.8
^{57}Co	270.0	42.2	115.0
^{75}Se	127.0	26.1	71.2
^{85}Sr	64.0	14.9	40.7×10^{-6}
^{90}Y	2.67	0.658	1.795
^{99m}Tc	0.25	0.0678	0.185
^{125}I	60.0	20.5	56.0
^{131}I	8.1	2.91	7.95
^{192}Ir	74.4	39.1	106.5×10^{-6}
^{198}Au	2.70	1.465	4.0
^{197}Hg	2.71	1.46	3.99
^{203}Hg	47.0	26.2	71.6
^{222}Rn	3.83	2.33	6.36
	Long Half-Life		
^{3}H	12.3 yr	36.9	0.000101
^{44}C	5,560.0 yr	77,800.0	0.212
^{60}Co	5.24 yr	314.0	0.000858
^{85}Kr	10.3 yr	876.0	0.00239
^{90}Sr	27.7 yr	2,490.0	.0068
^{137}Cs	26.6 yr	3,640.0	0.00994
^{226}Ra	1,622.0 yr	366,500.0	1.000
^{238}U	4.5×10^{9} yr	1.07×10^{12}	2.92×10^{6}

* In days except as noted.

† A, atomic mass number; T, half-life in years.

Appendix Table 4. Physical Data for Certain Radionuclides

Element	Atomic number	Mass number	Half-life	Type of radiation	Energy of principal gamma ray (kev)	$\overline{E}\beta$ mev per disintegration	HVL Pb cm	R/Γ mCi/hr at 1 cm
Carbon (C)	6	11	20.0 min	β^+		0.38	0.4	2.5
Chromium (Cr)	24	51	27.8 days	ec, γ	320	0.005	0.2	0.15
Cobalt (Co)	27	57	270.0 days	ec, γ	122	0.023	0.3	0.99
		60	5.27 yr		1332	0.093	1.2	13.0
Fluorine (F)	9	18	110.0 min	β^+, ec		0.279	0.4	4.4
Gallium (Ga)	31	67	78.0 hr	ec, γ		0.009		1.0
		68	68.0 min		511		0.4	
Gold (Au)	79	198	2.7 days	β^-, γ	412	0.315	0.3	2.3
		199	3.15 days			0.10		0.59
Hydrogen (H)	1	3	12.26 yr	β^-		0.0055		
Indium (In)	49	113m	1.73 hr	IT, γ	393	0.11		1.75
Iodine (I)	53	123	13.0 hr	ec, γ	159	0.028	0.04	2.2
		125	60.0 days	ec, γ	35	0.021		1.23
		131	8.05 days	β^-, γ	364	0.180	0.3	2.20
Iron (Fe)	26	52	8.2 hr	β^+, ec, γ	165	0.195	1.2	4.6
		59	45.0 days	β^-, γ	1095	0.116	1.1	6.4
Mercury (Hg)	80	197	65.0 hr	ec, γ	77	0.079	0.04	0.31
		203	46.9 days	β^-, γ	279	0.100	0.2	1.20
Molybdenum (Mo)	42	99	66.7 hr	β^-, γ		0.400		1.29
Oxygen (O)	8	15	2.0 min	β^+		0.72		0.25
Phosphorus (P)	15	32	14.2 days	β^-		0.694		
Potassium (K)	19	42	12.4 hr	β^-, γ	1524	1.42	1.2	1.4
Selenium (Se)	34	75	120.0 days	ec, γ	265	0.019	0.2	1.76
Strontium (Sr)	38	85	64.0 days	ec, γ	514	0.014	0.4	3.0
		87m	2.8 hr	IT, γ	388	0.082	0.3	0.7
Technetium (Tc)	43	99m	6.0 hr	IT, γ	140	0.014	0.03	0.73
Xenon (Xe)	54	133	5.3 days	β^-, γ	81	0.12		1.3

ec, electron capture; IT, isomeric transition; Γ, specific gamma constant

Appendix Table 5. Relative Importance of Different Types of Absorption

Photon energy (kev)	Type of absorption: Water	Type of absorption: Lead
	τ	τ
10 – 50	$\tau = \sigma$	τ
50 – 100	$\sigma > \tau$	τ
100 – 500	Mostly σ	$\tau \gtreqless \sigma$
500 – 1000	σ	$\sigma > \tau$
1000 – 10,000	$\sigma >> \kappa$	$\sigma \geqq \kappa$
Higher than 10,000	$\sigma \lesseqgtr \kappa$	$\kappa >> \sigma$

τ, photoelectric, linear absorption coefficient;
σ, Compton, linear absorption coefficient;
κ, Pair production, linear absorption coefficient.

Appendix Table 6. Energies of Compton Scattered vs Incident Photons for Various Deflection Angles (θ)

Initial kev	Scattered photon energy in kev for $\theta = 30°$	$\theta = 90°$	$\theta = 180°$	Average energy* of Scattered photon	Recoil electron
10	9.9	9.8	9.6	9.85	0.15
20	19.9	19.25	18.52	19.38	0.62
50	49	45.5	41.8	46.0	4.0
100	99	83.6	71.8	86.0	14.2
200	190	143.5	114.2	156.5	43.5
500	442	252.5	169.0	335.0	165.0
1000	790	338.0	203.0	560.0	440.0
2000	1310	404.0	726.0	900.0	1100.0
Extremely great	3830	514.0	257.0	——	——

* All angles of scatter included.

Appendix Table 7. Radiation Dose from Commonly Performed Nonimaging Procedures

Procedures and agents	Usual administered dose (μCi)	Radiation dose (rads)	
		Target organ	Whole body
Thyroid study			
Uptake I 131	5.0	6.5–9.0 (thyroid)	0.02
Renal study			
Orthoiodohippurate I 131	30.0	0.03 (kidney)	0.0009
Diatrizoate I 131	30.0	– (kidney)	>0.0009
Iothalamate I 125	50.0	0.004 (kidney)	0.0002
Body Space study			
HSA I 131	5.0	0.07 (blood)	0.01
HSA I 125	5.0	<0.07 (blood)	<0.01
Cloride K 42	100.0	0.13 (muscle)	0.008
Sodium chromate CR 51	50.0	0.1 (lung)	0.02
Hematology study			
Sodium chromate Cr 51	100.0	0.2 (lung)	
Vitamin B_{12} Co 57	0.5	0.08 (liver)	
Chloride Fe 59	5.0	1.75 (testes)	
Blood Flow study			
^{133}Xe	1000.0	0.05 (lung)	0.0002
Gastrointestinal study			
Oleic acid I 131	25.0	0.05 (intestine)	0.016
Triolein I 131		0.05 (intestine)	0.016

Appendix Table 8. Radiation Dose From Commonly Performed Imaging Procedures

Procedure and agents	Usual administered dose (mCi)	Radiation dose (rads)			
		Target organ		Whole body	
Brain scan					
Chlormerodrin Hg 203	0.7–0.9	70–90 (kidney)*		1.2	
Chlormerodrin Hg 197	0.7–1	8–10 (kidney)		0.083	
Pertechnetate Tc 9m	5–10	1–2 (colon)		0.2	
DTPA In 113m	5–10	2.5–5 (bladder)		0.05–0.15	
HSA I^{131} Cisternography					
Normal	0.1	7.2 (sp. cord)		0.05–0.1	
Hydrocephalic	0.1	12.3 (sp. cord)		0.05–0.1	
Cervical block	0.1	58.7 (sp. cord)		0.05–0.1	
Lung scan					
MAA I 131	0.3	1–3 (lung)		0.12	
MAA Tc 99m	1–3	0.4–1 (lung)		0.01	
Albumin microspheres Tc 9m	1–3	0.4–1 (lung)		0.01	
$(OH)_3$ particles In 113m	1–3	0.75–2 (lung)		0.012–0.036	
^{133}Xe	5–10	0.25–0.5 (lung)		0.001–0.002	
Cardiovascular blood pool scan					
HSA I 131	0.2–0.3	2.9–5 (blood)		0.2–0.4	
HSA Tc 99m	1–3	0.04–0.12 (blood)		0.01–0.03	
Transferrin In 113m	1–3	0.04–0.12 (blood)		0.01	
Placental localization		**Mother**	**Fetus**	**Mother**	**Fetus**
HSA I 131	0.005–0.010	0.073 (blood)	0.005	0.01	0.004
Albumin Tc 99m	1			0.01	0.01
Pertechnetate Tc 99m	05.–1	0.1 (colon)	———	0.01	0.03
Transferrin In 113m	1	0.12 (blood)	0.008	0.01	0.008
Thyroid scan					
^{131}I	0.05	65–90 (thyroid)		0.2	
^{125}I	0.05–0.1	45–90 (thyroid)		0.06	
^{123}I	0.05–0.1	1–2 (thyroid)		0.003	
Pertechnetate 7c 99m	1	0.2 (thyroid)		0.01	
Liver scan					
Colloid gold Au 198	0.1–0.15	4–8 (liver)		0.1–0.25	
Sulfur colloid Tc 99m	1–3	0.3–1 (liver)		0.008–0.02	
Colloid In 113m	1–3	0.5–1 (liver)		0.015–0.03	
Rose bengal I 131	0.15–0.3	0.2–1.4 (liver)		0.2–0.4	
Spleen scan					
Sulfur colloid Tc 99m	1–3	0.3–1 (liver)		0.008–0.03	
Colloid In 113m	1–3	0.5–1 (liver)		0.015–0.03	
Heated RBCs Cr 51	0.1–0.3	4–10 (spleen)		0.05–0.07	
Pancreas scan					
Selenomethionine Se 75	0.25	3.5 (pancreas) 7 (liver) 1.3–2.6 (gonads)		0.9–2.5	
Bone scan					
^{85}Sr	0.1	3.1–4.6 (bone)		0.68–1.6	
^{87m}Sr	1–3	0.1–0.5 (bone)		0.02–0.06	
^{18}F	1–2	0.12–0.4 (bone)		0.03–0.07	
Kidney scan					
Chlormerodrin Hg 197	0.1–0.15	1.2–1.8 (kidney)		0.01–0.02	
Iron ascorbate Tc 99m	1–2	0.5–1 (kidney)		0.008	
DTPA Tc 99m	1–2	0.05–0.1 (kidney)		0.03	
Orthoiodohippurate I 131	0.2–0.4	0.2–0.4 (kidney)		0.006–0.12	

* May be reduced 40 to 50% by a prior blocking dose of nonradioactive chlormerodrin.

Self-Evaluation Section

1 The atomic number of an atom equals
   a the number of protons in the nucleus
   b the number of neutrons in the nucleus
   c the number of protons plus neutrons

2 Photons are attenuated in matter by
   a photoelectric effect
   b Compton effect
   c pair production
   d all of the above

3 The half-life of a radionuclide is always less than the average life.
   a true
   b false

4 Beta particles have the mass of an electron and carry either a positive or negative charge.
   a true
   b false

5 The effective half-life of a radionuclide is
   a always greater than both the physical and biological half-lives
   b always less than either the physical or biological half-life
   c always less than both the physical and biological half-lives
   d none of the above

6 The relation between distance from a point source and the intensity of the source is
   a $1/r^3$
   b $1/r^2$
   c r^2
   d 1

7 Isotopes are atoms which have the
   a same number of neutrons but a different mass number
   b same number of protons but a different mass number
   c same mass number but a different proton and neutron number

8 A photon is a quantum of energy which exhibits both wave and particle characteristics.
   a true
   b false

9 ^{99m}Tc decays by
   a electron capture
   b positron emission
   c electron emission
   d gamma emission

10 The absorbed dose unit is
   a the roentgen
   b the rad
   c either of the above

11 The Anger camera operates best for radioisotopes having energies in the range
   a < 100 keV
   b 100-200 keV
   c > 200 keV

12 ^{99m}Tc has a half-life of
   a 8 days
   b 6 days
   c 6 hours
   d 13.2 hours

13 The parallel-hole multichannel collimator is used with the
   a Anger camera
   b scanner
   c well counter
   d uptake probe

14 The rectilinear scanner is
   a a stationary device
   b a non-stationary imaging device
   c used to measure background radiation
   d uncollimated

15 Both the rectilinear scanner and the Anger camera use a sodium iodide crystal to detect gamma-rays.
- **a** true
- **b** false

16 Gamma-rays can be focused with a lens much the same as light rays.
- **a** true
- **b** false

17 The standard Anger camera consists of a scintillation crystal viewed by
- **a** 1 phototube
- **b** 12 phototubes
- **c** 19 phototubes
- **d** 7 phototubes

18 Which of the following materials would be suitable for collimator construction?
- **a** aluminum
- **b** copper
- **c** lead
- **d** uranium

19 The purpose of the pulse height analyzer in both the camera and the scanner is
- **a** to reject scattered radiation from the image
- **b** to set the intensity for film exposure
- **c** to pre-select a given energy range
- **d** both (**a**) and (**c**)

20 The Anger camera has an advantage over the rectilinear scanner in that a rapid dynamic study, such as passage of radionuclide through the heart chambers, may be performed.
- **a** true
- **b** false

21 Which of the following may be used for readout from the camera?
- **a** Polaroid film
- **b** 35mm or 70mm film
- **c** x-ray film
- **d** all of the above

22 A radio-iodine thyroid uptake study is performed with
- **a** scanner
- **b** camera
- **c** simple shielded probe
- **d** none of the above

23 Radioimmunoassays are performed with
- **a** scanner
- **b** camera
- **c** well counter systems
- **d** uptake probe

24 The Anger camera utilizes a cathode ray tube (CRT) for display.
- **a** true
- **b** false

25 Radiopharmaceuticals are classified chemically as
- **a** compounds and complexes
- **b** colloids
- **c** generators
- **d** all of the above

26 A radiopharmaceutical is a diagnostic aid.
- **a** true
- **b** false

27 A non-isotopically labeled compound means that the carrier compound does not normally contain atoms of the same species as the radionuclide.
- **a** true
- **b** false

28 The colloid particle size is generally
- **a** 1μ to 500μ
- **b** 0.1 mm
- **c** a few microns
- **d** none of the above

29 A radionuclide generator
- **a** is simply a shielded container for isotopes
- **b** consists of a long-lived radioactive parent which decays to a radioactive daughter
- **c** has limited use in nuclear medicine

30 To be useful, a radiopharmaceutical must be organ specific.
   a true
   b false

31 $NaTcO_4$ is highly ionic and is carried by the blood as a plasma protein complex. Hence, $NaTcO_4$ is a good agent for
   a observing blood flow to an organ
   b static liver imaging
   c lung scanning
   d none of the above

32 Radiocolloids are used to detect space-occupying lesions in
   a the kidney
   b the liver
   c the thyroid
   d the brain

33 Lung scanning is generally performed with
   a ^{99m}Tc albumin microspheres
   b macroaggregated iodinated albumin I 131
   c macroaggregated albumin ^{99m}Tc
   d all of the above

34 ^{131}I orthoiodohippuric acid is the agent for studying tubular function in the kidneys.
   a true
   b false

35 The disadvantage(s) of ^{131}I labeled compounds compared to ^{123}I labeled compounds is (are)
   a relatively long half-life
   b relatively high energy gamma-ray
   c patient dose
   d all of the above

36 A computer may be either digital or analog.
   a true
   b false

37 Digital data is
   a discrete
   b continuous

38 An electronic computer typically consists of
   a 1 basic unit
   b 2 basic units
   c 3 basic units
   d 4 basic units

39 The number system used by the computer for processing is
   a decimal
   b binary
   c octal
   d hexadecimal

40 The magnetic tape unit is
   a a sequential access system
   b a random access system
   c both of the above

41 A magnetic disc system is
   a a sequential access device
   b a random access device
   c both of the above

42 The control unit interprets and forwards instructions to all other components in the system.
   a true
   b false

43 The interface between the camera and the computer is the
   a DAC
   b ADC
   c I/O unit
   d none of the above

44 The system software is
   a a compilation of all the programs which facilitate operation of the computer
   b the internal circuitry
   c the peripheral storage
   d unalterable

45 The image displayed by the computer
   a is in the form of a matrix of dots
   b has a gray scale
   c may be manipulated
   d all of the above

46 Software, as it applies to nuclear medicine, may be put in two categories, acquisition and processing.
- a true
- b false

47 The simplest type of image enhancement with the computer involves adjusting the linear region of the gray scale.
- a true
- b false

48 Smoothing data generally increases resolution.
- a true
- b false

49 Correcting the response of the camera over the field of view is
- a smoothing
- b uniformity correction
- c averaging
- d not useful

50 The most frequent site of obstruction of the internal carotid artery seen on dynamic brain flow studies is
- a at its end
- b at its mid-portion
- c just beyond the bifurcation
- d just before the bifurcation

51 The first scintigraph demonstrating absence of activity on one side of the carotid region is the most important of the series.
- a true
- b false

52 A solitary defect in the column of activity in the carotid artery is *not* caused by
- a the orbit
- b the mandible
- c gold teeth fillings

53 A positive static brain scan present on admission in a stroke patient is not suggestive of a preexisting brain tumor.
- a true
- b false

54 A normal dynamic and static brain study rules out the presence of a cerebrovascular accident.
- a true
- b false

55 An infiltrating lesion seen on a static brain scan is most suggestive of
- a infarction
- b cyst
- c glioblastoma
- d necrosis

56 A 70-year-old chronic smoker, male, with shortness of breath and back pains of two months duration, developed sudden generalized convulsive seizures. His chest x-ray revealed a large lung tumor. His brain scan most probably will show
- a absent right carotid flow
- b absent right middle cerebral flow
- c multiple lesions on static scans
- d abnormal arterial flow

57 Half of all meningiomas appear as an area with increased activity on the early arterial frames of a dynamic brain study. This finding is due to
- a vascular shunting in the lesion
- b increased vascularity of the tumor
- c venous obstructions associated with the lesion

58 An intracranial rim on a brain scan is most suggestive of
- a brain tumor
- b brain abcess
- c subdural hematoma
- d infarction

59 Paget's disease can result in decreased activity in the involved area of the brain scan.
- a true
- b false

60 Increased extracranial activity on a brain scan is *not* suggestive of
- a arteritis
- b sinusitis

c trauma
d meningiomas

61 The normal range for the 24-hour radioactive iodine uptake is
a 20–50%
b 10–40%
c 5–35%
d 1–25%

62 An increase in the 24-hour radioactive iodine uptake from 8% to 16% after TSH stimulation indicates secondary hypothyroidism.
a true
b false

63 A 23-year-old woman with a goiter and bulging eyes was found to be euthyroid after clinical evaluation. Her 24-hour radioactive iodine uptake dropped from 34% to 32% after cytomel suppression. The most probable diagnosis is
a simple nontoxic goiter
b early toxic goiter
c thyroiditis
d congenital goiter

64 A carotid thyroid transit time (CTTT) of zero is diagnostic of
a hypothyroidism
b euthyroidism
c hyperthyroidism

65 Which one of the following thyroid function tests, if elevated in pregnancy, is most suggestive of hyperthyroidism?
a PBI
b BEI
c T_3 test
d T_4 test

66 The normalized serum thyroxine test T_4N gives an elevated result in normal pregnancy.
a true
b false

67 Tertiary hypothyroidism has
a low TRH and high TSH
b low TRH and low TSH
c high TRH and low TSH

68 A negative selenomethionine ^{75}Se thyroid scan does *not* suggest
a thyroid cyst
b thyroid hemorrhage
c large mixed thyroid carcinoma
d adenomatous goiter

69 The "owl eye" sign in a thyroid nodule on scanning is highly suggestive of neoplasia.
a true
b false

70 Lack of suppression of the thyroid helps localize the parathyroid glands after selenomethionine ^{75}I injection.
a true
b false

71 Iodocholesterol ^{131}I is a useful radiopharmaceutical for scanning adrenal tissue because
a it stimulates the adrenals
b it avoids the liver
c it is a precursor of the adrenal steroids
d has a long biological half-life

72 A patient suspected of Cushing's syndrome is given large doses of corticosteroids for 2 days. In the morning, his ACTH blood level is 160 pg/ml. It is likely that he has the disease.
a true
b false

73 The average pulmonary capillary diameter is about
a 2μ
b 15μ
c 8μ
d 20μ

74 On a lung scan, a segmental area of perfusion defect without corresponding radiographic changes is suggestive of
a asthma
b embolism

c pneumonia
d emphysema

75 Hypoperfusion along the major fissure on a lung scan without demonstrable radiographic abnormalities strongly suggests pulmonary embolism.
a true
b false

76 A perfusion deficit on a lung scan with a corresponding area of radiographic density with absence of ventilation on ^{133}Xe study is typical of
a asthma
b embolism
c pneumonia
d emphysema

77 A 23-year-old woman presented with chest pain, cough, shortness of breath, and hemoptysis. A chest x-ray was clear and a ^{133}Xe study was normal, but she had an area of perfusion defect in her left lung. She most probably has
a pneumonia
b tuberculous
c embolism
d cancer of the lung

78 An abnormal retention of ^{133}Xe was found in the washout phase of a ventilation study. This is typical of
a embolism
b pneumonia
c emphysema
d none of the above

79 Bronchial obstruction causes marked abnormalities in perfusion and ventilation on lung scanning.
a true
b false

80 Fifty percent of radiopharmaceuticals for lung scanning of 10μ to 50μ, when injected intravenously, are removed from circulation by the lung during their first passage.
a true
b false

81 A hot spot on a lung scan is caused by
a lung tumor
b pneumonia
c defective radiopharmaceutical
d lung abscess

82 Lugol's solution must be given prior to lung scanning with ^{99m}Tc macroaggregated albumen.
a true
b false

83 Acute bronchial asthma can cause perfusion defects.
a true
b false

84 Our present technique for liver scanning depends on the function of which cell?
a reticuloendothelial
b fibroblast
c polygonal

85 The best method to determine liver size is
a physical examination
b x-ray
c scanning

86 Radiopharmaceutical colloid size is irrevelent as far as liver localization is concerned.
a true
b false

87 The best technique to separate an intraheptic cyst from a solid lesion is
a RES scan
b physical examination
c ^{67}Ga scan
d ultrasound scan

88 A discrepancy between the superior margin of the dome of the liver and the right diaphragm suggests the presence of
a tumor
b cyst
c hemorrhage
d abscess

89 Ascites and obesity enhance the liver RES scan.
- **a** true
- **b** false

90 A scan of the pancreas revealed increased radioactivity concentration in the tail. The patient most probably suffers from
- **a** cancer of the head of the pancreas
- **b** pancreatitis
- **c** no pancreatic disease
- **d** cancer of the tail of the pancreas

91 The passage of the aorta behind the pancreas creates a scanning defect in the body of the pancreas. This finding can easily be confused with
- **a** chronic pancreatitis
- **b** acute pancreatitis
- **c** cancer of the head of the pancreas
- **d** cancer of the body of the pancreas

92 The most common scanning abnormality observed in cancer of the body of the pancreas is a segmental defect in the midportion of the organ. Patients with this abnormal scan are *not* likely to have
- **a** weight loss
- **b** pain
- **c** jaundice
- **d** thrombophlebitis
- **e** epigastric mass

93 A normal pancreatic image is commonly seen in chronic pancreatitis.
- **a** true
- **b** false

94 Reduced or absent visualization of the pancreas can result from interference by other gastrointestinal diseases.
- **a** true
- **b** false

95 A well imaged pancreas head with an absent body is diagnostic of
- **a** pancreatitis
- **b** cystic fibrosis
- **c** cancer of the body of the pancreas
- **d** cancer of the stomach

96 In angiocardiography, the normal peak-to-peak time between right and left ventricles is about
- **a** 5–10 sec
- **b** 4–5 sec
- **c** 1–3 sec

97 A reflux into the inomenate vein and inferior vena cava on angiocardiography suggests
- **a** valvular lesion
- **b** lowered right heart pressure
- **c** elevated right heart pressure
- **d** elevated left heart pressure

98 A well defined area of radionuclide retention in the left ventricle during washout suggests
- **a** myxoma
- **b** clot
- **c** shunt
- **d** aneurysm

99 A high count density in the right heart, with no radioactivity within superimposed vascular structures, in the early phases of an angiocardiography suggests a myxoma of the right heart.
- **a** true
- **b** false

100 The appearance of radioactivity within the heart or aorta prior to pulmonary perfusion indicates the presence of
- **a** left to right shunt
- **b** right to left shunt
- **c** valvular defect
- **d** pericardial effusion

101 Left to right shunts are best detected on angiocardiograph by
- **a** image subtraction
- **b** analysis of isotope dilution curves
- **c** differential scanning

102 A recirculation curve peak in the time activity curves placed over various heart chambers and lungs is indica-

tive of right-to-left shunt on an angiocardiogram.
a true
b false

103 Aneurysm of thoracic aorta appears as a localized area of luminal widening on an angiocardiogram with an abnormal flow pattern.
a true
b false

104 The effective lumen of an abdominal aneurysm is best demonstrated by
a dynamic isotope examination
b ultrasonography
c none of the above

105 Isotope dilution curves obtained over lungs and cardiac chambers provide other means of establishing the presence of
a right to left shunt
b valvular insufficiency
c left-to-right shunt
d heart failure

106 Visualization of renal activity following the injection of intravenous ^{99m}Tc labeled MAA generally indicates a right-to-left shunt in excess of 35%.
a true
b false

107 In pericardial effusion, the separation between the cardiac from that within the pulmonary and hepatic activity is
a normal
b decreased
c increased
d diminished

108 The degree of radionuclide uptake at the site of a bone lesion depends on blood flow and reactivity of the newly forming bone.
a true
b false

109 ^{99m}Tc labeled polyphosphate and diphosphonate localize in bone by
a osmosis
b chemisorption
c competitive binding
d all of the above

110 The main advantage of ^{85}Sr as a bone scanning agent is its
a energy
b cost
c shelf-life

111 ^{18}F-Floride as a bone scanning agent has numerous disadvantages except
a short half-life
b high cost
c availability
d prompt uptake by bone
e increased radiation to the bladder

112 Metastasis must be larger than 3 cm in diameter to become visible radiologically.
a true
b false

113 False negative bone scans are *not* seen in
a multiple myeloma
b thyroid carcinoma
c breast carcinoma
d recent fracture

114 A bone fracture may show increased concentration of ^{99m}Tc polyphosphate as late as 3 years from the time of fracture.
a true
b false

115 Positive bone scans can be seen in osteoarthritis.
a true
b false

116 A positive bon scan is pathognomonic of specific disease.
a true
b false

117 In a 70-year-old man complaining of headaches of 2 weeks duration, a history of skull fracture after a fall 4 years earlier was obtained. A bone scan revealed two areas of increased

radionuclide concentration in the skull. The patient most probably has
a nonhealing skull fracture
b osteoarthritis
c osteomylitis
d metastatic tumor

118 Serial bone scans can be used to monitor the response of metastatic prostatic carcinoma to ^{32}P therapy.
a true
b false

119 Radiochlormerodrin is used to image the kidney because it localizes in
a distal tubules
b collecting tubules
c proximal tubules
d glomeruli

120 85% to 90% of radiohippuran is secreted promptly by the proximal renal tubules following an intravenous injection.
a true
b false

121 The renogram is useful in the evaluation of renovascular hypertension.
a true
b false

122 Radionuclide uptake within a renal bulge is suggestive of fetal lobulation.
a true
b false

123 Reduced radionuclide concentration in a renal bulge is *not* suggestive of
a cyst
b tumor
c infarct
d fetal lobulation

124 A 30-year-old drug addict with fever and shortness of breath developed sudden left flank pain. An IVP was normal. Radiohippuran scan revealed focal segmental loss of radionuclide uptake. A bolus ^{99m}Tc pertechnetate flow study revealed reduced perfusion to the area. The most likely diagnosis is
a pyelonephritis
b cystic kidney
c renal infarction
d ruptured kidney

125 The characteristic changes in renal vascular hypertension on a renogram are a delay in the peak of the curve and impaired second and third phases.
a true
b false

126 A high renal flow rate enhances the renogram findings in renal vascular hypertension.
a true
b false

127 A ^{99m}Tc pertechnetate renal flow study showing asymetrical perfusion patterns is suggestive of
a renal vascular hypertension
b pyelonephritis
c renal reflux

128 Renal transplant rejection, when evaluated with ^{99m}Tc pertechnetate flow study, shows
a increased perfusion
b normal perfusion
c reduced perfusion

129 Radiochlormerodrin is useful in evaluating vesicoarterial reflux.
a true
b false

130 The renal scan is useful for differentiating obstructions from prerenal and renal cases of uremia in patients with renal failure.
a true
b false

131 Placental transport of substances is not developed until the 50th day of life.
a true
b false

132 ^{99m}Tc sulfur colloid crosses the placental barrier.
- **a** true
- **b** false

133 The placenta appears as an area of decreased radioactive uptake in the abdomen on ^{99m}Tc pertechnetate placentography.
- **a** true
- **b** false

134 A falling HPL level with vaginal bleeding indicates
- **a** cyst rupture
- **b** abortion
- **c** neoplasia
- **d** all of the above

135 HCG level is important in the diagnosis and follow-up of patients with
- **a** bleeding problems
- **b** trophoblestic disease
- **c** tubal pregnancy

136 At term, a 24-hour estriol value of less than 2mg/24h suggests
- **a** abortion
- **b** fetal death
- **c** diabetes
- **d** hydramnious

137 In a normal pregnancy, LH rises 12 to 24 hours prior to ovulation.
- **a** true
- **b** false

138 HPL level in toximia of pregnancy is
- **a** increased
- **b** normal
- **c** decreased

139 The placental bed is first seen on dynamic imaging in
- **a** 1–5 sec
- **b** 10–15 sec
- **c** 30–40 sec

140 1.5% of an intravenous dose of ^{75}Se selenomethionine crosses the placenta and is accumulated in the fetus.
- **a** true
- **b** false

141 The splenic vein hematocrit in a normal man is 70%.
- **a** true
- **b** false

142 ^{51}Cr has become the standard for measuring blood volume because
- **a** it is cheap
- **b** it has a reasonable half-life of 27.8 days
- **c** it gives low body radiation dose

143 ^{51}Cr attaches itself to the RBC by binding itself to the
- **a** heme
- **b** α chain of globuin
- **c** β chain of globuin

144 The most common error in technique in performing a blood volume is
- **a** pipetting
- **b** inadvertent injection of part of a sample into the cutanious tissue
- **c** counting

145 Vitamin C intake can result in an unreliable blood volume determination.
- **a** true
- **b** false

146 A normal donor has normal red cell survival when his labeled red blood cells are injected into a patient with hereditary spherocytosis.
- **a** true
- **b** false

147 A patient with a high spleen-to-liver ratio is likely to improve following spleenectomy as a treatment of his hyperspleenism.
- **a** true
- **b** false

148 Bone marrow can increase productivity on need by a factor of
- **a** 1-5 times
- **b** 7-10 times
- **c** 10-20 times

149 In a normal individual 70% to 100% of the administered ^{59}Fe activity will appear in the circulating red cell mass by 7 to 14 days after the intravenous administration.
a true
b false

150 A normal individual will, in 60 minutes, excrete in the urine more than 8% of the absorbed labeled Vitamin B_{12} following a flushing dose of B_{12}.
a true
b false

151 ^{111}In chloride administered intravenously can define the erythron just as reliably as technetium sulfur colloid.
a true
b false

152 The mechanism of concentration of gallium in tumors is known.
a true
b false

153 Serum transferrin is the carrier protein for gallium.
a true
b false

154 The following organ normally has a high concentration of gallium.
a stomach
b colon
c uterus
d bone

155 Chronic renal disease results in increased gallium concentration in
a kidneys
b bladder
c bone
d parathyroids

156 Which one of the following diseases does *not* have an increase in gallium concentration in the involved area?
a sarcoidoses
b osteomyelitis
c pneumonia
d lymphoma

157 A major advantage of ^{111}In is its minimal concentration in the gut.
a true
b false

158 ^{67}Ga and ^{111}In scanning can detect all cases of proven involvement with neoplastic disease.
a true
b false

159 A bone tumor appears as a hot spot on an ^{111}In scan.
a true
b false

160 A patient with Paget's disease can give a positive Ga scan.
a true
b false

161 Carcinoembryonic antigen (CEA) found in some adenocarcinomas is a
a polypeptide
b glycoprotein
c mucopolysaccaride

162 In a double antibody radioimmunoassay, the antigen–antibody complex is precipitated by a second antibody directed against the immunoglobulin of the species engendering the first antibody.
a true
b false

163 The following are tumor associated antigens *except*
a alpha fetoprotein
c gamma fetoprotein
c B globulin
d fetal sulphoglycoprotein antigen
e T-globulin

164 A large colonic tumor gives a higher CEA titer than a small colonic tumor.
a true
b false

165 The CEA test detects recurrent metastatic colonic carcinomas with a high degree of reliability.
- **a** true
- **b** false

166 Surgical removal of a colonic cancer will result in a drop in the CEA level.
- **a** true
- **b** false

167 Alpha fetoprotein is a tumor-associated antigen present in the serum of over 70% of patients with
- **a** carcinoma of the pancreas
- **b** carcinoma of the lung
- **c** hepatomas
- **d** nephromas

168 A gastric carcinoma can give a positive alpha fetoprotein test.
- **a** true
- **b** false

169 Smoaking can result in a positive CEA test.
- **a** true
- **b** false

170 A good antigen must have a molecular weight of at least 10,000.
- **a** true
- **b** false

171 Antigens have 2 reaction sites.
- **a** true
- **b** false

172 In a radioimmuno reaction, the concentration of labeled antigen
- **a** is variable
- **b** increases
- **c** decreases
- **d** remains constant

173 Antibodies are
- **a** monovalent
- **b** bivalent
- **c** trivalent

174 The most important quality of an antibody in an RIA is
- **a** purity
- **b** specific activity
- **c** specificity
- **d** short biological half-life

175 The quantity of labeled antigen–antibody complex formed in an RIA reaction is inversely proportional to the quantity of standard present.
- **a** true
- **b** false

176 A solid phase RIA means that the antigen–antibody reaction becomes solid.
- **a** true
- **b** false

177 Serum insulin levels are better for following the diabetic state of a patient than blood sugar measurements.
- **a** true
- **b** false

178 Angiotenson I is converted into Angiotension II in the
- **a** liver
- **b** kidney
- **c** lung
- **d** adrenals

179 Serum gastrin level of 350 $\mu\mu$/ml is suggestive of ZE syndrome.
- **a** true
- **b** false

180 When Plummer's disease is treated with $Na^{131}I$ the dose should range from
- **a** 1–10 mCi
- **b** 10–50 mCi
- **c** 50–100 mCi

181 The most accurate test for hyperthyroidism is
- **a** the RAIU test
- **b** the T_3 uptake test
- **c** total serum thyroxine T_4N
- **d** thyroid scan

182 An unusual complication of $Na^{131}I$ therapy is
- **a** stomatitis
- **b** parotitis
- **c** pancreatitis
- **d** gastritis

183 The incidence of hypothyroidism following $Na^{131}I$ therapy after 10 years of follow-up is
- a under 25%
- b over 50%
- c over 75%
- d 100%

184 $Na^{125}I$ therapy for hyperthyroidism markedly reduces the incidence of hypothyroidism following therapy.
- a true
- b false

185 Thyroid nodules are malignant in children in what percentage of cases?
- a 10%
- b 25%
- c 50%
- d 75%

186 The use of diuretics in cases of thyroid carcinoma prior to $Na^{131}I$ therapy results in
- a reduced concentration of radioiodine in the tumor
- b increased concentration of radioiodine in the tumor
- c no change in the concentration of radioiodine in the tumor

187 A history of head and neck irradiation in childhood reduces the probability of malignancy in the thyroid later.
- a true
- b false

188 There is an increased incidence of malignancy of the thyroid following NaI^{131} therapy for the thyroid.
- a true
- b false

189 Thyroidectomy prior to $Na^{131}I$ ablation in a case of thyroid carcinoma results in a lower concentration of the isotope in the tumor.
- a true
- b false

190 ^{131}I labeled rose bengal is used to study liver function by placing a stationary probe in the temporal region and measuring the clearance as a function of time.
- a true
- b false

191 Glucagon depresses human growth hormone levels.
- a true
- b false

192 Ideally, a radioisotope for imaging purposes should be a monoenergetic gamma emitter.
- a true
- b false

193 Gamma camera resolution is on the order of
- a 1 mm
- b 1 cm
- c 5 cm
- d none of the above

194 The pinhole collimator is more sensitive than the parallel hole multichannel collimator.
- a true
- b false

195 The tube-coated antibody used in the RIA for the Australian antigen makes the assay a
- a direct solid phase
- b direct liquid phase
- c indirect solid phase

196 Which thyroid cancer has the most frequent functioning metastasis?
- a follicular
- b papillary
- c mixed
- d medulary

197 The most effective therapy for thyroid cancer is
- a surgery
- b radioactive iodine
- c surgery and radioactive iodine
- d external irradiation
- e hormone therapy

198 The present day assay for vitamin B_{12} is by
- a RIA
- b CPBA
- c both

199 RAI can be used to assay
- a thyroxine
- b T_3
- c morphine
- d all of the above

200 The most common therapy for hyperthyroidism is radioiodine.
- a true
- b false

Answers

1–a	35–d	69–b	102–b	135–b	168–a
2–d	36–a	70–b	103–a	136–b	169–a
3–a	37–a	71–c	104–a	137–a	170–a
4–a	38–d	72–a	105–c	138–c	171–b
5–b	39–b	73–c	106–b	139–b	172–d
6–b	40–a	74–c	107–c	140–a	173–b
7–b	41–b	75–a	108–a	141–a	174–c
8–a	42–a	76–c	109–b	142–b	175–a
9–d	43–b	77–c	110–c	143–c	176–b
10–b	44–a	78–c	111–d	144–b	177–b
11–b	45–d	79–a	112–b	145–a	178–c
12–c	46–a	80–b	113–d	146–a	179–b
13–a	47–a	81–c	114–b	147–a	180–b
14–b	48–b	82–b	115–a	148–b	181–c
15–a	49–b	83–a	116–b	149–a	182–b
16–b	50–c	84–a	117–d	150–a	183–b
17–c	51–a	85–c	118–a	151–a	184–b
18–c	52–a	86–b	119–c	152–b	185–c
19–d	53–b	87–d	120–a	153–a	186–b
20–a	54–b	88–d	121–a	154–b	187–b
21–d	55–c	89–b	122–a	155–c	188–b
22–c	56–c	90–c	123–b	156–c	189–b
23–c	57–b	91–d	124–c	157–a	190–a
24–a	58–c	92–c	125–a	158–b	191–b
25–d	59–b	93–b	126–b	159–b	192–a
26–a	60–d	94–a	127–a	160–a	193–b
27–b	61–c	95–c	128–c	161–b	194–b
28–a	62–b	96–b	129–b	162–a	195–a
29–b	63–b	97–c	130–a	163–c	196–a
30–b	64–c	98–d	131–a	164–a	197–c
31–a	65–c	99–a	132–b	165–a	198–c
32–b	66–b	100–b	133–b	166–a	199–d
33–d	67–b	101–b	134–b	167–c	200–a
34–a	68–c				

Index

Acquisition software, camera-computer, 15–16
Adrenal scanning, 51–52
AFP (alpha fetoprotein) detection, 160, 161, 162
Albumin ^{131}I, 9
Albumin microspheres ^{99m}Tc, 10, 54, 55
Alpha fetoprotein (AFP) detection, 160, 161, 162
Amniocentesis, placental localization and, 119
Amniography, 119
Analog-to-digital converter (ADC), 12, 15
Anger camera, *see* Gamma camera, Anger type
Angiocardiography, *see* Radionuclide angiocardiography (RAC)
Angiography, *see* Radionuclide angiography (RA)
Antibodies, radioimmunoassay and, 169
Antigens
    radioimmunoassay and, 168–169
    tumor-associated, *see* Tumor-associated antigens, detection of
Arterial phase circulation, brain scanning and, 24–30, 31, 33
Arteriovenous malformation scintigraphs, 34
Arteritis detection, 33
Aseptic necrosis diagnosis, 115
Ashkar, Fuad S., 38–52, 63–79, 168–181
Asthma, lung scanning and, 57–58
Atelectasis, lung scanning and, 59–60
Autofluoroscope, digital, 80

Barium-131, 108
Barium-135, 108
Bezjian, Alex A., 118–129
Blood pool scanning, 86, 89
Blood tests, 141–149
    blood volume calculation, 141–143
    external imaging, 147–148
    future prospects, 149
    in vitro procedures, 141–147
    marrow tumor detection, 148
    platelet survival time estimation, 147
    radiopharmaceuticals for, 142–144, 147–149
    red cell metabolism evaluation, 148–149
    red cell production estimation, 145–147
    red cell production sites identification, 147–148
    red cell survival time estimation, 143–144
    Schilling test, 147
Bone scanning, 108–117
    application of, 113–116
    aseptic necrosis and, 115
    bone islands and, 116
    indications for, 113–116
    inflammatory disease and, 115–116
    metabolic disorders and, 116
    neoplastic disease and, 113–115
    principles of, 108–110
    radiopharmaceuticals for, 108, 110–113, 150
    summary, 116
    trauma and, 115
Brain abscess detection, 24, 30, 31
Brain scanning, 23–37
    abnormal dynamic, abnormal static, 30–36
    abnormal dynamic, normal static, 25–30
    advantages of, 23–24
    disadvantages of, 23–24
    interpretation of, 24–36
    normal dynamic, abnormal static, 25, 30
    normal dynamic, normal static, 24
    procedures, 23
    radiopharmaceuticals for, 8–9
Bronchogenic carcinoma detection, 60

Calcium-47, 108
Cameras, scintillation, 4–5
Capillary phase of circulation, brain scanning and, 24, 30, 31, 33
Carbon-47, 118
Carcinoembryonic antigen (CEA) detection, 160, 161, 162–164
Cardiac blood flow studies, computer and, 20–21
Cardiac function evaluation, 95–101
Cardiac mass detection, 90–95
Cardiovascular system, *see* Radionuclide angiocardiography (RAC); Radionuclide angiography (RA)
Carotid artery, brain scanning and, 24, 25–27, 31, 33
Carotid-thyroid transit time (CTTT), 40–41
CEA (carcinoembryonic antigen) detection, 160, 161, 162–164
Central nervous system, *see* Brain scanning
Central processing unit (CPU), digital computer, 14
Cerebral arteries, brain scanning and, 26–29
Cerebral vascular accident scintigraphs, 27, 28
Chlormerodrin ^{197}Hg, 11, 130–133, 135, 136
Chlormerodrin ^{203}Hg, 9, 11
Chromic phosphate ^{32}P, 181
Chromium-51
    blood volume calculation with, 142
    placental localization with, 120
Collimators, 2, 4, 75, 110
Colloids, 6, 8
Competitive protein-binding analysis (CPBA), 41, 42, 168
Complexes, 6, 8
Compounds, 6, 7–8
Computer, *see* Digital computer
Congestive heart failure, lung scanning and, 60
Core storage, digital computer, 12–13
Cow, radioisotope, 6–7

CPBAC (competitive protein binding analysis), 41, 42, 168
CTTT (carotid-thyroid transit time), 40–41
Cyclotron, 149
Cystic astrocytomas, brain scanning and, 29
Cystic fibrosis detection, 60

Diabetes, radioimmunoassays and, 172
Digital autofluoroscope, 80
Digital computer, 12–22
- acquisition software, 15–16
- camera-computer hardware system, 14–15
- camera-computer software system, 15–21
- central processing unit (CPU), 14
- definitions, 12
- enhancement, 17–19
- frame arithmetic, 20
- input/output devices, 12, 15
- processing software, 16–21
- quality control, 16–17
- region of interest assignment, 19
- smoothing, 19–20
- storage devices, 12–13
- time-activity histograms, 20–21
- uniformity correction, 16

Diisopropyl fluorophosphate (DFP 32), 142, 147
Diphosphonate ^{99m}Tc, 112–113
DTPA ^{113m}In, 130
DTPA ^{99m}Tc, 11, 130
DTPA ^{169}Yb, 130
Dynamic scintigraphs, 16, 23
- abnormal, and abnormal static scintigraphs, 30–36
- abnormal, and normal static scintigraphs, 25–30
- normal, and abnormal static scintigraphs, 25, 30
- normal, and normal static scintigraphs, 24
- placental localization and, 122–123
- thyroid function and, 39–41

Dysprosium-157, 108

Echocardiography, 81, 95
Enhancement program, 17–19
Erythropoiesis, 148–149
Estrogen, radioimmunoassays for, 123, 125–127
Ewing's sarcoma detection, 113

Ferrokinetics, 145–147
Fetal sulfoglycoprotein antigen (FSA) detection, 160, 161, 162, 166–167
Fibrous dysplasia detection, 33, 35
Five-point smoothing, 19–20
Fluorine-18, 108, 110–112, 150
Frame arithmetic program, 20
FSA (fetal sulfoglycoprotein antigen) detection, 160, 161, 162, 166–167
FSH (follicle stimulating hormone), radioimmunoassays for, 123, 127–128

Gallium-67, 151–158
Gallium-68, 108
Gallium-72, 150–151
Gamma camera, Anger type
- -computer hardware system, 14–15
- -computer software system, 15–21
- *See also* Imaging procedures, instruments for

Gamma fetoprotein (GFP) detection, 160, 161, 162, 166–167
Gastrointestinal system, *see* Liver scanning; Pancreas scanning; Spleen scanning
Generators, 6–7
GFP (gamma fetoprotein) detection, 160, 161, 162, 166–167
Gilson, Albert J., 23–37
Glioblastoma detection, 28, 30
Glioma detection, 30, 31, 33
Goiter evolution, thyroid scanning and, 46–47
Gold-198
- intracavity use of, 181
- liver scanning and, 63, 118
- pregnancy and, 118

Gottlieb, Stuart, 80–107
Grave's disease, therapy for, 176–178
Gynecology, 118–119, 123–128
- *See also* Placental localization

Hardware system, camera-computer, 14–15
HCG (human chorionic gonadotropin), radioimmunoassays and, 123, 125
Heal, Albert V., 168–175
Heart failure, lung scanning and, 60
Heart scanning, *see* Radionuclide angiocardiography (RAC)
Hematoma detection, 24, 28, 33
Hepatitis detection, 174
Hepatomegaly detection, 66, 69, 71
HMG (human menopausal gonadotropin), 127
Hormones, identified by radioimmunoassay, *see* Radioimmunoassay
HPL (human placental lactogen), radioimmunoassays and, 123, 124–125
HSA ^{99m}Tc, 82
Human chorionic gonadotropin (HCG), radioimmunoassays and, 123, 125
Human growth hormone (HGH), radioimmunoassays and, 172
Human menopausal gonadotropin (HMG), 127
Human placental lactogen (HPL), radioimmunoassays and, 123, 124–125
Hupf, Homer B., 6–11
Hydrated ferric oxide ^{113m}In, 54
Hydrated ferric oxide ^{99m}Tc, 54
Hypertension
- radioimmunoassays and, 172, 174
- renovascular, 135–136

Hyperthyroidism
- radioactive iodine and, 38–41
- radioisotope therapy for, 176–178

Hypoglycemia detection, 172

Imaging procedures, instruments for, 1–5
- bone scanning, 110, 112
- collimators, 2, 4, 75, 110
- digital autofluoroscope, 80
- electronics, 2–3
- image data processing, 5
- liver scanning, 63–64
- lung scanning, 61
- pancreas scanning, 75
- radionuclide angiocardiography (RAC), 80, 81–82

readouts, 3
rectilinear scanners, 1–3
scintillation cameras, 4–5
Immunodiffusion tests, 162
Indium-111, 150–151, 155–158
Indium-113m
liver scanning with, 63
placental localization with, 121
Input/output devices, *see* Digital computer
Iodinated serum albumin, 120
Iodine, radioactive, 47, 50
thyroid physiology and, 38
uptake test, 38–39
Iodine-125, 120
Iodine-131
blood volume calculation with, 142
hyperthyroidism and, 177–178
placental localization with, 120
pregnancy and, 118
Iodocholesterol ^{131}I, 51
Iron complex ^{99m}Tc, 130

Kenny, Peter J., 1–5
Kidney scanning, *see* Renal scanning
Kupffer cells, 9–10

LH (luteotropic hormone), radioimmunoassays and, 123, 127–128
Liver scanning, 63–71
abnormal liver, 65–68
diagnostic accuracy of, 69–71
errors, 68
indications for, 68–69
instrumentation for, 63–64
interpretation of, 65–68
normal liver, 65
principle of, 63–65
radiopharmaceuticals for, 9–10, 63, 64–65, 67–68, 71, 118, 150
results, 64–65
safety of, 71
Lung scanning, 10
See also Perfusion lung scanning; Ventilation lung scanning
Luteotropic hormone (LH), radioimmunoassays and, 123, 127–128
Lymphocyte cytotoxicity assay, 165–166
Lymphocyte transformation assay, 164–165

Macroaggregated albumin ^{131}I, 54
Macroaggregated albumin ^{99m}Tc, 54, 55
Macroaggregated iodinated albumin ^{131}I, 10
Marrow tumor detection, 148
Mediastinum, radionuclide angiography of, 105–106
Megaloblastic anemias, radioimmunoassays and, 174
Meningioma detection, 31, 32
Miale, August, Jr., 63–69
Multiple-point counting, 121

Neoplastic disease detection, 113–115
Neurofibroma detection, 29
Nine-point smoothing, 20

Obstetrics, 118–119, 123–128
See also Placental localization
Obstructive pulmonary disease detection, 58–59, 60
Organ specificity, radiopharmaceuticals and, 7, 9
Organic compounds, preparation of, 7–8
Orthoiodohippuric acid ^{131}I, 11, 130–134, 136–138
Osteogenic sarcoma detection, 114
Ouchterlony immunodiffusion, 167

Paget's disease
bone scanning and, 116
brain scanning and, 33, 35–36
Pancreas scanning, 74–79
abnormal pancreas, 77
acute hemorrhagic pancreatitis and, 77–79
contraindications for, 75
indications for, 74–75
instruments for, 75
interpretation of, 75–79
normal pancreas, 75–77
principle of, 75
procedure, 75
radiopharmaceuticals for, 75, 118, 150
Parathyroid scanning, 50–51
Pelvic angiography, 119
Peptic ulcer, radioimmunoassays and, 174
Perchlorate discharge test of thyroid function, 39–40
Perfusion lung scanning, 53–60
bronchogenic carcinoma and, 60
chronic obstructive pulmonary disease and, 58–59, 60
cystic fibrosis and, 60
normal scan, 55
patient preparation, 55
principle of, 53–54
procedure, 55
pulmonary embolism and, 53, 55–60
radiopharmaceuticals for, 54–55
safety of, 54
Pericardial effusion, radionuclide angiocardiography and, 86–89
Pernicious anemia diagnosis, 147, 148
Pertechnetate ^{99m}Tc
brain scanning with, 9
renal scanning with, 11, 130, 132–137
thyroid scanning with, 47, 50
Pituitary disorders, radioimmunoassays and, 172
Placental localization, 119–123
amniocentesis and, 119
dynamic imaging, 122–123
indications for, 119
methods for, 119–120
multiple-point counting, 121
procedures, 121–123
radiation dosage, 121
radiopharmaceuticals for, 120–121
scanning, 121–122
Plasma volume determination, 142
Platelet survival time estimation, 147
Pleural effusion, lung scanning and, 59
Plummer's disease, radioisotope therapy for, 176–178
Pneumonia, lung scanning and, 59, 62
Polycythemia vera, radioisotope therapy for, 181
Polyphosphate ^{99m}Tc, 112
Porencephalic cyst detection, 29
Pregnancy, *see* Placental localization; Radioimmunoassay, reproductive hormones and

Progesterone, radioimmunoassays and, 123, 127
Pulmonary emphysema, lung scanning and, 62
Pulmonary embolism
 perfusion lung scanning and, 53, 55–60
 ventilation lung scanning and, 62

Quality control program, 16–17

Radioactive iodine uptake (RAIU) test, 38–39
Radioimmunoassay, 168–175
 of adrenals, 51, 52
 for alpha fetoprotein (AFP), 164
 antibody and, 168, 169
 antigen and, 168–169
 carcinoembryonic antigen (CEA) determination, 162–164
 characteristics of common, 172
 clinical applications, 171–174
 data derivation, 171
 diabetes and, 172
 digitalis levels in cardiac disease and, 174
 estrogen determination, 123, 125–127
 follicle-stimulating hormone (FSH) determination, 123, 127–128
 gonadotropin determination, 123, 127–128
 hepatitis and, 174
 human chorionic gonadotropin (HCG) determination, 123, 125
 human placental lactogen (HPL) determination, 123, 124–125
 hypertension and, 172, 173
 hypoglycemia and, 172
 labeled antigen, 169
 luteotropic hormone (LH) determination, 123, 127–128
 megaloblastic anemias and, 174
 of parathyroid, 51
 peptic ulcer and, 174
 pituitary disorders and, 172
 principles of, 168–171
 progesterone determination, 123, 127
 reproductive hormones and, 11, 123–128
 separation, 169, 171
 special applications, 171
 techniques, 168–171
Radioisotope cow, 6–7
Radioisotope therapy, 176–181
 hyperthyroidism, 176–178
 intracavitary use of radioactive colloids, 181
 polycythemia vera, 181
 thyroid carcinoma, 178–180
Radionuclide angiocardiography (RAC), 80–105
 cardiac masses and, 90–95
 cardiac function and, 95–101
 indications for, 81
 interpretation of, 82–105
 intracardiac shunting and, 101–105
 method of, 81–82
 normal heart, 82–86
 pericardial effusion and, 86–89
 radiopharmaceuticals for, 82
 valvular disease and, 95
 ventricular aneurysm and, 89–90
Radionuclide angiography (RA), 80
 of mediastinum and great vessels, 105–106
Radiopharmaceuticals, 6–11
 for adrenal scanning, 51
 blood tests and, 142–144, 147–149
 for bone scanning, 108, 110–113, 150
 for brain scanning, 8–9
 characteristics of, 6
 classification of, 6–7
 clinical applications, 8–11
 as colloids, 6, 8
 as complexes, 6, 8
 as compounds, 6, 7–8
 as generators, 6–7
 for liver scanning, 9–10, 63, 64–65, 67–68, 71, 118, 150
 for lung scanning, 10, 54–55, 61
 medical cyclotron and, 149
 physical properties of, 7
 for placental localization, 120–121
 preparation, methods of, 7–8
 for radionuclide angiocardiography (RAC), 82
 for renal scanning, 10–11, 130–132
 specificity of, 7
 for spleen scanning, 71
 for thyroid scanning, 9, 38–41, 44, 45, 47, 50, 51
 transport of, 7
 for tumor localization, 151–158
Rectilinear scanners, 1–2, 63
Red blood cell
 mass determination, 142–143
 metabolism evaluation, 148–149
 production estimation, 145–147
 production sites identification, 147–148
 survival time estimation, 143–144
Renal scanning, 130–140
 chlormerodrin ^{197}Hg and, 11, 130–133, 135, 136
 cross-fused kidneys and, 134
 horseshoe kidneys and, 134
 indications for, 132–139
 infarction and, 134
 morphologic evaluation, 132–133
 orthohippuric acid ^{131}I and, 11, 130–134, 136–138
 outlet obstruction and, 136–137
 pertechnetate ^{99m}Tc and, 11, 130, 132–137
 radiopharmaceuticals for, 10–11, 130–132
 renovascular hypertension and, 135–136
 space-occupying lesions and, 133–134
 transplants and, 137–138
 trauma and, 134–135
 triple scanning, 130–132
 vesicoureteral reflux and, 138–139
Reproductive system, *see* Placental localization; Radioimmunoassays, reproductive hormones and
Respiratory system, *see* Perfusion lung scanning; Ventilation lung scanning
Roentgenography, 119
Rose bengal ^{131}I
 liver scanning and, 9, 10, 63, 64–65, 67–68
 pregnancy and, 118
Rosenberg, Eugene B., 160–167

Sankey, R. Roger, 12–22
Scalp hematoma detection, 33, 35
Schilling test, 147
Scintillation cameras, 4–5
Selenomethionine ^{75}Se
 pancreas scanning with, 75, 118, 150

parathyroid scanning with, 50, 51
pregnancy and, 118
thyroid scanning with, 44, 45
Serafini, Aldo N., 108–117, 130–140
Shunting, intracardiac, 101–105
Sinusitis detection, 33
Skeletal system, *see* Bone scanning
Smith, Patricia M., 160–167
Smoak, William M., III, 23–37
Smoothing program, 19–20
Sodium chromate ^{51}Cr, 142–144, 147
Sodium iodide ^{131}I, 9, 44, 45
Sodium pertechnetate ^{99m}Tc
dynamic imaging and, 122
radionuclide angiocardiography (RAC) and, 82
thyroid scanning with, 9, 39–41, 44, 45, 150
tumor localization with, 150
Software system, camera-computer, 15–21
acquisition software, 15–16
enhancement, 17–19
frame arithmetic, 20
quality control, 16–17
region of interest assignment, 19
smoothing, 19–20
time-activity histograms, 20–21
uniformity correction, 16
Spirometers, 61–62
Spleen scanning, 71–74
accessory spleen and, 73
interpretation of, 71–74
left upper quadrant masses, 73
liver-spleen uptake and, 74
radiopharmaceuticals for, 71
spleen size and, 72
spleen tissue, absence of functioning, 72–73
splenic rupture and, 71–72
splenosis and, 73–74
Static scintigraphs, 15, 16, 23
abnormal, and abnormal dynamic scintigraphs, 30–36
abnormal, and normal dynamic scintigraphs, 30
normal, abnormal dynamic scintigraphs, 25–30
normal, and normal dynamic scintigraphs, 24
of thyroid, 41
Storage devices, digital computer, 12–13
Strontium-85
bone scanning with, 108, 110, 150
pregnancy and, 118
Strontium-87m, 108, 110
Sulfur colloid ^{99m}Tc
liver scanning with, 10, 150
radionuclide angiocardiography (RAC) and, 82
spleen scanning with, 71

T_3 resin uptake test of thyroid function, 43, 44
T_3 suppression test of thyroid function, 39, 40
T_4 test of thyroid function, 43, 44, 45
T_4N test of thyroid function, 43–44, 45
Technetium-99m
blood tests with, 147–148
bone scanning with, 108, 150
liver scanning with, 63
placental localization with, 120–121
T-globulin detection, 160, 161, 162, 166–167
Thermography, 119
Thyroid carcinoma, radioisotope therapy for, 176–180
Thyroid scanning, 38–50
conditions identifiable by, 45–50
dynamic study, 39–41
functioning nodule, evaluation of, 48–50
goiter evolution, evaluation of, 46–47
in vitro function tests, 41–44
in vivo function tests, 38–41
iodine cycle and, 38
nonfunctioning nodule, evaluation of, 50
perchlorate discharge test, 39, 40
radioactive iodine uptake (RAIU) test, 38–39
T_3 resin uptake test, 43, 44
T_3 suppression test, 39, 40
T_4 test, 43, 44, 45
T_4N test, 43–44, 45
thyroid regulation, evaluation of, 45–46
TSH stimulation test, 39, 40
Thyrotropin (TSH) stimulation, 39, 40
Thyrotropin-releasing hormone (TRH) stimulation, 38
Time-activity histograms, 20–21
Todd's radioimmunoassay, 163
Tracers, *see* Radiopharmaceuticals
Transferrin ^{113}In, 82
TRH stimulation, 38
Triple renal scanning, 130–132
TSH stimulation test of thyroid function, 39, 40
Tumor localization, 150–159
organ scanning, 150
principles of, 151
procedures, 151
scan evaluation, 151–156
total-body scanning, 150–156
Tumor-associated antigens, detection of, 160–167
anticipated progress, 166–167
lymphocyte cytotoxicity assay, 165–166
lymphocyte transformation assay, 164–165
methods, 160–166
radioimmunoassay for alpha fetoprotein (AFP), 164
radioimmunoassay for carcinoembryonic antigen (CEA), 162–164
24-hour radioactive iodine uptake (RAIU) test, 38–39

Uniformity correction program, 16

Valvular disease, radionuclide angiocardiography (RAC) and, 95
Venous phase of circulation, brain scanning and, 24, 29, 31, 33
Ventilation lung scanning, 60–62
inspiratory capacity method, 61–62
instruments for, 61
interpretation of, 62
intravenous method, 61
principle of, 61
procedure, 61
radiopharmaceuticals for, 61
Ventricular aneurysm, radionuclide angiocardiography (RAC) and, 89–90
Vesicoureteral reflux, 138–139

Weinstein, Morton B., 141–149, 160–167

Xenon-133, 53–54, 61–62

Yunus, Mohammed, 53–62